Raw Can Roll
More power
to you.
John McCabe

Sunfood Living
Resource Guide for Global Health

John McCabe

With a Foreword by
David Wolfe
Author of *The Sunfood Diet Success System*

North Atlantic Books
Berkeley, California

Sunfood Living: Resource Guide for Global Health

Disclaimer

ISBN 13: 978-1-55643-733-5
ISBN 10: 1-55643-733-1
First Edition: July 4, 2007
Web site: SunfoodLiving.Com
Cover photos by Rich Marchewka Photography (Marchewka.Com). Front cover photo taken during winter solstice of Sun reflecting in droplets of water on leaf. Cover design by John McCabe. Graphics by Steve Minard (minarddesign@yahoo.com). Manuscript editing by Brenda Koplin. Indexing by Irv Hershman.

Published by **Sunfood Publishing**, 11653 Riverside Drive, Lakeside, CA 92040, USA; Sunfood.Com; 800-205-2350; 888-RAW-FOOD; International: +001-619-596-7979
Distributed by **North Atlantic Books**, P.O. Box 12327, Berkeley, California 94712 (www.northatlanticbooks.com)

"*Sunfood Living* is a lifesaving book. Its abundance of documented facts demonstrates how our current way of living and eating rapidly destroys the environment and our health. John McCabe offers a wide spectrum of sustainable solutions from around the world. I consider this book a timely eye-opener for individuals, families, businesses, and governments."
— **Victoria Boutenko, author of the books** *Green for Life; 12 Steps to Raw Food;* **and co-author of** *The Raw Family: A True Awakening;* **RawFamily.Com**

"This is one of the most comprehensive educational tools available on the market today. John McCabe is doing the world a great service, helping others help themselves through education. *Sunfood Living* is carefully researched and covers every topic you need to know in order to thrive in excellent health and make conscious choices in everyday life."
— **Cherie Soria, owner of Living Light Culinary Institute; author of** *Angel Foods: Healthy recipes for Heavenly Bodies; The Raw Food Diet: Feast, Lose Weight, Gain Energy, Feel Younger!;* **co-author of** *Comiendo Pura Vida;* **RawFoodChef.com**

"*Sunfood Living* is a heroic compilation that every household will benefit from. A key catalyst for action and responsible living is access to information, and these pages provide an encyclopedia of resources for just that.
Sunfood Living is a steadfast tool to reclaim the power of choice each of us wields in shaping the future of global health. In a time when consumerism and lifestyle have an unparalleled, momentous impact on our planet, this book offers information, options and solutions for shaping the change we wish to see in the world."
— **Renée Loux, author of** *Living Cuisine: The Art and Spirit of Raw Foods;* **celebrity chef and TV personality; EuphoricOrganics.Com**

"John McCabe's *Sunfood Living* is very timely and important. It is the researcher's resource for gaining inspiration, insight, and information for learning how to actively participate on a personal level in cleaning up our individual and collective pollution by being a part of the sustainability solution.
Accessible and down-to-earth, *Sunfood Living* offers not only resources but also commentary loaded with facts from the dangers of eating 'flesh food' and its byproducts, to the importance of organic foods, to eating solely a plant-based diet and living healthfully by returning to Nature. He also gives a plethora of crucial how-to informa-

tion from battery and cell phone recycling, to heart disease, hemp, environmental protection, sprouting, solar energy, money and investing, and much more.

Are you ready for massive personal and planetary transformation? This invaluable resource guide is more than food for thought; it could actually change and save your life, the lives around you, and many species facing extinction. It is true that the truth sets you free. Roll up your sleeves, McCabe has given us a powerful and potent hands-on source of truth and empowerment."

— **Amy Rachelle, author of** *Transformation: A 33 Day Self-Empowerment Program for Cleansing Body, Mind, & Spirit; AmyRachelle.Com*

This book is dedicated to you, the reader.
May yours be a Sunfood life filled with health and protecting wildlife, Nature, and Earth.

I would like to sincerely thank Brenda Koplin for her editing; David Wolfe for his inspiration and drive; Rich Marchewka for his photography skill; Dianne Onstad for helping to move this book project along into the publishing phase; and to all the people fighting to make the world a better place for wildlife.

NEW LEAF PAPER®

ENVIRONMENTAL BENEFITS STATEMENT
of using post-consumer waste fiber vs. virgin fiber

Sunfood Living saved the following resources by using New Leaf Opaque 100 (FSC), made with 100% post-consumer waste, and New Leaf Primavera Gloss, made with 80% recycled fiber and 40% post-consumer waste, both manufactured with electricity that is offset with Green-e® certified renewable energy certificates, and processed chlorine free.

trees	water	energy	solid waste	greenhouse gases
172 fully grown	75,205 gallons	124 million Btu	8,313 pounds	16,220 pounds

Calculations based on research by Environmental Defense and other members of the Paper Task Force.

©2007 New Leaf Paper   www.newleafpaper.com

Table of Contents

It's up to us

"The future of the Earth is in the balance. It's up to us –
who else? There is no one big fix. It involves everything we do,
permanently, forever."
 – David Attenborough

Foreword

By David Wolfe

If you have always wanted to do the right thing, to make sustainable, environmentally conscious, as well as relevant decisions and purchases, but you have been too busy and/or uncertain where exactly to track down all the greatest resources... then this is the book for you. Please pick it up now and take it home. Or, if you have this book at home or are browsing it at a friend's house, look deeper into these pages.

Sunfood Living is a resource for global health and well-being par excellence. No one I have previously met in the entire movement for sustainable ecologically friendly living on Earth has produced as valuable and useful a resource book as this. The collection of resources within these pages allows one to create a vortex of order out of an explosion of chaos. Specifically, these pages instruct us where to go for information, products and resources that are in alignment with sustainable planetary systems and environmental ethics.

In addition, *Sunfood Living* empowers you with unique and startling information on a wide range of relevant subjects including: online health resources, eco-friendly baby care, the importance of fat in our diet, vitamin B12 sources, the air-pollution impact of cooking, what flowers to eat (and which to avoid), where to buy your tissue paper, where to buy heirloom seeds, how livestock tending endangers wildlife, the ethics of plant-based foods, and much, much more!

Not only does John McCabe's book *Sunfood Living* provide us with massive amounts of resources and choices, he also injects ethical concerns into these pages. As an outspoken proponent of plant-based nutrition, John McCabe leads the field in his breadth of knowledge about how our food choices affect the planet. This is critical information. No longer can the environmental discourse continue without a profound and major revision of our views and habits concerning food.

Sunfood Living overturns the usual "problem, reaction, solution" protocol delivered to us by the powers that be; where the "problem" is manufactured (created), the "reaction" is managed through the manipulation of mass media, and the already prepared "solution" is implemented to take away whatever freedoms are left. Instead of the "problem, reaction, solution" protocol, John McCabe delivers "challenge, action, resolution" where the "challenge" is identified and awareness is created, a positive "action" is implemented immediately and a "resolution" is delivered that embodies a complete, total and, in fact, elevated solution.

Our world is in a state of utter transformation. Things could suddenly take a sharp turn for the better as we find ourselves aligned moment-to-moment with thoughts, words, and actions that are congruent with the lifestyles discussed in *Sunfood Living*.

Overall, this book will make it simple and convenient for you to become part of the solution. Reading this book and taking action means that you can join forces with a legion of people who are excited about healing ourselves and our environment with the best planetary choices ever. Yes, paradise on Earth is possible.

I met John McCabe under a unique circumstance in some small corner of the Anaheim Natural Products Expo in 1997. We shared stories and quickly took a liking to each other. Since then John has been the chief editor of all my books, has supported me with shelter when necessary, and has supported the entire movement that I am personally involved in which helps assist people with vegetarian, vegan, and raw-food nutrition.

John McCabe has been there for me and others through thick and thin. He has persevered through many personal trials and has created a great life for himself. He has always spoken positively about everyone as much as anyone could. And John has an exceptional amount of wisdom. To me this is someone I can learn something from.

When I first read the manuscript for *Sunfood Living* I knew that this book was going to be a great companion to my book *The Sunfood Diet Success System*. The two books have now been designed to support each other, to help educate everyone with choices, to create real freedom in our lives through healthy, happy, spiritual living.

By creating such a great reference book John McCabe makes it easier for all of us to make excellent choices in how we spend our money, which has literally become our vote for the future. In the current plutocratic system of governance we live under, our money is our vote. Voting with one's money is a vote that counts.

My friend and radio personality, Riley Martin, has juiced all philosophy down to one statement: "Do the right thing."

In *Sunfood Living*, John McCabe has done the right thing.

This book is meant to be used. Travel with it, lend it to friends and family, or keep it close at hand. And remember, when you take action on the content of material in this book, you will have the best day ever!

David "Avocado" Wolfe, JD
Author of *The Sunfood Diet Success System*; *Eating for Beauty*; and *Naked Chocolate*
Founder of nonprofit The Fruit Tree Planting Foundation (wwwftpf.org)
Co-founder of the online healthfood store: www.sunfood.com

June 2007

Our task

"A human being is part of a whole, called by us the 'Universe,' a part limited in time and space. He experiences himself, his thoughts and feelings, as something separated from the rest – a kind of optical delusion of his consciousness. This delusion is a kind of prison for us, restricting us to our personal desires and to affection for a few persons nearest us. Our task must be to free ourselves from this prison by widening our circle of compassion to embrace all living creatures and the whole of nature in its beauty."
— **Albert Einstein**

Within our lifetime

"Ecologists assert that the only large mammals to survive the near future will be those which humans allow to live. Biologists predict the Earth could lose one quarter to one third of all known species within our lifetime."

— EarthFirst.Org

Dream Another Dream

"All that we see or seem, is but a dream within a dream."
— Edgar Allan Poe

Consider that you are living in a dream. You say that may be a silly thought. But, similar to a dream, many people lead their daily lives making decisions based on perceptions that they believe to be true, but that actually are not. Some perceptions are made up in their minds, and some are taught to them by others who may have created them, or passed along myths formed over the years by their culture, or by those with an agenda.

You know that there were things you believed at one time that you eventually realized were untrue. Now think back and realize that you made decisions, and may have lived your days, based on those falsehoods. Consider that some of these falsehoods may have limited your life.

One example of what people are capable of doing based on false information is what happened when Orson Welles broadcast a reading of H.G. Wells' *The War of the Worlds* on Mercury Theatre Radio on October 20, 1938. Many thousands of people who heard this broadcast believed that Martians were attacking the world. People became engulfed in fear. Massive panic happened in and around New York City. People ran from their homes, abandoned their workplaces, and clogged the streets to escape the Martians. Their decisions were based on imagination.

Consider that you are currently making decisions in your daily life based on things that are not true.

Think of the possibility that all you believe about the past, from what you think you know about world history, to what you consider to be the truth about the people around you, and even about yourself, may all be nothing but created perceptions.

What if everything you have believed in and learned up to this point has been based on false information fashioned by the dreams or clever minds of others?

Maybe it is time to realign your perceptions.

Perhaps it is time to begin to dream another dream.

"Never doubt that a small group of thoughtful, committed citizens

can change the world; indeed, it's the only thing that ever has."
— **Margaret Mead**

"Our lives begin to end the day we become silent about things that matter."
— **Martin Luther King, Jr.**

"Nothing will benefit human health or increase the chances for survival of life on earth as the evolution to a vegetarian diet."
— **Albert Einstein**

"If you want something you've never had, you have to do something you've never done!"
— **Kimnesha Benns**

"Everything happening around you is only a reflection of what is going on inside you. If you want the world to change, you have to change."
— **David Wolfe**

Begin It Now

If all of the destruction done by humans to Earth since men started large-scale petroleum drilling in the 1800s had instead happened within a month, humanity would be astounded. But because the destruction has taken place over such a stretch of years, people seem to have been unable to grasp the enormity of the tragedy.

It seems some people are becoming aware of what we have done. Some are realizing what we can do.

"Why are we here?... The quality of water and the quality of life in all its infinite forms are critical parts of the overall, ongoing health of this planet of ours, not just here in the Amazon, but everywhere... The hardest part of any big project is to begin. We have begun. We are underway. We have a passion. We want to make a difference."
— **Sir Peter Blake, Wednesday, December 5, 2001**

Sir Peter Blake, a 53-year-old, two-time America's Cup winner and environmentalist from Auckland, New Zealand, was on his 119-foot vessel, *Seamaster*. It was docked near the mouth of the Amazon River.

He had traveled there as part of his worldwide expedition to document the impact of global warming and pollution.

Later that night, eight armed and hooded robbers boarded the *Seamaster* and held the crew at gunpoint. Shots were fired. Blake was killed.

Blake's murder was a great loss for his wife and their two young children. It was also a great loss for the environmental movement.

Blake's intention was to document humanity's destruction of Nature so that we might realize the problem and get to work on a solution.

Blake was trying to make a difference.

Allow his intention to be an inspiration.

> "Concerning all acts of initiative and creation, there is one elementary truth, the ignorance of which kills countless ideas and splendid plans: That the moment one definitely commits oneself, then Providence moves too. Whatever you can do or dream you can do, begin it. Boldness has genius, power, and magic in it. Begin it now."
> — Johann Wolfgang von Goethe

Tuning In

You don't have to be a world-famous yachtsman to work on improving the health of Earth.

As we are increasingly being bombarded by massive marketing, technomania, economic globalization, industrial agriculture, factory farming, nonstop road building, traffic, genetic engineering, threats of nuclear disasters, radioactive waste, perpetual war, and an extinction crisis like no other, it seems that humans have become to Earth as disease is to humans.

The human experience has become increasingly distressed because society has disconnected from Nature. Business and governments are attempting to control natural systems for short-sighted consumption that favors corporate interests rather than global health. Most often this is done while abusing and misusing all natural resources — and creating extreme amounts of pollution on and in the land and water, and in the air. Much of this is done to feed the people of North America and Western Europe, the most gluttonous societies of the world.

We may perceive comfort and convenience in our "modern" and corporate-dominated way of living, but the waste and destruction of

Nature we are creating on this planet degrades the quality of all life and inflicts a great deal of suffering on the other forms of life with which we share Earth.

To realize this, we should become more attuned to our natural surroundings and with protecting the other beings with whom we share the planet.

When we recognize our kinship with wildlife we rediscover our connection to, and reliance on all life forms.

Currently the way most people are living is not in tune with Nature. The way they are leading their lives is in direct opposition to the needs of a healthy planet and contributes to the loss and extinction of species. It doesn't help that governments are creating situations of danger, which they then claim they can protect us from, perpetrating the hero syndrome while doing little to nothing about the real problems facing the planet. Often the governments are creating the problems, allowing them to happen, or being the enabler in the most dysfunctional of all relationships, those between corporations and governments as the neglected citizens and wildlife suffer the consequences.

"Nearly one-third of the timber cut from national forests is used for paper production. Half of that paper ends up in landfills. Is this making your ears red? Thousand-year-old Doug firs from the Great Bear Rainforest are clearcut to make paper..."
   — Malus and John Lorax, Attention Shoppers, Lockdown in Aisle Three!, *Earth First! Journal*, December-January 2002; EarthFirstJournal.Org

"All too many politicians are corporate-owned and operated, and do whatever their loudest constituents and richest campaign contributors tell them to. All too few show any genuine outrage at the destructive immorality of a small portion of corporate America – the industries that rape and pillage Nature, the very lungs of our planet – to make a buck, regardless of what it costs the rest of us.
   The honest truth is that humanity needs trees to survive. Trees shade our ground, create topsoil, clean the air and help the land attract, hold and filter water. The trees and their roots purify the water as the rains fall. Clean streams keep millions of aquatic and other species alive. The cycle is perfect."
   — Tim Hermach, President Native Forest Voice; *Forest Voice*, Spring 2006; ForestCouncil.Org

Each day thousands of acres of trees are cut down to make such items as chopsticks, toothpicks, disposable furniture, and paper for junk mail, newspapers, magazines, paper bags, paper plates, take-out food containers, napkins, and tissue. Every year the people of China use about 45 billion pairs of disposable chopsticks, which amounts to about 25 million trees being cut down. Around the world there are several hundred billion paper napkins used every year. Billions of paper bags, all made from trees, are used every year, and hardly any of the paper is recycled.

> "Since 1937, about half the world's forests have been cut down to make paper. If hemp had not been outlawed, most (of those forests) would still be standing, oxygenating the planet."
> — **Alan Bock, Columnist,** *Orange County Register,* **1988; as quoted in the documentary** *Emperor of Hemp,* **EmperorOfHemp.Com**

> "These mountain lands, which boast some of the most spectacular natural beauty on Earth, are now being devastated to briefly quench the needs of a single generation."
> — **Al Gore, on the deforestation of the Himalayas**

> "In a brief moment in the life of our planet, we have destroyed all but a remnant of Earth's ancient forests. The United States has already lost a stunning 97 percent of its native forests. Worldwide, 80 percent of native forests have been cut down, and 25 percent of mammals, 20 percent of reptiles, 25 percent of amphibians, and 34 percent of fish are in danger of extinction. Water around the world is polluted with the soil that washes off bare mountains. The biological inheritance of humanity is being forever diminished, reducing potential sources of medicines, foods, and fibers. Destruction of forests is a leading cause of global environmental breakdown, including global warming."
> — **AncientTrees.Org, 2006**

Every day thousands of rare trees are being cut down and sold on the international market for use in furniture, flooring, and construction. At the same time, countries have no laws banning the import of wood from trees that were cut down illegally. Here in North America, where much of that rare tree lumber is used, lumber companies continue to cut down some of the oldest trees on the planet. Meanwhile, law enforcement works to protect the lumber companies while arresting protesters working to block the lumber companies from decimating the forests and the variety of wildlife that exist in them.

Because of both legal and illegal logging in forests around the planet, many species of plants, animals, and other living things are endangered and many have become extinct. That is because each tree and every forest are host to a number of plants, insects, amphibians, reptiles, mammals, birds, fungi, and microscopic organisms that play a role in the network of life on Earth. Because many forests are where the streams and rivers begin, trees and forests support water life of all varieties. When a forest is destroyed, so too are the homes to some combination of life, such as butterflies, lichens, amphibians, mushrooms, songbirds, voles, fish, crustaceans, and flowers that may exist only in a small region of the planet.

In Africa, where forests are open to Asian and European logging companies, gorillas are losing their last remaining homes. Because of the logging, eating wild African animal meat of all sorts is more common than ever. Gorillas are still being hunted. Gorillas are also experiencing an Ebola outbreak that scientists estimate has killed about one fourth of the world's gorillas in the last 12 years. The hunting, the illness, and the loss of forest habitat are likely to result in the extinction of gorillas in the wild.

On Borneo the logging and farming industries have destroyed 90 percent of the forests. This has placed the orangutans there on the road to extinction that is expected to come to a dead end within ten years. As I write this there have been forest fires burning there for months. Intentionally set to expand the palm oil plantations, the fires cause orangutans to flee, often to places where humans live. Some of the people torture the orangutans for entertainment. Other people consider the orangutans to be pests and shoot them. Some of the orangutans are captured and sold into the exotic pet, circus, and zoo markets. Some of the orangutans die from burns and injuries suffered in the forest fires, and their babies die of starvation.

Every day thousands of trees in the Central and South American forests are cut down to provide grazing land for cattle. Many thousands of other trees are cleared to make room to grow soybeans that are then fed to farm animals. The soybeans grown there are also used to make fried chicken products sold by such massively environmentally destructive companies as McDonald's and Kentucky Fried Chicken.

Throughout coastal areas of the world the mangrove swampland forests have been and continue to be destroyed to make way for resorts and marinas, and for shrimp and other types of seafood farms. This destruction contributed greatly to the damage done by the tsunami that swept away villages and towns throughout the Indian Ocean region in December 2004. Clearing of coastal forests and damage to barrier islands to create fish farms and to drill for oil also contributed to the strength of Hurricane Katrina that decimated the New Orleans region in 2005.

> "The end of the human race will be that it will eventually die of civilization."
> — Ralph Waldo Emerson

> "The frogs are sending an alarm call to all concerned about the future of biodiversity and the need to protect the greatest of all open-access resources – the atmosphere."
> — Andrew Blaustein, of Oregon State University, and Andy Dobson, of Princeton University in New Jersey, in a commentary in *Nature*, about global warming and the extinction of hundreds of species of amphibians; February 23, 2006. According to the Global Amphibian Assessment, about one third of the amphibians remaining on the planet are classified as threatened.

Every day thousands of acres of wildlands from the mountains to the coasts and on the islands of the seas are being cleared to make way for roads, stores, restaurants, resorts, golf courses, factories, houses, parking lots, mining operations, office buildings, marinas, airports, military bases, prisons, and power plants.

On every continent there are dams built, and more being built, that alter landscapes that took unknown amounts of time for Nature to form, and where varieties of wildlife have lived since the beginning of their species.

Throughout the world large mining operations are altering the landscape. They are digging holes deep into Earth in places like Indonesia, Africa, and Alaska, and leaving behind toxic heavy metal sediment that poisons water, killing generations of wildlife.

Coal mining companies are cutting down Appalachian mountain tops in Tennessee, West Virginia, Virginia, and Kentucky. They then fill valleys where rivers and streams ran, killing millions of fish, frogs, toads, snakes, insects, birds and other wildlife. Instead of the ancient mountains and pristine valleys, the people and the remaining wildlife of Appalachia are being left with poisoned rivers that are unfit for swimming, and many wells that are too poisoned to drink from. The denuded land is subject to mud slides that do more damage to creeks and rivers and the wildlife that depend on them (UnitedMountainDefense.Org).

Those who have protested the works of the coal companies involved with removing mountaintops have not only been presented with lawsuits for interfering with business, but have also found themselves to be the focus of the Department of Homeland Security. Nowadays those involved with protesting huge companies that destroy the planet can find themselves being labeled as "domestic terrorists." Others have been put in prison for years, and even for life because they protested corporate destruction of the environment. This sort of thing is happening in countries around the world. For instance, when villagers in Sudan gathered to discuss a dam project that would displace farmers and others who lived on the land for generations, they were shot at by police. This killed three villagers, and others were arrested and charged with waging war against the state (EarthFirstJournal.Org).

As I write this there is a large coal mining operation being planned for the pristine Happy Valley area of New Zealand, home to endangered species and fragile wetlands. The plan is to export coal to China for steel production. Environmental activists are working to stop this mine from opening (SaveHappyValley.Org.NZ).

Meanwhile, instead of providing useful information, the leading news sources are focused on babies being born to selfish movie stars; on which spoiled pop star is dating or divorcing the other; on the most popular fashion styles; and on what company is making the most money.

All of this pop culture news is presented while virtually little information about the state of the planet and what we can do about it is provided by any of the so-called major news sources. Instead we are presented with weak journalism that essentially appeases corporate interests by spreading corporate propaganda that elevates the deity of the dollar bill.

Commercial culture is inundating people with ads pushing the coolest things to purchase. Apparently corporations are doing a very good job at convincing kids that it is really awesome to become obese while eating toxic junk food and staring at computer games and repetitive television shows. In the past 20 years the proportion of overweight adolescents has more than tripled. The obesity of children is part of the result of the $10 billion per year that the junk food industry spends on marketing disease-inducing products to children. The sugary, salty, fatty, fried, and artificially dyed and flavored junk that is marketed as "food" is propagating a lazy generation with high rates of Type 2 diabetes, weak bones, attention problems, and early-onset cardiovascular disease. It doesn't help the children when the government keeps reducing funding for sports, music, and arts programs. To make up these funding cuts, the schools are increasing the number of vending machines on their campuses, and many schools have signed exclusive marketing contracts with soft drink and fast-food companies that pay for access to sell their junk drinks and garbage foods to the students. Meanwhile, every year the government gives billions of dollars in subsidies to corn growers whose crop is turned into disease-inducing corn syrup. Since it was first derived from corn in the 1960s, corn sweetener has become the most popular sweetener in the things children eat. The inundation of hydrogenated "trans fats" in many of the most commonly consumed foods is also damaging to the health of all those who eat them. Often the children consume this junk while staring at the TV that exposes them to more junk food commercials. In May 2005 the Grocery Manufacturers Association released a study concluding that the average American child sees 4,900 food commercials per year. About half of American children are overweight, and one in four is considered to be obese.

In the adult marketing sector millions of dollars are spent on ad campaigns to convince people that their lives would be better and they would be much sexier if they drove the right kind of car, if they ate the right kind of artery-clogging dessert, and if their hair coloring looked natural. The lifestyle that mass marketing promotes has helped increase the demand for electricity more than 70 percent in 20 years and has resulted in an adult population that is 65 percent overweight. It is a population that consumes about 100 pounds of sugar additives per year in a diet saturated with hydrogenated fats and farming chemicals that cause a variety of ailments. It is a population that is increasingly obese, and that has made liposuction one of the most popular surgeries.

For the moment the societal norm is to attempt to look like you belong in a clothing commercial while you create a façade to make it look like everything is okay.

But it isn't.

"Today, the mainstream media is only concerned with profits and ratings, paparazzi, and propaganda. They fail in their responsibility as journalists to report the unbiased truth and present the world as it actually is. For years, most of the scientific community has believed that we're on the verge of an ecological crisis – the 6th mass extinction. They're predicting that within 100 years HALF of all (non-human) species on Earth will be wiped out."
— **ZeroImpactProductions.Com**

The devastation humans have caused, and are causing, to the planet is difficult to ignore.

> "Americans are producing more and more waste with each passing year. In 1960, the average American threw away 2.7 pounds of trash a day. Today, the average American throws away 4.4 pounds of trash every day."
> — Energy Information Administration, EIA, DOE, Gov/Kids/EnergyFacts

Every day millions of fish and other sea creatures are dying from pollution, from fishing, and from damage done by recreational, cruise line, and industrial and military watercraft. In 2005 there were nearly 20,000 beach closings on U.S. shores triggered by pollution. Throughout the coastal areas of the planet, on beaches in the middle of the oceans, and in areas far from major cities, tons of plastic pollution gathers on the sand and rocky shores.

Every day unknown numbers of wild animals are being caught and used for entertainment, for caged hunting, for fur, for zoos, for scientific experimentation, for pet store profits, and for ways to transport drugs.

Every day thousands of animals and millions of plants and other life forms in the mosaic of Nature are being killed by human activity in the quest for the suicidal progress we call global industrialization.

> "The second step toward making America less dependant on foreign oil is to produce and refine more crude oil here at home in environmentally-sensitive ways.
> By far the most promising site for oil in America is the Arctic National Wildlife Refuge in Alaska."
> — George W. Bush, 16th Annual Energy Efficiency Forum; June 15, 2005

> "America is addicted to oil."
> — George W. Bush, State of the Union Address; January 31, 2006

The biggest threat to the world is the environmental desecration being carried out by corporate and government interests. One of the most notorious global polluters on the planet is the U.S. military, which is addicted to oil, war, misspending, and the abuse of power.

As of this writing the U.S. has spent an estimated $350 billion on the war in Iraq. The Pentagon is seeking an additional $99.7 billion to fund the wars in Iraq and Afghanistan. An estimated 75 percent of that is for Iraq. According to the Congressional Research Service, both wars have already cost $500 billion. If less than half of that money had been spent to wean the U.S. off of fossil fuels and into a future of plant-based fuels and on restarting the industrial hemp farming industry the nation could have been transformed.

How much has the current administration spent to protect the environment? The Bush administration has a history of not protecting the environment, including not signing the Kyoto Protocol; working to get rid of zero emissions vehicles by killing California's electric car mandate; opening wetlands, grasslands, and protected lands to development, drilling, and mining; degrading protection of endangered species; reducing the size of wildlife habitat; opening U.S. forestland to lumber companies; disregarding science relating to damage caused by cattle grazing on public lands; increasing beef production for export; pushing for more nuclear power plants; opening wildlands to off-road vehicles; weakening cancer safeguards; continuing to miss deadlines for updating health standards; taking action to demolish the hemp industry; cutting deals that favor the petroleum industry; shortening science review processes that regulate industrial polluters; and weakening pollution standards.

It does not help that the White House administration continues to behave as if they are working as a concierge service for businesses and industries with horrible environmental records.

As this book was going into editing the Bush administration's latest move against protecting the environment involved slashing the budget for the Environmental Protection Agency research libraries. The EPA is closing its headquarters library as well as regional libraries. Other branches of the government are doing the same, including NASA. The libraries have been used by scientists and others to conduct research with the goal of protecting the environment through the creation of new laws as well as the enforcement of established laws.

The World Meteorological Organization has recorded 2006 as the sixth warmest year since records began 150 years ago. The ten warmest years on record have occurred in the past 12 years.

As I write this the polar ice packs are thinning and the far reaches of Earth are under attack by those seeking to exploit resources on land newly exposed by the melting ice. There is a fight going on in Alaska to protect the Arctic National Wildlife Refuge from oil drilling to help provide some of the 5.7 billion barrels of crude oil Americans consume every year.

A separate and no less important fight is going on to protect the Bristol Bay Alaska headwaters region from gold and hard rock mining that could end up polluting pristine waters with toxic chemicals. This will kill millions of fish that are also the food for the surrounding bear and eagle populations, which in turn fertilize the surrounding forests.

In the Antarctic waters where the ice is melting, the tiny organisms called phytoplankton are dying, which in turn damages the populations of the tiny marine animals called zooplankton, including the shrimp-like crustaceans called krill, which feed on the phytoplankton. A reduction in both phytoplankton and zooplankton is taking place in many of the world's oceans. This is resulting in a loss of food sources for seabirds, fish, and marine mammals. The resulting loss in food for seabirds has caused a great reduction in the number of nesting birds and a great increase in the number of dead seabirds washing up on the coasts. In Antarctica the reduction in food for wild animals has been turning more of them toward cannibalism.

The predator animals living on and near the ice caps are also under threat from a silent danger that is biomagnifying in their food chain. Because the predator animals are at the top of the food chain, they are collecting all of the pollutants in their bodies that exist in the fatty tissues of the smaller creatures they eat. Although they live far from industrial society the body tissues of these creatures have been found to contain fire retardants, pesticides, perfluorinated compounds used to make Teflon, and other industrial chemicals. Seabirds, forest birds, seals, foxes, bears, whales, and fish living in the southern and northern regions of the planet have all been found to contain these chemicals.

One of the most common chemicals found in polar bears is a fire retardant used in furniture, carpeting, plastics, and electronics. These chemicals are known to disrupt thyroid and sex hormones, impair mental abilities and motor skills, and to alter brain development. Bears are being found with weak bone structures and weakened immune systems, and the milk of lactating bears has been found to contain enough of these chemicals to jeopardize the health of cubs. These are problems directly attributed to the pollution the bears are accumulating in their body tissues. With only 20,000 to 25,000 polar bears left in the wild, facing problem chemical pollutants and melting ice caps along with the threat of being hunted, their existence on the planet may soon come to an end.

The melting of the ice caps of the planet, which is caused by pollutants, is also one of several factors leading to the warming of the oceans. Ice reflects the heat of Sun. Where the ice has melted, the ocean water and the newly bare land are absorbing that heat. Because the polar oceans are becoming far less fresh and more acidic, and the tropical oceans far more salty, the global atmosphere is accumulating more water vapor, which is accelerating the problem.

That is just a small part of the story of what modern human lifestyles are doing to Earth.

Every minute enormous amounts of toxic pesticides, fertilizers, fungicides, insecticides, and other agricultural chemicals are being spread over farmland throughout the world. All of these chemicals are known to cause birth defects, hormonal imbalances, learning disabilities, cancers and other disease in both humans and wildlife. Farming and industrial chemicals also accumulate in water and result in large areas of the seas that are void of natural life. Inland, there are people who are told not to drink the tap water because it contains such high levels of chemical fertilizers that drinking the water can cause brain damage.

Low-paid farm laborers are exposed to these chemicals, and often get sick from them. Many of the workers have no idea what the dangers are of the chemicals they are being exposed to. For example, the fumigant chloropicrin that is used on farms contains the same active ingredient as tear gas. A chemical called Nemagon had been used for decades on sugar cane, pineapple, and banana farms. It caused cancers and a variety of terrible ailments in the farm workers. Women repeatedly exposed to it had miscarriages and stillbirths, and their babies that lived often were born with horrible deformities. Today there are similar chemicals being used that are poisoning workers on farms around the planet. When farm workers who are exposed to toxic chemicals do get sick they may not know what caused it. If they are able to visit a nurse or doctor they may be misdiagnosed, or their concerns dismissed or lost in translation. Long-term exposure can result in numerous health problems in the workers and in their children.

Farming chemicals damage soil organisms, such as mycorrhizal soil fungi, that play a large role in soil health and help plant root systems obtain nutrients and water from the soil. There are many hundreds of billions of chemical reactions that go on in a handful of soil as various forms of microorganisms live and interact through their life processes. If the genetically engineered plants and/or various toxic chemicals produced by industries begin to kill soil organisms or lead to a bacteria that largely damages or kills soil organisms, it could stop all plants from growing. If the obscene development of genetically engineered food plants isn't bad enough, there are companies that are developing genetically engineered bacteria. This should be stopped.

There are many people on this planet fighting over land; and the last remaining wildlands are being grabbed up and controlled by governments and corporations that exploit Nature's resources. Because of this, many animals and plants have become extinct while others are on the edge of becoming so.

> "There is but one ocean though its coves have many names; a single sea of atmosphere with no coves at all; the miracle of soil, alive and giving life, lying thin on the only Earth, for which there is no spare."
> — David Brower, first executive director of the Sierra Club; founder of Friends of the Earth; founder of Earth Island Institute; father of the modern environmental movement

Wherever a piece of land is changed from its wild state to that of roads, houses, buildings, pavement, timber "management," and farming, all life on that piece of land is changed — from that of free-living wild animals and plants to that of an unnatural state often unsuitable for most or all of the wildlife that has existed there for many thousands of generations.

> "It has long been apparent that every large, land-based animal on this planet is ultimately fighting a losing battle with humankind."
> — Charles Siebert in his excellent article, Are We Driving Elephants Crazy?: Their behavior in the wild has grown strange and violent in recent years. Researchers say our encroachment on their way of life is to blame; New York Times Magazine, October 8, 2006; NYTimes.Com/2006/10/08/Magazine/08Elephant.html

As I write this another story appeared telling of yet another study concluding that Earth is warmer now than it has been in thousands of years. This study also states that the cause of the warming is human activity, and specifically the burning of fossil fuels. According to several studies from various parts of the world, the meat industry causes more pollution on the planet than any other industry. Intensive livestock farming and the cooking of meat cause more pollution on the planet than automobiles.

> "The livestock sector generates more greenhouse gas emissions as measured in CO2 equivalent than transport [cars and trucks]."
> — Food and Agriculture Organisation, Rome, Italy; 2006

Meanwhile, vegetation is growing higher on the world's mountains than we can find record of. Certain species of insects are appearing in places where they have never been seen, including billions of beetles that are destroying hundreds of millions of trees in the mountain forests of North America. Tropical fish are swimming to parts of the oceans that are closer to the poles. Forms of bacteria and fungi are being found in parts of the world where it was thought they couldn't survive. Tropical diseases are spreading to new regions. Amphibians are increasingly being found with extra legs and other physical deformities. Algae overgrowth is becoming a problem in the world's largest bodies of fresh water as well as throughout swamplands and saltwater marshes and reefs. Flowers and trees are blooming out of season. Birds are building nests during parts of the year that aren't their traditional breeding season.

What is happening on the land is only a fraction of what is happening to wildlife on the planet. What is going on in the oceans, which make up the majority of the surface of the planet, is reflective of what is happening on the land.

The oceans continue to show signs that they are dying. Thousands of miles of coral reefs that were filled with life just a decade ago sit almost empty of life because of bleaching, dynamite fishing, overfishing, and rising levels of water acidity, or are being strangled by algae overgrowth caused by pollution. Kelp and sea grass beds are vanishing, as are the forms of life that depend on them.

Sonar technology being used by the military and fuel industries is killing thousands of sea mammals in excruciating ways by destroying their ears. The Marine Mammal Protection Act continues to be overridden by the U.S. Department of Defense so that the use of the sonar equipment can keep being used by the U.S., by Britain, and by several other nations.

Other sea mammals are absorbing so much pollution that their young feeding off mother's milk suffer and die from the poisons. Both pollution and industrial sea noise are to blame for the Puget Sound orca whales being declared an endangered species; joining them are their neighbors, dozens of varieties of salmon and steelhead trout are on the edge of extinction.

The worldwide fishing industry is playing a major role in destroying the oceans. Fish species are becoming rare or extinct in regions where they were common just decades ago, every type of sea turtle is endangered, massive fishing operations are setting billions of hooks every year to capture large fish and kill sea life of all sorts. It is estimated that 25 percent of the sea life captured is not what the fishing fleets want, and toss these dead or dying sea creatures back into the water.

Massive nets are being dragged across the ocean floors at deeper and deeper levels to capture fish that were once abundant, but are becoming sparse or nonexistent in places where they had existed since their species began. This causes a destabilizing of sea life biodiversity, extinguishing populations that rely on others to survive. These deep-sea trawling operations are the equivalent of killing every bird, animal and bug in a forest during a hunt for several hundred deer. Many of these massively destructive fishing expeditions operate on government subsidies and are protected by laws formed to protect not the oceans or sea life, but the profits of the fishing industry. Because of industrial pollutants the fish that are left are becoming more and more toxic, resulting in fish that can poison both predator fish and the humans that eat fish.

The fishing industry continues to lobby for more protection of their fishing rights, for more government funding for fishing fleets, and spends more and more money to promote the consumption of sea life with no mention of the state of the oceans or the poisons that may exist within the fish. In many parts of the world people can go to their local restaurant or seafood market to get a piece of a sea creature that is a species at risk of extinction.

Additional damage is being caused by the hundreds of millions of pharmaceutical drugs that are being taken every day and that are ending up in the water bodies of the planet. According to the Centers for Disease Control and Prevention, 130 million Americans use prescription drugs every month. The drugs are urinated away, or expired and unwanted prescriptions are flushed down toilets. As the chemical drugs dissolve into the waterways they wreak additional havoc on water life.

"Right now is the time to act wisely – by getting wisely informed. The key to saving ourselves (and countless innocent bystanders) from ourselves is education. We must change our ways, or face the collapse of the ocean world... and life on this planet as we know it."
— ZeroImpactProductions.Com

Because of dead zones created by the accumulation of farming and industrial chemicals flowing into the ocean, and air pollution dropping from the sky, increasingly larger areas of the oceans are devoid of healthy populations of natural sea life. As the dead zones increase, so does the surface temperature of the water, resulting in an increasing number of intense storms.

Because of all this, it is of great importance that we work to preserve and protect what is left of Earth's original beauty, to restore whatever we possibly can, and to start living in a way that is less damaging to the natural cycles of Nature.

> "The Earth has been around for 4.6 billion years. Scaling this time down to 46 years, we have been around for four hours and our Industrial Revolution began just one minute ago. During this short time period we have ransacked the planet for ways to get fuels and raw materials, have been the cause of extinction of an unthinkable amount of plants and animals, and have multiplied our population to that of a plague."
> — **From Earth Day pamphlet of WorldFestEvents.Com; 2006**

Without a healthy planet we cannot survive.

We need to stop looking at what is best for the human condition for decades, and start considering what is best for all of Earth's life forms for millennia.

> "No one is useless in this world who lightens the burden of it for anyone else."
> — **Charles Dickens**

For ten years people have been trying to get me to write another book. I have helped a lot of other writers research, compile, and write their books. After doing that for a number of years, and getting more and more offers to do so, I put an end to allowing other writers to access my brain. I felt it was once again time to do my own book.

I didn't want to write just any book. I wanted to write something that I felt was worth both the time and energy I would put into it as well as for the time and energy spent on and with it by those who held it in their hands. With this book I felt I wanted to do something that would help to reverse this terrible downfall we are experiencing. I dug through nearly two decades of my writing to find what I wanted to say. This book is the result of that work.

It is time to realize that each of us can work to make a difference in bringing Earth to a healthier state, for now, and for the future.

Donate money to an organization that works to protect wild animals or that aims to improve the condition of Earth. Get involved in other ways to improve the state of the planet. Get closer to Nature through your food choices, and through the ways you spend your time, energy, and resources. Clean up your act.

"Picketing and policing in the name of peace, can there be an end to planetary destruction without first acknowledging and accepting responsibility and accountability for the internal war?"
— Amy Rachelle, AmyRachelle.Com

If you are not actively working to make the world a better place, then you are working to make the world a worse place.

"The only thing necessary for the triumph of evil is for good men to do nothing."
— Edmund Burke

GET INVOLVED in protecting the environment, in protecting animals, and in restoring Nature.

"There are two primary choices in life: To accept conditions as they exist, or accept the responsibility for changing them."
— Dr. Denis Waitley

"Let every individual and institution now think and act as a responsible trustee of Earth, seeking choices in ecology, economics and ethics that will provide a sustainable future, eliminate pollution, poverty and violence, awaken the wonder of life and foster peaceful progress in the human adventure."
— John McConnell, founder of International Earth Day

It seems to me that we are all part of a bigger picture. That we are all connected in a way – whether we like it or not. The more the human population of the planet explodes, the more this seems to be evident. It also seems that we can all decide whether we are going to be part of the solution, or part of the problem.

Stop being part of the problem.

Make your daily life part of the solution.

Eating: It's What's Eating Us

"Creatures shall be seen upon the earth who will always be fighting one with another, with very great losses and frequent deaths on either side. These shall set no bounds to their malice; by their fierce limbs a great number of the trees in the immense forests of the world shall be laid level with the ground; and when they have crammed themselves with food it shall gratify their desire to deal out death, affliction, labours, terrors and banishment to every living thing. And by reason of their boundless pride they shall wish to rise towards heaven, but the excessive weight of their limbs shall hold them down. There shall be nothing remaining on earth or under the earth or in the waters that shall not be pursued and molested or destroyed, and that which is in one country taken away to another; and their own bodies shall be made a tomb and the means of transit of all the living bodies which they have slain. O Earth! what delays thee to open and hurl them headlong into the deep fissures of thy huge abyss and caverns, and no longer to display in the sight of heaven so savage and ruthless a monster?"

  — *Of the Cruelty of Man*, **Leonardo da Vinci, a vegetarian and outspoken protector of animals and Nature**

Food As Entertainment in Commercial Society

When you look at the pop culture of today, it treats food as a form of entertainment. Food is no longer eaten for nutritional needs, but is eaten for want and for some sort of imagined enjoyment. It has been turned into a hip adventure. And it has become all so dangerously silly. The commercials have talking pizzas, dancing cupcakes, gangsta' burritos, and people who fall in love at the bite of a potato chip. Selling food has turned into a pile of putrid nonsense. And people are buying it.

But the processing, packaging, marketing, and consumption of unhealthful food products also has turned into something more serious than simple blatant commercialism. From the commercials to the packaging, from the theme restaurants to the product giveaways, the marketing of food is something that causes an enormous amount of gluttony, pollution, and environmental damage all over the planet.

On average those people who watch television are fatter than those who do not watch television. Those who spend more time in front of a television are likely to weigh more. Probably the chief reason for this is that, in addition to being a sedentary activity, watching television exposes a person to an enormous number of images of processed and cooked foods that are made to look appealing, exciting, filled with flavor, and sexy. Much of the stuff in the commercials shouldn't be considered food. Most of it has significantly less nutritional content than an equal amount of garden soil.

When the money spent on corporate food is taken into consideration, the consumers are paying about 80 percent of their food dollar for processing, packaging, shipping, and other marketing-related costs. In 2000 the U.S. Department of Agriculture estimated that less than 15 percent of the food dollar is going to the farmer. In other words, what most people are eating from the supermarket barely consists of real food, and what they spend on it is also not for food, but for the commercialism.

Corporate food is not an efficient use of resources, and does not provide a body with what it needs to experience vibrant health.

"Food is an important part of a balanced diet."
— Fran Lebowitz

"The average American child sees 20,000 junk food ads per year on television. That is their nutritional education. That is how children are being taught about food."
— Eric Schlosser, author of the books *Fast Food Nation: The Dark Side of the All-American Meal, and Chew on This: Everything You Don't Want to Know About Fast Food*, appearing in the McLibel documentary; SpannerFilms.Net

Commercials are designed to ignite the passions, to play with the emotions, and to get people to feel a need or a want for a product or service. Commercials are designed to seduce money out of pockets. And food commercials promote substances that you have no need for. Other than a few commercials that promote fruits and vegetables, the vast majority promote foods that are damaging to health. From burgers to sodas to desserts and fast-food and TV dinners, all the foods in the commercials are not healthful — even if the commercials say the products are healthful. Big surprise: advertising lies.

"Our poor eating habits and lack of activity are literally killing us, and they're killing us at record levels."
— **US Health and Human Services Secretary Tommy G. Thompson; March 9, 2004**

A study released in 2003 by the Santa Monica-based Rand Corporation predicted that within 20 years the diseases related to unhealthful food and lack of exercise will cancel out health improvements seen in other areas. This is because the extent of obesity being experienced in industrialized countries is unlike any that has been experienced in human history. It is leading people down a path toward heart disease; high blood pressure; hardening of the arteries; diabetes and diabetes-related nerve damage; cirrhoses of the liver; macular degeneration; arthritis; cancers of the colon and other organs; kidney disease; bone structure and joint injuries; and early death.

In September of 2006 it was reported that Americans are watching more television than ever, spending a large chunk of their time in front of the TV, and many times in front of numerous TVs that are stationed in various rooms of their homes.

Television is collectively a negative and greed-based energy that provides almost nothing worthy of watching and it has a negative impact on society. The television news digs up the freakiest stories of the day to keep people tuned in, adds an alarmist spin on terrible events, plays with emotions, instills fear, creates havoc, and rarely offers solutions. Television and other pop media are mostly tools for companies to advertise their products to turn people into consumers. A majority of the advertising has to do with unhealthful foods sold in supermarkets.

When you consider the ingredients, nutritional value, and advertising of foods that people purchase in supermarkets, they are often not buying food. They are buying entertainment. They don't need the fancy packaging and the sugar coating and the pop sexiness to feed their bodies. All they really need are pure foods that are highly nutritious. But instead they are buying cookies and cakes, chips, candy, processed dinners, processed snacks, fried foods, and generally foods that squash health. In addition, most of the foods in supermarkets contain chemical dyes, flavors, scents, preservatives, and emulsifiers. All of this garbage works against health. It clogs body tissues, it wastes money, and it causes health problems that limit lives.

What drives the purchase and consumption of commercial foods is the emotion the marketers have successfully attached to the products. People eat sugar-coated breakfast toasty things because that is what they ate in the morning when they were little. They eat potato chips because the commercial tells them how crunchy and desirable the chips are. They drink soda because that is what cool people drink, and the sugar and caffeine are addictive and destroy health, including their bones (which are damaged by the phosphoric acid). They fill themselves up with cooked starches because they are dense and give them that filled feeling that replaces the emptiness they have in their lives from the disconnection from Nature and the lack of love that they may not even know they are experiencing. And children stuff themselves with all sorts of junk associated through marketing with their favorite cartoon characters.

Disney just finished a ten-year business relationship with McDonald's to familiarize children with various Disney film characters. After the pact with Disney ended, in 2006 McDonald's signed a deal with another film studio, DreamWorks Animation. Another fast-food chain, Burger King, has a deal with Warner Brothers. But fast-foods are not the only foods being used to market to children. Makers of the most unhealthful breakfast cereals often have business arrangements with major studios to market films on cereal boxes. What better time to get into the minds of children than by having them see your cartoon characters on their cereal box every morning? When the children go to school they are likely to see a vending machine on their school campus. On the labels of the junk snacks there are likely to be more images associated with film or TV characters.

Taking into consideration that the foods the film studios advertise are the worst types of things children can eat, it appears that the studios don't care about the health of children. What seems to be the only concern of the studios is that the stockholders stay happy with the returns on their investments. Let the environment suffer and the rates of obesity, diabetes, and heart disease in young people rage – the greedy film studios need to make money!

"The scientific evidence of risk to your heart from eating the standard American diet rivals in depth, breadth, and uniformity the evidence that smoking causes cancer...

People who merrily eat their cheeseburgers and pepperoni pizzas while putting their faith in drugs and medical technology to keep them alive might as well cheerfully beat themselves over the head with an anvil while keeping a first-aid kit handy."
— Former Montana cattle rancher Howard Lyman, in his book *No More Bull: The Mad Cowboy Targets America's Worst Enemy: Our Diet*; MadCowboy.Com

After people eat commercial processed foods for months and years, they end up going to the doctor to deal with all the health problems they have when their body doesn't function right because it can't function healthfully when all of the cells in their body are saturated with toxic junk food residues. But the doctor doesn't tell them to stop eating junk. Instead, the doctor prescribes medications made of toxic chemicals that some international drug company is selling successfully, filling their stockholders' pockets with money. The doctor may also suggest risky surgeries that bring money into the hospitals and medical centers.

As far as a business, the prescription drug industry is very successful. Pharmaceutical companies consistently earn billions of dollars every year. Allopathic doctors aren't so poor, either.

Meanwhile, people in industrial and high-tech societies throughout the world keep eating massive amounts of junk food, continue to gain weight, and persistently experience record numbers of diet-induced health problems. The average weight of commercial society has increased so much that furniture and automobile companies are creating wider seating to accommodate the plump bodies.

I can go on and on and quote all sorts of studies and statistics about how fat people are getting, and the subsequent health problems, but the point is that obesity is a problem, and it is getting worse. And it is tied in with the spiritual health of the culture we are living; in the damage people are doing to the planet; and in their disconnection from Nature.

Eating a bad diet perpetuates a vicious circle. The diets people in modern society are following are ruining their health, damaging the environment, and playing a major role in disrupting wildlife to the point that extinction of many species is accelerating.

Fighting the Beast

When London Greenpeace activists Helen Steel and Dave Morris stood outside a London McDonald's handing out fliers headlined *What's Wrong with McDonald's*, they triggered events that would lead to the longest court battle in the history of England.

As is told in the *McLibel* documentary, McDonald's hired two different investigative firms to spy on the London Greenpeace group. Several different spies began attending London Greenpeace meetings, and some participated in handing out fliers on the streets.

The fliers covered the topics of the unhealthful food served by the fast-food chain, the working conditions of the employees, the animal cruelty involved in raising meat, the environmental impact the company had on the world, and how the company focused their junk food advertising on children.

The court case began in June 1994. Steel and Morris were denied a jury and they represented themselves. They spent 314 days in court.

In June 1997 the judge ruled that McDonald's is deceptive in its advertising, exploits children, pays low wages, is anti-union, does cause cruelty to animals, provides bad working conditions, and that eating McDonald's food can lead to heart disease.

The court also ruled that Morris and Steel owed McDonald's damages of £40,000, which Morris and Steel have bravely and rightly refused to pay.

Additionally, in 2005, the European Court of Human Rights ruled that England's legal system violated the freedom of expression of Morris and Steel.

Because the media kept distorting the story, or at least reporting it in a way that was more fantastic than fact, Steel and Morris started their own Web site, McSpotlight.Org, so that they could tell their side of the story. The court case also resulted in the International Day of Action Against McDonald's, which takes place every October 16, and which is detailed on McSpotlight.Org. The Web site contains downloadable copies of the current *What's Wrong with McDonald's* leaflet that people are welcome to copy and distribute.

It wasn't only McDonald's that Morris and Steel were fighting, but the whole concept of the way multinational corporations operate: damaging wildlife and animals; purchasing huge swaths of the planet and making them off-limits to others; practically enslaving people at unlivable wages while limiting their ability to unionize and improve their conditions; and resulting in a culture that serves corporations over people, with half the world living in poverty while only an extremely small percentage live with the majority of the wealth, which they use to manipulate government policy around the planet.

Part of what the McLibel lawsuit exposed is this sort of activity. Often when the so-called "world leaders" meet, they don't talk about what is best for the population at large; they often conduct business in a way that makes the seemingly elected officials ambassadors for the corporations, and not for the people. An example of this is when

George W. Bush met with Japan's president in Washington in June 2006. What they discussed was not global warming; or the Japanese practice of killing whales, porpoises, and dolphin (SeaShepherd.Org); or how to improve the conditions for organic farmers; or how to ban toxic chemicals; or how to reduce the threat of species extinction; or how to protect the environment and ancient forests. What they discussed was how Japan and the U.S. could improve the beef trade. Weeks later Japan began importing more U.S. beef.

"We want a society that's not run for the benefit of shareholders, but that's run for the benefit of everybody."
— Helen Steel, in the *McLibel* documentary; SpannerFilms.Net

"It's not just what goes on at McDonald's itself that's the problem. It's that key practices that they've pioneered over the last 50 years are spreading throughout society and becoming the norm...
Human beings are amazing. Look at our inventiveness and creativity, in all the great things, art, music. Surely we could come up with something better than this current economic system – which allows a few people to become obscenely rich while half the planet has to live in poverty."
— Dave Morris, in the *McLibel* documentary; SpannerFilms.Net

There are about 30,000 McDonald's "restaurants" in 119 countries. The company has been the focus of protests in many of these countries.

When McDonald's planned to open a McDonald's near the Piazza di Spagna in Rome in 1986, a man named Carlo Petrini organized a protest. As their weapons the protesters used bowls of penne. Petrini wrote a manifesto against the fast-food culture and he founded the Slow Food Movement. The movement promotes traditional and regional foods as well as agricultural biodiversity, small farms, and sit-down dinners. Many affiliate groups have been started around the world.

"I'm very into the development of communities of producers and farmers, and it's only if we develop and enforce these communities that we can overcome an industrial logic."
— Carlo Petrini, founder of the Slow Food movement

Also notable is the 2004 film *Super Size Me* in which filmmaker Morgan Spurlock documents the health problems he experienced by eating McDonald's for breakfast, lunch, and dinner for 30 days. The film was nominated for an Academy Award for Best Documentary Feature. Spurlock thought of the idea for the film when he heard a news story about a lawsuit filed by two teenage girls who blamed McDonald's for their obesity. During Spurlock's filmed experiment he gained 25 pounds and experienced liver dysfunction. His doctor warned him to stop the experiment before he suffered a health crisis.

Localizing Your Food

"There are many reasons to buy locally grown food. You'll get exceptional taste and freshness, strengthen your local economy, support endangered family farms, safeguard your family's health, and protect the environment.

... Getting to know the farmers who grow your food builds relationships based on understanding and trust.

... Fruits and vegetables shipped from distant states and countries can spend as many as seven to fourteen days in transit before they arrive in the supermarket."
— **FootRoutes.Org**

"Supporting local, ecologically sound agriculture is one step we can take toward achieving a more sustainable lifestyle. Buying locally grown food conserves fuel and reduces pollution by shortening shipping distances. Local food is also fresher, and therefore tastier and more nutritious. Choosing organically grown food provides for the conservation of our valuable agricultural soils. Supporting local farmers contributes toward preservation of the rural character of the New England landscape."
— **FarmDirectCoOp.Org**

The primary way you can help to restore and protect not only Nature, but also the world as a whole, is through your food choices.

The way we live in modern society depends on airplanes, boats, and other forms of transportation to ship food products around the world.

Why are you eating apples grown five thousand miles from where you live? Why are you eating spinach grown three thousand miles away? Why are you drinking orange juice from oranges grown in Italy when you live in Australia? Why are you using grapeseed oil from

France when you live in California? Why are you eating grapefruit grown in Australia when you live in Arizona? Why are you eating almonds grown in California when you live in Italy, where almonds also grow? Why are you eating grapes from California when you live in China? Why are you eating cherries from Canada when you live in Japan? Why are you eating lettuce grown in California when you live in Florida? Why are you drinking wine from South Africa when you live in France, or California wine when you live in Argentina? Why is most of the food you eat arriving in containers consisting of paper made from trees, and plastic made from crude oil? Why are you filling a trash bag with food packaging every two days? Why are you eating food that was grown using toxic chemical fertilizers, pesticides, defoliants, fungicides, biocides, herbicides, and insecticides, and that contains food dyes, preservatives, and flavorings made from petroleum, coal, and other fossil fuels? Why are you eating fruits and vegetables that have been coated with wax and/or shellac? Why are you buying food that you can grow yourself?

Consider what it takes to grow, ship, package, and market the food you eat. Then think of ways along the entire path your food takes in which you can play a part in making less toxic and more Earth-friendly.

Begin seeking foods that are grown within your foodshed.

Your foodshed isn't a little room, it is the region of the world where you live – generally a circle of about one to six hundred miles that surrounds you.

With many types of food shipped thousands of miles before they are eaten, it only makes environmental sense to choose to make the largest part of your diet consist of foods that are grown within a few hundred miles of where you live. Some people describe this way of eating as being a "localvore."

Choosing to purchase and consume locally grown foods will reduce fossil fuel use as well as contribute to your community. This is because you will be supporting local farms.

Large food companies have been taking over the food industry as people rely more on commercial foods and become less involved with growing their own food. If you also grow some of your food, which you should, you can further reduce dependence on fossil fuels as well as on multinational corporations.

Another way to improve the quality of your food is to avoid produce that has been genetically engineered.

The documentary *The Future of Food* points out in frightening detail what genetic engineering can lead to, and is leading to. I encourage people to watch that documentary in group settings so that everyone can learn about the dangers of genetic engineering of plants. I also encourage everyone to read *The Food Revolution*, by John Robbins. Then you will begin to understand why you should look for the term "non-GMO" on food labels. GMO is the abbreviation for genetically modified organism. Companies that label their foods as non-GMO are aiming to supply food that has not been genetically modified. A good source for information on this is the National Family Farm Coalition, a group working with many other farm organizations to stop the spread of GE (genetically engineered) agriculture (NFFC.Net/Issues/GEIssues.html).

The activities of the companies that are genetically engineering food plants are a danger to everyone. Some of the companies include Aventis (France), BASF (Germany), DOW Chemical (U.S.), DuPont (U.S.), Monsanto (U.S.), Novartis (Switzerland), and Zeneca (Britain). The very same companies are also involved in the manufacture of dangerous farming chemicals that poison our food, water, soil, and air.

Refrain from eating foods that were grown using toxic chemical fertilizers, insecticides, herbicides, pesticides, fungicides, defoliants, and other farming chemicals. Refuse genetically engineered foods. Seek organically grown foods and you will be reducing the use of toxic chemicals while supporting the growing organic foods industry.

While you may not be able to localize all of your food choices, you can certainly do so with most of the foods you eat. The more you eat organically grown and locally grown food, and the less you eat foods that were transported from distant lands, the more you will be improving the level of your nutrition while protecting wildlife and the ecosystems of both your region and the rest of the planet.

Becoming a "food artisan" by growing your own organic food garden is one of the best things you can do for the environment. You will reduce packaging, because there won't be any on the food you grow. You will improve your level of nutrition, because freshly grown food is more nutritious than food that has been shipped and stored. You will save money. You will get exercise. You can give away the food that is more than you can eat. And you will be opting out of the globalized, industrialized, supermarketized, corporatized, and increasingly genetically engineered food industry.

An interesting book on the topic of corporate food and how it is produced and transported is *Tangled Routes: Women, Work, and Globaliz-ation on the Tomato Trail*, by Deborah Barndt. The book details the route of a corporate-grown tomato from a Mexican farm to a consumer in Canada.

See the *Gardening* section of this book for more information about gardening, seed saving, heirloom seeds, farming and sustainable food culture groups like Food Not Lawns, and Eat the View.

An interesting book on the topic of localizing your food is Brian Halweil's *Eat Here: Homegrown Pleasures in a Global Supermarket*.

The Food Shortage Myth

The contemptible companies that genetically engineer food crops are bombarding us with messages that there is a food shortage, and that this food shortage can be solved through genetic engineering. That is a combination of lies.

As mentioned, I encourage people to watch the documentary *The Future of Food* so that they can get a better understanding of what the genetic engineering companies have been up to.

Genetic engineering is a dangerous activity that will not result in more food, it will result in less food. The genetically engineered sterile and suicide seeds that these companies have developed are an assault on Nature, on family farming, on organic foods, and may lead to a food shortage.

There is no food shortage. Even though an estimated one in six people is going hungry, there are more people suffering from obesity than from starvation. The food shortage that does exist in certain parts of the planet, including in some of the wealthiest areas, has to do with what food is being produced, how it is being produced, and what is being done with it.

Over ten percent of the food grown on U.S. farms is plowed under to help control pricing. In the cities, supermarkets often lock their trash bins or use trash compacters to discard food that has expired or is slightly blemished. Much of this food is trashed even thought it is still edible. Some stores throw bleach into their dumpsters to discourage people from "dumpster diving." More than ten percent of food purchased for home use also is thrown away.

The chemically grown and mass-marketed food industry is a source of massive quantities of pollution that has spread and is spreading throughout not only the surface of the planet, but also into its underground water banks, into its crust, and into the atmosphere surrounding the planet. In fact, more pollution is created as a result of the fast-food, cooked food, and animal-eating diet than any other source. It starts with the farmlands.

The consumption of meat by the affluent people of the planet has a negative impact on the poor because the land used to grow food for people is being taken over by companies involved in growing food for livestock. It is being done by international corporate agricultural businesses. This is helping to create the system and culture of dependency on corporations and on the small number of people who control the global flow of money. It is widening the gap between the rich and the poor. Global trade, free trade, and exclusive contracts in the growing, processing, and distribution of food is negatively impacting family farmers around the planet, often demolishing their way of life.

Over half of the beef from Latin America is exported to more affluent countries. In the U.S., Australia, and Europe more money is spent on one dairy cow per day than what many people in Third World countries live on per month.

> "Hunger afflicts more than 800 million people worldwide and kills 24,000 per day. Three fourths are children under five. Chronic hunger causes stunted growth, poor vision, listlessness, and susceptibility to disease.
>
> A major factor is the waste of foodstuffs fed to animals raised for food, rather than to starving people. This was documented in Frances Moore Lappé's 1972 classic *Diet for a Small Planet* and was reaffirmed at the 2002 World Food Summit in Rome.
>
> A meat-based diet requires 10 to 20 times as much land as a plant-based diet.
>
> An acre of prime land can produce 40,000 pounds of potatoes, 30,000 pounds of carrots, 50,000 pounds of tomatoes but only 250 pounds of beef."
>
> — Citizens for Healthy Options in Children's Education, CHOICE.USA; 2006

Most food grown on the planet is fed to farm animals. Over two thirds of the land in Central America is used to grow livestock feed. About two thirds of the grain in Russia is fed to farm animals. Grain grown for livestock is the primary crop on every continent.

If the companies that genetically engineer food crops are so concerned about feeding the world's hungry, then why are they focusing so much on crops that are to be fed to farm animals? On the same note, a lot of the food that is grown at taxpayer expense in the form of tax subsidies (corporate welfare) paid to large farming conglomerates is food for farm animals. Corn is the most subsidized crop in the U.S., and the large majority of the corn is fed to farm animals.

> "The amount of grain that we grow in the West is mostly used to feed our cattle. Eighty percent of the corn grown in this country is to feed the cattle to make meat. Ninety-five percent of the oats produced in this country is not for us to eat, but for the animals raised for food. According to this recent report that we received of all the agricultural land in the U.S., eighty-seven percent is used to raise animals for food. That is forty-five percent of the total land mass in the U.S."
> — John Robbins, author of the books *The Food Revolution; May All Be Fed; Diet for a New America; and Reclaiming Our Health*; FoodRevolution.Org

On the land used to produce the beef that would provide the daily food needs of one person, the daily food needs of more than 15 people could be met by growing fruits and vegetables. As John Robbins points out in *The Food Revolution*, if Americans would reduce their beef consumption by about 15 percent, the land used to produce the beef could feed all of the hungry people on Earth — if that land were planted with fruits and vegetables, herbs, and edible grains and beans.

> "ECONOMIC IMPERIALISM
> Some 'Third World' countries, where most children are undernourished, are actually exporting their staple crops as animal feed, i.e., to fatten cattle for turning into burgers in the 'First World.' Millions of acres of the best farmland in poor countries are being used for our benefit — for tea, coffee, tobacco, etc., while people there are *starving*. McDonald's is directly involved in this economic imperialism, which keeps most black people poor and hungry while many whites grow fat.
> GROSS MISUSE OF RESOURCES
> GRAIN is fed to cattle in South American countries to produce the meat in McDonald's hamburgers. Cattle consume ten times the amount of grain and soy that humans do: one calorie of beef demands ten calories of grain. Of the 145 million tons of grain and soy fed to livestock, only 21 million tons of meat and by-products are used. *The waste is 124 million tons per year at a value of 20 billion U.S. dollars.* It has been calculated that this sum would feed, clothe and house the world's entire population for one year."
> — From the original *What's Wrong with McDonald's* leaflet distributed by London Greenpeace, which resulted in McDonald's suing for libel, and the longest

court case in England's history; McSpotlight.Org

The concept that there is a food shortage on the planet is a huge mistruth. In 2005, the U.S. alone had more than 95 million cattle, several billion chickens (including 347 million egg-laying hens), 100 million hogs, 300 million turkeys, millions of lambs, and many other types of animals, such as buffalo, and even ostrich, ducks, and an increasing number of farmed fish – all being fed enormous amounts of food so they can be killed and fed to humans, and a smaller portion going to pet food and farm feed.

It is estimated that today there are over 20 billion farm animals on the planet, and that is a low estimate. These animals consume tremendous amounts of food. In fact there is such a need for farm animal feed that companies are now creating animal feed out of such things as the feces of chickens, cows, and pigs; the leftover dead animal parts, including massive quantities of blood, from slaughterhouses; killed animals from city and county animal "shelters"; and the road kill that cities and counties remove from their streets.

According to the Department of Agriculture, in 2006 there were about 35 million Americans who were "food insecure" – a phrase describing a diet that lacks enough nutrition to keep a person healthy. It said that over 13 million of those people consisted of children. According to the U.S. Conference of Mayors, 56 percent of the emergency food outlets in America turned away hungry families in 2003 because there was not enough food to feed them. When this report was released, it brought about news reports of church groups, food banks, and soup kitchens struggling to provide food for hungry people. Politicians and welfare organization leaders spoke out about how, because America is the wealthiest nation, there should be no people going hungry, especially when millions of pounds of food is being thrown away every day by restaurants, supermarkets, cafeterias, and catering companies. Unfortunately, when people do get food from food banks they are often given food of low-quality that has been overly processed, and that contains many unhealthful ingredients that are directly linked to diabetes, heart disease, cancers, and other degenerative diseases.

The words of the politicians sound very convincing, and likely help them at reelection time, but if they and those who work to "feed the hungry" are using meat and dairy foods to fill stomachs, they are simply contributing to the problem of hunger.

If politicians and welfare organizations are truly looking for a solution, they can start with supporting groups like Food Not Bombs and Food Not Lawns.

Food Not Bombs began in 1981 and grew out of a movement in Boston to protest the government's nuclear energy programs. Food Not Bombs now has branches in many countries. It provides free vegetarian meals from unsold and donated produce, and works to make people food independent. Food Not Bombs activists in San Francisco have been arrested for feeding the homeless. That's a real good use of tax dollars and the police force, don't you think? (See the book *Food Not Bombs* by C.T. Lawrence Butler and Keith McHenry.)

Food Not Lawns teaches people how to grow food, and it is also the title of a book by Heather Coburn Flores wherein she explains the concept.

I found it quite absurd when I saw a newspaper announcement in the spring of 2004 that told of how Tyson foods, an animal farming and meat distribution company, was donating meat to groups working to feed hungry Americans. If all the land and resources used to grow the food fed to those animals were converted into farms growing fruits, vegetables, herbs, nuts, and seeds for human consumption, they would do a much better job of feeding the hungry, while also protecting the environment, wildlife, Nature, and Earth.

Make no mistake, there are children going hungry, and many are starving. Not only in the poor countries of Africa, but also in the wealthiest countries. There is a serious lack of quality nutrition, including among the children who are fat. One reason for the lack of nutrition is that the foods the children are being fed are of a very low nutritional quality, weak in vibrancy, and contain harsh and poisonous substances, such as sweeteners and chemical dyes and flavors that harm body tissues.

The children who are starving from lack of food and the children who are not getting quality nutrition both are in a sad situation. Their bodies need nutrients to form healthy cells in their bones, muscles, nerves, skin, brains, and in every organ of their bodies. Lack of good nutrition in a growing body leads to organ dysfunction, including brain growth problems, which affects all areas of learning and life because the neurological system does not grow in the way it should. When the children suffer through lack of quality nutrition and education, everyone suffers.

There is no food shortage. There is an enormous misunderstanding of what food is. There is a mismanagement of the system. There is a misappropriation of funds. There is more than enough food grown on the planet to feed every human. Humans could not even consume all the food that is grown on this planet. But farm animals are being fed a majority of the food. The real reasons that there are people starving on this planet are ridiculous. Blame the meat eaters, the junk food eaters, and the farming, marketing, packaging, shipping, and advertising engines required to feed their desires for the flesh of dead animals.

There is also a stupendously immense and growing dependence on supermarkets, fast-food outlets, and on international companies to supply food. As people have become more dependent on an industrialized and commercialized society, they have become more removed from Earth, from being self-sufficient, from the connection they once had to taking care of their own needs through growing much of their own food in garden plots, and in harvesting food from the wilds of Nature.

People would do a great service to themselves, to their community, and to the planet if they would begin to once again grow their own food, even if it results in only a small portion of what they eat.

If companies, charities, and governments are interested in feeding the world's hungry, they would be focusing on shutting down the animal farming industry, destroying genetically engineered plants, supporting organic food farming and gardening, and legalizing industrial hemp farming.

Currently the U.S. government gives multiple billions of dollars in corporate welfare every year to the meat, dairy, and egg industries and the companies that grow food to feed to farm animals. That money, properly used, would easily cure the world's human nutritional problems.

Eating Animals

"Of the mouth of man which is a tomb there shall come forth loud noises out of the tombs of those who have died by an evil and violent death."
— **Leonardo da Vinci, a vegetarian who was outspoken about protecting animals from harm. He considered the bodies of meat eaters to be the tombs of the animals they ate.**

"Throughout history, many great religious leaders, spiritual teachers,

yogis, and many of the world's religions have recommended a vegetarian diet, and they have done this for a good reason. The karmic consequences of eating animals dampen the spiritual powers while raising
the emotions of fear and doubt in the mind."
  — **David Wolfe**

"I consider them fellow living creatures with certain rights that should
not be violated any more than those of humans."
  — **Jimmy Stewart**

"The greatness of a nation and its moral progress can be judged by
the way its animals are treated."
  — **Mahatma Gandhi,** *The Moral Basis for Vegetarianism*

"More animals are being subjected to more torturous conditions in
the United States today than has ever occurred anywhere in world history…
Today, because of the way animals are raised for market, the question of whether or not it's ethical to eat meat has a whole new mean-
ing and a whole new urgency. Never before have animals been treated
like this. Never before has such deep, unrelenting, and systematic cruelty been mass produced."
  — **John Robbins, The Food Revolution**

"Pale yellow chickens were flying past us by the thousands, propelled
through the cavernous factory by a dizzying maze of belts and pulleys
and hooks and chains and gears. Everything was wet – drenched in
water, fat, blood, and offal – dripping down gutters and gushing down
drains. The smell of flesh, although not fetid, was raw and gamy… The
chickens flowed faster than any of us could hook them. They piled up
on the conveyor belt until they spilled onto the floor… Greasy water
splashed in my face.
  — **1,000 Miles of Hope, and Heartache, by Jesse Katz, a** *Los Angeles Times* **writer**
    who went undercover to work in a Missouri chicken slaughterhouse;
    November 10, 1996

"Chickens and other birds are not protected by the U.S. Humane
Slaughter Act."
  — **A Voice for Animals, VoiceForAnimals.Net**

"In his book, *Diet for a New America*, John Robbins describes in
detail the correlation between human disease and eating animals.
Heart disease, the number one killer in the United States, is directly

attributed to eating animals. The incidence of cancer has been statistically correlated to the consumption of milk, meat, and eggs. Colon cancer and other diseases of the digestive tract are directly caused by the overconsumption of animals, and the under-consumption of raw plant foods. Environmental toxins accumulate in animals, especially in animal fats. All the toxins being poured into the atmosphere collect in the tissues of animals. Eating those animals, whether they are insect, fish, or mammal, will give one a strong does of toxins. In his book, Robbins mentions that meat contains 14 times the pesticide level that an equivalent amount of commercial plant food would contain; dairy products contain 5 1/2 times as much. The more animals people eat, the more likely they are to experience all sorts of health problems. That is a fact. The opposite is true as well. The more people subsist on raw plant foods and the less they rely on cooked and processed foods, animal flesh, and dairy, the more likely they are to experience all sorts of health benefits."
— David Wolfe

As Wolfe points out in *The Sunfood Diet Success System*, some people make the argument that "plants have a higher consciousness than animals, and therefore should not be eaten." But when you look at the diet of most of the types of animals that people eat, most of the animals are consuming plants. The animals are plant elements transformed. When a person eats an animal, they are eating both the consciousness of the plants the animal has consumed, as well as the consciousness of the animal.

Much of the plant matter that people consume does not kill the plant. Especially with fruit, the person is eating only the fruit, and not killing the plant. All plant structures grown in Nature consist of soil nutrients, water, Nature energy, and sunshine transformed into a plant. When you are eating plants you are eating these elements as they have been transformed. When you eat living plants, you are transferring that energy into your system.

I am not advocating a diet that consists only of fruit, but only giving that example as a way to discuss the issue.

Other plants that people eat are harvested only at the end of their life cycle. This includes many types of vegetables, as well as fruit and seeds. If they are not eaten, they rot into Earth, which keeps presenting Nature energy back to us in the form of plants.

"Cooking led to the animal and seed diet. The most frequent way

people interact with animals is by eating them. The most frequent way
people interact with seeds is by eating them."
— **David Wolfe**

All food carries energy. Meat has the energy of suppression and the
fear, violence, illness, and horror of the slaughterhouse. Dairy has the
energy of animals that are incarcerated. Plants have the energy of Sun
and Nature.

Meat also carries the energy of fright chemicals. These stress hormones are released into the body tissues of the animals as they are
aware that they are about to be murdered.

It is interesting that those parts of the cities where there are the
most fast-food restaurants, and citizens whose diets consist largely of
meat and dairy, also experience the highest rates of murder. The mix
of bad karma from the food, as well as the stress chemicals in the
meats, plays out in the drama of the inner cities. Oppressed poor people, eating the meat of incarcerated, distressed, and diseased animals,
absorb the drama of that energy, which fuel the anger, violence, and
crime.

When the human body is put into a stressful situation the body
cells respond by releasing stress hormones into the tissues. The hypothalamus sends signals through the sympathetic nerves near the
spinal cord and trigger the adrenal glands to release epinephrine and
norepinephrine. The pituitary gland releases a chemical signal into
the blood that triggers the adrenal glands to release other hormones,
including cortisol. The body under stress also produces higher levels
of hormones labeled inflammatory cytokines, which cause inflammation, pain, and swelling. A similar scenario happens within the bodies of animals when they are exposed to stressful situations.

Animals raised in the stressful, unhealthful, and unnatural situations of today's factory "confinement" farms are filled with illness.
Stress and bad diet destroy the health of farm animals in the same
way that stress and bad diet destroy the health of humans.

"Modern meat production, modern dairy production, treat the animals with a level of cruelty, brutality, that if you saw how severe it is –
you wouldn't have to be a vegetarian, you wouldn't have to be an animal rights activist – to be appalled. I'm not talking about the fact that
the animals are killed. I don't want to deny that, but what I'm talking
about is how they live, how they are treated in a factory farm by corpo-

rate agribusiness, and it is really ugly. And you don't have to support it."
— **John Robbins**, author of *The Food Revolution*, FoodRevolution.Org

Stress hormones damage brain cells and impair memory. They also raise the blood pressure and trigger the endocrine system to produce and release inflammatory hormones, which leads to damaging plaque buildup in the arteries. The hormones thicken the blood, increasing the likelihood of stroke and heart attack, and of irregular heartbeat. The hormones also cause fat to build up in the abdominal area, which is a risk factor in a slew of health conditions, such as heart disease, hypertension, and diabetes. In fact there is no part of the body that is not damaged by long-term stress, from the skin, hair, and nails, to the lungs and stomach, to the intestines, bones, joints, and nerves. Mental function is altered as stress ages the brain and brings about depression, psychosis, and other types of mental derangement. The immune system is degraded and the stage is set for bacteria, viruses, inflammation, and cancers to gain hold within the tissues.

When people consume animals raised in an unhealthful atmosphere, animals that are unhealthy because of the way they are treated, and the bad food and toxic drugs and poisonous farming chemicals they are exposed to, they are eating tissues that contain all of the elements these animals have in their system. The meat they are eating contains residues of all of the poisonous farming chemicals the animal has been exposed to, and all of the toxic drugs it was given, which cause disease. They are eating the fright chemicals that are released into the animal's body tissues when the animal knows it is about to be slaughtered, and the hormones that trigger their blood flow, breathing patterns, and senses surge with alarm. When people eat meat, they are eating the energy of illness, abuse, incarceration, suppression, violence, and slaughter.

"The thinking man must oppose all cruelties, no matter how deeply rooted in tradition or surrounded by a halo."
— **Albert Schweitzer**

You can decide what sort of energy you will allow into your body simply by selecting the types of foods you eat. You can either bring into your system the destructive energy that exists in slaughtered meat, which is the product of sickly and incarcerated farm animals, or you can bring in the good energy of Nature through following a diet that consists of plant matter: veganism.

When people or animals are mistreated, the pain they feel in their mind creates energy waves that travel through their body tissues, and into the surrounding atmosphere and elements. This creates a karmic ripple effect that travels through the energy fields of the planet, and affects all of humanity. This is the horror spread through war, through animal farming, through animal slaughter, through child abuse, through the destruction of and misuse of Nature, and all of the other ugly, unkind, and cruel behaviors of humans.

If a person disrespects other life forms and Nature, they will not be able to tune in to the spiritual power to be gained by respecting life. Spiritual truths will be closed off to them. The abuse of farm animals, the mass breeding of them into the tens of billions, the vile factory farming of them, the slaughter and consumption of them, and the destruction of Nature in relation to raising billions of farm animals are damaging to the collective spiritual health of all life.

People should use only what they need from Nature; otherwise the misuse and destruction of Nature can create energy that leads to destruction and illness. When people live in tune with Nature, they absorb the good energy that Nature has to offer, and this energy can help those people be healthy and happy.

Meat, Dairy, Eggs, and Human Disease

Imagine being kept in a box your entire life, indoors, fed an unnatural diet, and surrounded by and slathered with your own excrement. This is how factory farm animals live their lives. Then their flesh, milk, and eggs are sold in packaging that feature drawings of happy animals living in pleasant, pristine country farm settings.

The meat, dairy, and egg industries work very hard to promote their products. One way they do this is by hiring top celebrities and sports stars to appear in funny little slick commercials promoting the consumption of meat, eggs, and dairy products.

Most every American is familiar with one or more of the phrases, "Got milk?" "Milk does a body good," "Every body needs milk," "The other white meat," and "The incredible edible egg." We have been bombarded with a slew of ads from the National Fluid Milk Processor Promotion Board featuring "super" models, singers, sports stars, and cast members from popular TV shows wearing milk mustaches.

The animal farming industry also spends millions of dollars every year to influence government and industrial nutrition programs, and to produce and distribute free school materials to misinform children that eating meat, dairy products, and eggs is a good thing to do for the body.

Who pays for a large portion of this advertising from the meat, milk, and egg industries, including those mustache ads? Taxpayers. The government provides funding in the form of corporate welfare that we nicely refer to as "subsidies." The government does this to help various industries promote business. The dairy industry gets federal money to advertise milk. The cheese industry gets federal money to advertise cheese. The egg industry gets federal money to advertise eggs. The beef industry gets federal money to promote beef. The chicken industry gets federal money to advertise chicken. The hog industry gets federal money to promote pork. And all that money advertises foods that promote heart disease, diabetes, arthritis, colon cancer, obesity, strokes, heart attacks, breast cancer, osteoporosis, prostate cancer, blindness, kidney disease, and perhaps Alzheimer's disease.

The publicity and advertising campaigns of the animal farming industries present the image that Americans are not eating enough animal products and that eating more of those products rather than less promotes better health. The truth is that the amount of animal products Americans already eat is unhealthful, and increasing the amount of the products would be even more unhealthful.

A closer look at meats, dairy products, and eggs shows why this is so.

"Most people have no idea at all that animals are being fed to animals; have no idea that we are feeding arsenic to chickens; that we end up recycling manure back through the animals; that we feed them [farm animals] cement dust. Most of us have no idea in the world who produced our food, or what they used on it, what it will do to us, the environment, or the animals."
— Howard Lyman, author of *Mad Cowboy and No More Bull: The Mad Cowboy Targets America's Worst Enemy: Our Diet*; MadCowboy.Com; appearing in the McLibel documentary; SpannerFilms.Net

What the commercials and promotional materials do not tell you is that the more meat, dairy products, and eggs a person consumes, the more likely he is to get cancer and experience other degenerative diseases. Studies have shown over and over that the less meat people consume and the more their diets are based on fruits and vegetables, the less likely they are of experiencing heart disease.

In addition to heart attacks, a person's risk of experiencing strokes, kidney disease, diabetes, arthritis, obesity, and various types of cancer corresponds with the amount of meat, eggs, and milk products that person consumes.

The foods that contain heart-choking cholesterol – meats, dairy, and eggs – also contain an unhealthful substance: saturated fat. Cholesterol and saturated fat clog the blood systems in the body and this causes heart disease and strokes. Heart attacks and strokes are leading causes of death in the U.S., Argentina, and Finland, and these countries are the world's top consumers of meats. Using 2005 statistics from the American Heart Association, heart disease in the U.S. accounts for about 900,000 strokes and heart attacks per year.

For men, the consumption of meat and dairy and the cholesterol imbalances these substances cause increases the incidence of prostate cancer. Researchers at Johns Hopkins University conducted a study that showed how men with low cholesterol are one-third less likely to get high-grade prostate cancer. This aggressive cancer is likely to recur after the prostate has already been removed. The study used statistics from an ongoing Harvard University study that involves 18,000 health professionals. The prostate cancer study took the blood samples of 700 men in the study with prostate cancer and compared those to blood samples of 700 men who had not experienced the cancer. Numerous other studies have concluded that men who are overweight are more likely to experience prostate cancer, and that men and women who are overweight are more likely to experience cancers of the colon, kidney, liver, and pancreas. People who are vegetarian or vegan are less likely to be overweight.

Eating animals also includes the risk factor of experiencing other illnesses.

Along with the cholesterol that is contained in meat, there are contaminants that can cause illness.

People often associate the salmonella and Escherichia coli (E. coli [there are hundreds of strains of E. coli]) bacteria with getting poisoning from flesh foods. The reality is those are only two types of contamination found in flesh foods. Other bacteria include clostridia, campylobacter, staphylococci, and lysteria. Other than a variety of bacteria, some of the more common contaminants found in beef include urine, dirt, feces, vomit, bovine immunodeficiency virus, bovine leukemia virus, pus, rodent contaminants, insects, and parasites. Pork and poultry also contain some of these and other contaminants. Basically the slaughter of the animals spreads their blood, urine, feces, and undigested food among the meats. This should be no surprise; cutting the bodies of animals into pieces is a messy activity.

Some of the carcinogens that meat eaters are exposed to are the residues of the toxic pesticides, insecticides, and other chemicals that are used on and around the livestock, and on the grains and other things fed to them. Additionally, the antibiotics, breeding drugs, and other drugs fed to and injected into farm animals, as well as the fertilizers in the feed often are present in the flesh and dairy foods that humans consume. According to the EarthSave Foundation, 55 percent of the antibiotics used in the U.S. are given to livestock.

If that isn't enough, chickens are often given feed additives containing arsenic. These "arsenicals" are growth-promoting and antimicrobial substances for chickens. In humans arsenic is known to cause or contribute to diabetes, heart disease, cancer, and brain function disorders.

In April 2006 the Institute for Agriculture and Trade Policy released a study that looked into the arsenic levels of chicken commonly sold in supermarkets and fast-food outlets. Over half of the supermarket chicken and all of the fast-food chicken they had tested contained arsenic. It doesn't stop there; the arsenic from chicken farms also contaminates the surrounding environment and water sources.

"The conservative estimate is that bad chicken kills at least 1,000 people each year and costs several billion dollars annually in medical costs and lost productivity."
— *Time Magazine*, October 17, 1994

One of the worst incidents of food poisoning occurred in 1993 when E. coli bacteria-contaminated beef sold in California, Idaho, Nevada, and Washington killed five people, sickened more than 500, sent 144 to the hospital, and caused thirty to experience kidney failure. When this type of thing happens the U.S. Department of

Agriculture gets involved because that branch of the government is responsible for meat, poultry, and processed eggs; and the Food and Drug Administration gets involved because that department oversees fresh produce and other foods. And a lot of fingers get involved because everyone starts pointing fingers at each other, and at what they think may be source of the pathogen.

Even when food poisoning results from eating fruits and vegetables it is often traced back to water or farming equipment contaminated by farming animals.

The occurrence of food poisoning from meat, dairy, and eggs is not rare. In the 1990s the Centers for Disease Control and Prevention reported that there were 6.5 million cases of illnesses and 9,000 deaths caused by food poisoning every year. Most of these cases of food poisoning are from contaminated meat, eggs, milk, and seafood products.

In July 1996, when President Clinton announced sweeping changes in the government's meat and poultry inspection system it was reported that salmonella bacteria kills more than 4,000 people a year and meat and poultry containing pathogens (microorganisms that cause disease) sickens as many as ten million.

Anyone who has ever experienced salmonella bacteria poisoning can attest to how sick it can make a person. Typical signs of salmonella poisoning include diarrhea, chills, lethargy, vomiting, and fever. Occasionally a person dies from salmonella poisoning.

People may think that it is difficult to be exposed to salmonella bacteria. But more than 20 percent of broiler chickens are contaminated with the bacteria. Eating undercooked chicken is thought to be the most common way to be exposed to the bacteria. Exposure also occurs when the bacteria are spread around on kitchen utensils and surfaces while chicken carcasses are being prepared for consumption.

> "E-coli 01 57:H7 a meat-borne pathogen is responsible for approximately 73,000 cases of infection and 60 deaths in the United States each year."
> — A Voice for Animals, 2006; VoiceForAnimals.Net

The U.S. government began its USDA meat inspection program in 1907 after the filthy and hazardous conditions of Chicago stockyards and slaughterhouses were exposed in Upton Sinclair's book *The Jungle*.

Though the Department of Agriculture would like the public to think otherwise, meat inspectors do not inspect every nook and cranny of every dead hog, cow, chicken, turkey, lamb, and other farm animal to find diseases and contaminants before the meats from these animals are sold in markets. The dead animals pass by the inspectors at very high rates of speed at meat processing plants.

The inspectors, who are supposed to rely on touch, smell, and visual inspection of meats are hardly likely to detect much of anything that can poison humans who eat dead animals. The cow carcasses in the IBP beef processing plant in Dakota City, Nebraska, accelerated 125 percent from 1969 to 1994 and in 1996 the carcasses whizzed by at 330 per hour (*The New Jungle,* by Stephen J. Hedges, Dana Hawkins, and Penny Loeb; *News & World Report,* September 23, 1996).

In his book *Beyond Beef,* Jeremy Rifkin explains, "Under the new FSIS (Food Safety Inspection Service) program, federal inspectors no longer have the authority to even stop the line if they spot a problem... Unless the company itself agrees that a problem exists or a violation of law occurred, the federal inspector is helpless to take a remedial action." Stopping the inspection line to pull a carcass slows down the packaging plants, and slowing down the work costs money. Regulators have suggested making inspectors use microscopes to detect bacteria on the dead animals, but the industry has opposed such measures.

> "The inspection system is only marginally better today at protecting the public from harmful bacteria than it was a year ago, or even 87 years ago when it was first put into place. FSIS' recent efforts have neither dealt with the inspection system's inherent weaknesses, nor fundamentally changed the system's predominant reliance on sensory inspection methods. These methods cannot identify microbial contamination, such as harmful bacteria, which is the most serious health risk from meat and poultry. Although FSIS has known about this problem for fifteen years or more, its major initiative in response – creating a new inspection system – is still years away."
> — **U.S. General Accounting Office assessment of meat inspection in the U.S., presented to the Senate, May 24, 1994**

The changes that have been made to the meat inspection process are implemented slowly and randomly. They may reduce the risk of becoming sick from contaminated meat, but no matter how many changes are made in the inspection process, meat will continue to make people sick.

> "A considerable body of scientific data suggests positive relationships between vegetarian diets and risk reduction for several chronic degenerative diseases and conditions, including obesity, coronary artery disease, hypertension, diabetes mellitus, and some types of cancer."
> — The American Dietetic Association

It is interesting that after the fast-food restaurants have made billions from selling disease-inducing food, they donate money to open places like Ronald McDonald House (headquartered in Chicago) and the Burger King Cancer Caring Center (headquartered in Pittsburgh). As if they care about our health — as they sell large orders of French fries that contain more fat and calories than their burgers, and oversized soda drinks containing the corn syrup that leads to obesity, intestinal inflammation, and diabetes, and phosphoric acid that weakens bones.

> "Worldwide, if you look at the rise in fast-food consumption, it's very closely linked to the rise in obesity."
> — Eric Schlosser, author of *Fast Food Nation*, appearing in the *McLibel* documentary; SpannerFilms.Org

The fast-food companies know that it is best to hook consumers when they are young. That is why they use cartoon characters in their commercials, design their restaurants to appeal to children, and build playgrounds next to the dining areas. They also do commercial tie-ins with Hollywood movies that appeal to children and sign exclusive marketing agreements with Hollywood studios to give out movie-related toys. All this is done to get children hooked on the disease-causing stomach filler sold at the counters and to make eating dead animals and junk look like an ecstatic rush.

The film companies should refuse to participate in this unhealthy practice of luring children to meat, dairy, soda, and junk foods. But TV and film companies partially finance their productions with money paid to them by food companies that want their products seen in the hands of TV and movie stars.

When you watch a TV show or movie and you see the label on the can of soda the star is holding, it is no mistake that the label is facing the camera lens. That's what the food companies pay for. Maybe

later in their career you will see the same star featured in a commercial marketing pharmaceutical drugs prescribed to treat the osteoporosis partially caused by drinking soda.

Many studies have concluded that drinking soda beverages weakens bones, especially in women. They may do this by preventing the
absorption of calcium from food and by altering bone density-regu-
lating parathyroid hormones.

Weak bones from consuming soda is only one of the many damaging effects of eating what is typically sold at fast-food restaurants.

A 1995 study of 2,000 people published in the *Archives of Ophthal-
mology* suggested that eating a diet high in saturated fat and cholesterol increases the risk of age-related macular degeneration – the
leading cause of irreversible blindness among persons older than
sixty-five. This being so, perhaps many of these cases of blindness
should be diagnosed as "meat-eater-related macular degeneration."

> **"The U.S. Public Health Service has said that there is consistent evi-
> dence between the intake of saturated fat with the incidence of higher
> blood cholesterol, and increased risk of colon cancer, breast cancer, and
> coronary heart disease."**
> **– The Surgeon General's Report on Nutrition and Health, 1989**

People see the juicy meat on their plates but are not exposed to the
sight of the heart-stopping cholesterol and saturated fat that gets
slathered through their veins and arteries when they eat that meat.

The unhealthful animal flesh-based American diet contributes to
many of the ailments people experience and for which they seek medical help. Besides being major risk factors in the most common types
of heart diseases and strokes, meats are a major source of destructive
free radicals that damage body tissues. Eating animal products intro-
duces prostaglandin-2 into the body and increases the uric acid level,
and these both promote arthritic conditions.

In the U.S., osteoporosis causes more deaths than cancers of the
breast and cervix combined. Americans have the highest rate of
osteoporosis in the world. Americans consume more meat and dairy
products than anyone in the world. Osteoporosis is most common in
exactly those countries where dairy products are consumed in the
largest quantities – the United States, Finland, Sweden, and the
United Kingdom.

While many people believe they need to eat animal flesh to get protein and drink milk to get calcium, they would be better off getting their protein and calcium from plant sources. Trying to get calcium from milk to prevent osteoporosis actually does the opposite – it contributes to osteoporosis.

The protein in meats, dairy, and egg products is concentrated. Eating these animal products leads to bone calcium depletion. After the concentrated protein from animal products is consumed, it makes its way into the blood where it produces an acid condition. The blood then takes calcium out of the bones where the body stores calcium and uses the calcium to neutralize the acidity level of the blood. The kidneys then excrete this calcium and excess protein. This scenario (protein-induced hypercalcuria) leads to osteoporosis (bones lacking in calcium) and some types of kidney stones. Eliminating animal protein from the diet can cut urinary calcium loss in half (*American Journal of Clinical Nutrition*, 1994; 59:1356-1361). Osteoporosis and hip fractures are much less common in countries where meat, dairy, and egg consumption is low (*The China Diet and Health Study*, Colin Campbell, MS, Ph.D., director).

A high-protein diet is also not recommended for such ailments as Parkinson's disease (*Nutritional Considerations of Parkinson's Disease*, National Parkinson Foundation, 1995), and for kidney dialysis patients (*Journal of the American Society of Nephrology*, December 1995). For these and other reasons, the last thing people need to do is eat more animal-based foods. It would be more healthful to eliminate all animal-based foods – and instead, eat a plant-based diet.

After heart disease, the second-leading cause of death in the U.S. is cancer.

The second-leading cause of cancer-related deaths in the U.S. is colorectal cancer. This type of cancer is most common in people who eat meat and dairy products.

"Women ages fifty-five to sixty-nine who eat more than thirty-six servings of red meat a month appear to have a 70 percent greater risk of developing non-Hodgkin's lymphoma than those who consume less than twenty-two servings."
— Time Magazine, May 13, 1996

Advertising produced by the animal-farming industry can give a person the impression that meat, dairy, and eggs are health foods. The commercials mention the protein content of the products and say this is good. They tell us "milk is a natural."

This advertising is a pack of lies. Dead cow is not a health food. Cow milk is also not a health food for humans. Cow milk is best consumed by baby cows. Dead chicken is not a health food. Chickens, hogs, lambs, cows, turkeys, deer, ducks, and other dead animals and fowl that humans eat have the fat and cholesterol that cause a wide variety of human diseases.

Mad Cow

On March 20, 1996, British Health Minister Stephen Dorrell conceded that the incurable and deadly Creutzfeldt-Jakob disease (CJD) which had killed at least ten people in that country was being linked to bovine spongiform encephalopathy (BSE) – now more popularly known as "mad cow disease."

Dorrell told the British Broadcasting Corporation that the "risks associated with eating beef and beef products are extremely low." He also stressed that a conclusive link between BSE and CJD had not been established. His words did not reassure the public, especially after he added, "Is there a particular risk for beef eating among smaller children? That is a precise question to which we have not yet received a precise answer."

The deaths attributed to BSE infection in 1996 were reported by scientists in Scotland. These scientists found a new strain of CJD in teenagers and young adults. They theorized that the victims might have been infected by beef from the first stage of the BSE epidemic that happened in Britain between 1986 and 1990.

The earlier epidemic caused hundreds of schools in Britain to eliminate beef from cafeteria menus and prompted many British consumers to eliminate beef from their diet. The schools continued to keep beef off their menus even though the British government repeatedly stated that it was unlikely BSE would cause any risk to human health.

The CJD cases among younger people in Britain rose from 18 cases in 1990 to 56 cases in 1994 and dropped to 42 cases in 1995. The average age of the previous victims of CJD was 63 years. It was reported at the time that ten or more years might pass after infection before physical symptoms of the disease become apparent.

The $6-billion-a-year British cattle industry was turned upside down overnight as cattle prices immediately dropped 15 percent and eventually collapsed. Over 161,000 cattle in Britain had been identified as having BSE and were eventually slaughtered and then burned in incinerators. Beef was eliminated from school and restaurant menus in Britain. Restaurants serving beef lost their clientele. The McDonald's restaurant chain outlets in Britain, already unpopular with British consumers because of the company's brash business practices, suspended the sale of British beef products. McDonald's and other fast-food restaurants announced that they would supply their British restaurants with imported beef. Belgium, France, and five German states immediately banned imports of British beef. British Airways stopped serving beef. The $1 billion annual British beef export business collapsed within days. British scientists and veterinary experts met with officials of the European Union in Brussels and tried unsuccessfully to quell the public concerns and prevent the EU from taking action to alter the exporting of British beef products. (The EU is a multinational organization that regulates trade and agricultural policy in Western Europe.)

The British beef news was reported around the world and threw the entire global beef industry into a tailspin. U.S. military officials in Germany ordered British beef products removed from commissaries in Italy, Spain, Turkey, Greece, and Scotland. More damage was done to the beef industry when people found out that BSE was not confined to Britain, but that Switzerland had recorded more than 200 cases of BSE and Ireland reported 124 cases. Farmers all over the world complained that the demand for beef had dramatically declined within one week.

One week after the British beef frenzy started, EU Agricultural Commissioner Franz Fischler announced that the 20-member EU executive commission was banning exports of British beef. The EU applied the ban to all live animals, all beef and veal products made from animals slaughtered in Britain, cattle sperm and embryos, as well as beef products used in the pharmaceutical and cosmetic industries.

Britain's Agricultural Secretary, Douglass Hogg, said he thought the ban was an overreaction based on public fears rather than scientific evidence and that the ban should be removed. New Zealand, Africa, Singapore, and South Korea joined the EU in banning imports of British beef. Dutch authorities ordered the destruction of 64,000 calves imported from Britain. The Irish Food Board in Dublin reported drops in beef purchases of as much as 30 percent in Italy and Spain, 40 percent in France, and 55 percent in Germany.

Within days of the ban there was a day where only four cows were killed in British slaughterhouses nationwide. One slaughterhouse that normally killed 350 cows a week closed down its beef area. Europe's largest livestock market sold no cattle, but the prices of hogs and sheep increased to record levels.

In response to the British beef ban, U.S. beef industry leaders issued press releases and pressured U.S. health officials to announce that CJD was not a threat to U.S. residents. The Department of Agriculture announced that the U.S. stopped importing British beef in 1985, and stopped importing British cattle in 1989.

Though the U.S. Department of Agriculture announced that it checks every head of cattle brought to slaughterhouses for signs of neurological disorders, including BSE, rabies, and milk fever, anyone familiar with the meat inspection program in the U.S. knows that this claim is very far from the truth. Saying that inspectors can detect BSE in cows whizzing by inspectors in slaughterhouses is more than an unfounded claim, it is a blatant lie. Only post-slaughter laboratory examinations can detect BSE in cows that show no symptoms.

Radio talk show hosts around the world were deluged with calls from listeners wanting to know more about CJD.

Cattle industry stocks dropped in the U.S. and investors lost hundreds of millions of dollars the day Oprah Winfrey broadcast an episode of her show that questioned the safety of U.S. beef. Iowa legislators who were pressured by their state beef interests asked Winfrey to take back what was said on the show, but she defended the program.

In response to the concerns over BSE, the World Health Organizations held a two-day conference that drew 30 scientists from 14 countries. The team recommended that to keep the disease from spreading, all countries should immediately destroy all animals infected with BSE.

Though cattle in Britain had been dying of the disease for more than a decade, and CJD was linked to meat consumption in the July 7, 1990, issue of the *Lancet* (British medical journal), the news from the British prime minister that BSE could cause humans to die a slow and miserable death was the first time many people heard of the disease.

In April 1996, Britain began killing and incinerating nearly five million older cows at a rate of approximately 15,000 per week. This was done at a huge cost and used up tremendous amounts of resources.

Prosper de Mulder, the company entrusted with destroying cows suspected of harboring Mad Cow disease accidentally exported animal feed containing cattle to as many as 70 countries around the world.

> "In reality, out of 900 million U.S. cattle slaughtered in the last decade, the USDA only tested 12,000 for Mad Cow disease – roughly one in every 75,000 cattle."
> — **John Robbins, *The Food Revolution*; TheFoodRevolution.Org**

Scientists believe BSE in cattle is linked to ground-up sheep parts, ingredients cryptically referred to as "sheep offal," such as brains and spinal cords that were infected with scrapie and that had been blended into cattle feed to increase its protein content – a practice that was banned in Britain in 1989 – though some slaughterhouses violated the ban.

Based on the theory that BSE hides in the central nervous system, the British ban on using sheep offal in cattle feed also included a ban on the use of brains and spinal cords in human food. But it is easy to figure out that the presence of BSE is hardly limited to the brain and spinal column. Nerves exist throughout all the body tissues. It is highly unlikely that those people who experienced the horrible death caused by mad cow disease contracted the disease by feasting on cow brains.

Some understanding of the disease came about when Dr. Stanley Prusiner of San Francisco State University reported his belief that CJD is caused by a malfunctioning infectious misfolded protein called a prion (pronounced PREE-on). Prions deposit plaque on the brain and kill brain cells.

Other infectious diseases are caused by organisms containing either RNA or DNA, the materials that carry genetic information. Proteins do not contain RNA or DNA, and this made the discovery of prions a major new development in understanding the way diseases may be transported.

CJD is similar to a disease called *kuro* or *kuru* that was found in the 1950s in women and children who were members of the cannibalistic Fore tribe in New Guinea. It is also related to an ailment noticed in sheep and goats that causes the animals to lose their motor functions. The ailment in sheep and goats was noticed a couple hundred years ago in England and given the name "scrapie" because the ailing farm animals often rubbed against trees and other objects. In France it was given the name *tremblant* because the animals trembled. (The Prion Diseases, *Scientific American*, January 1995. Mad Cow Disease: Is It a Prion or a Virus?; *Los Angeles Times*, May 26, 1996.)

Both CJD and BSE eat away at the brain, resulting in microscopic holes, which give it a spongelike appearance. Cows with BSE lose weight, walk crookedly, become uncoordinated and aggressive, begin to shake and stare – essentially, they become incapacitated and go "mad." People with CJD become visually impaired, suffer from dementia, experience limb paralysis, lose the ability to formulate words, their thought processes become blurred, their memory fails them. It usually causes death within six months after the onset of symptoms.

After all this mad cow news in the 1990s, the U.S. Centers for Disease Control reported that there were an estimated 250 cases of CJD in the U.S. every year, but they were quick to add that they believed these cases were unrelated to diet. Some people believe the number is much higher, and that the CJD rate of infection will start to expose itself much in the same way that HIV has in the last 30 years.

Researchers at the Imperial College School of Medicine in London concluded that biochemical traces of an infectious agent from people with a rare form of CJD are identical to such traces found in cows. The researchers announced that they developed a test for prions. They found biochemical patterns of prions found in patients with the rare form of CJD to be identical to those of prions from laboratory animals infected with the disease. They found the "fingerprints" to be different from those of prion strains taken from patients who suffer from what is believed to be an inherited or what they call a "sporadic form" of CJD.

"I believe that in the U.S. up to 14 percent of cows are ground up and fed back to cows. I am very concerned that this will lead to the same sort of thing that is happening in the UK."

— Former Montana cattle rancher Howard Lyman, author of *Mad Cowboy*, and *No More Bull: The Mad Cowboy Targets America's Worst Enemy: Our Diet*, MadCowboy.Com; referring to mad cow disease in his testimony at the McLibel trial in London in April 1996. See the *McLibel* documentary, SpannerFilms.Net

Meanwhile, more and more cases of mad cow disease keep turning up in cattle in North America – followed by unconvincing press releases stating that American meat eaters have no need to worry, that the beef they are eating is safe.

On December 30, 2003, after a Holstein raised on a Washington state farm tested positive for mad cow disease, three dozen countries banned the import of American beef. That halted 90 percent of U.S. beef exports.

> "The system that we had in place, plus the additional safeguards that were announced, should continue to satisfy consumers in the U.S. that we have a very safe meat supply."
> – Dr. W. Ron DeHaven, USDA chief veterinarian; December 2003

The U.S. Meat Export Federation is an organization that is partially funded by the U.S. Department of Agriculture. They have been very busy working to convince other countries that U.S. beef is safe to eat. According to their Web site, the USMEF has offices in Seoul, Tokyo, Osaka, Hong Kong, Shanghai, Singapore, Taipei, Moscow, St. Petersburg, Mexico City and London. Yes, millions of American tax dollars help promote the sale of meat around the world.

During the last week of December 2003, the U.S. sent officials to Japan to convince them to continue their annual $1 billion importation of American beef. But Japan refused. The American beef industry was not happy. Japan only opened its doors to U.S. beef in the 1980s. It quickly became the number one importer of U.S. beef, which accounted for over 35 percent of the beef consumed in Japan.

The U.S. announced more stringent regulations to track cattle. But their tactics were somewhat unconvincing. The U.S. still only tests a small fraction of its cattle for BSE. It is estimated that the U.S. tests about one of every 90 cows for BSE. Since Japan discovered a cow with BSE among its own herds in September 2001, that country tests every single one of their cattle. Europe tests about one in four of their cattle.

A typical large beef processing plant in the U.S. grinds the meat of so many cows together that one hamburger could contain the meat from hundreds – if not thousands – of cows.

There is also the problem of what cows are eating. Cattle are naturally vegetarian. What they eat in the wild is plants. They don't eat animals. Although cattle aren't supposed to be eating dead cows, it is typical to have the remains of cows from slaughterhouses in feed that is given to other farm animals, such as chickens and pigs. It is also typical to use chicken manure in cattle feed.

Do you recognize the circle? Have you ever seen a group of chickens eat? Their food gets scattered. In a factory farm the food the chickens eat gets scattered below them, where their manure drops. The manure is gathered and sold to companies that use it as part of the ingredients in cattle feed. So cattle are still eating cattle. Also, baby cows are often fed a "milk replacer" that contains blood from slaughterhouses. Do you think that is disgusting? Baby cows don't normally consume the blood of cows. Baby cows drink cow milk. But the milk of their mothers is taken and sold for human consumption.

Meanwhile, Australia and some other "beef-producing countries" have increased their imports of beef to Japan and some of the other three dozen countries refusing U.S. beef.

Some countries have opened their doors to U.S. beef, and then shut them again after BSE has been found among U.S. cattle.

It didn't help the profits of the U.S. beef industry when the U.S. Department of Agriculture announced the death of a cow in June 2005 that had died from BSE seven months prior to the announcement. The department said that it wasn't trying to cover up the evidence. Oh, and they once again assured the public that U.S. beef is safe to eat.

The USDA's assurance isn't very assuring when it is taken into account that more cattle with BSE continue to be found in the U.S. Aside from the concerns of BSE, how safe is a product that leads to heart disease, heart attacks, strokes, colon cancer, arthritis, and a slew of other health problems?

In the dictionary it says that safe means free from risk, harmless, and secure from threat or danger. That word doesn't define the product we call "beef."

As I write this during the summer of 2006 there is another case of mad cow disease. This is something we should get used to. Maybe one day people will wake up and realize that the government has been misleading American consumers, that the government is acting out of the financial interests of the beef, restaurant, and supermarket industries, and that the government can't be relied on as a source for accurate information about food safety.

Diseases Jumping from Animals to Humans

Consider the threat to the human species that exists in breeding billions of farm animals on every continent, keeping them in cramped quarters, feeding them unnatural diets that weaken their immune systems, and giving them drugs that familiarize various germs and viruses to the same drugs that are used to protect the human species.

The number of diseases that have jumped from animals to humans is a long one, and includes some of the most recognizable disease names:

• AIDS: Autoimmune Deficiency Syndrome

• Bubonic plague

• CJD: Creutzfeldt-Jakob disease, the human form of mad cow disease. In cows it is called bovine (cow) spongiform (sponge-like) encephalopathy (brain disease): BSE.

• Influenza

• Leprosy

• Measles

• Smallpox

• Tuberculosis

• Typhoid fever

• Whooping cough

• Yellow fever

• and evidence suggests: Alzheimer's disease

Eating animal protein in the form of meat, dairy, and eggs increases the likelihood that you will experience:

• Acne

• Alzheimer's disease

• Arteriosclerosis

- Arthritis
- Asthma
- Back injuries
- Cancers of a wide variety, including that of the colon, bladder, breasts, prostate, and other organs
- Degenerative vision disease
- Diabetes
- Heart attack
- High blood pressure/hypertension
- High cholesterol
- Kidney disease
- Kidney stones
- Obesity
- Osteoporosis
- Stroke

Including trans fats and/or pasteurized/processed/heated/non-raw dairy (milk, cream, cheese, yogurt, kefir, butter, etc.) in the diet seems to magnify and/or contribute to a number of these conditions.

"In 1980 the FDA reversed a 1967 prohibition on feeding poultry waste to cattle, leaving the regulation of feeding animal wastes to the individual states. Downer cattle – dead, dying, diseased or disabled (what the Food and Drug Administration refers to as the 4-Ds) – have also been 'recycled' into feed, including poultry feed, as a source of protein.

While the case of mad cow disease in Washington State may have been from a Canadian herd prior to the 1997 ban on feeding ruminant proteins to cattle, it is equally plausible – though state and federal agencies have not discussed it with the public – that the case was caused by feeding contaminated poultry feces to cattle. The FDA did not ban the inclusion of ruminant proteins in nonruminant feed, as did the United Kingdom. Thus ruminant proteins from both healthy and 4-D animals continue to be 'recycled' into animal feed and pet foods, including poultry feed.

The problem is that poultry feces have routinely been used as cattle feed, keeping the prohibited cycle of 'feeding cattle to cattle' intact.

Perhaps the recent finding of mad cow will alert Americans who naively believe that the government is protecting the food supply."
— Safe Food and Fertilizer, *Earth Island Journal*, Spring 2006

That article in *Earth Island Journal* suggests that people be aware that contaminated poultry feces may end up in their yards via "organic" fertilizer. If you purchase fertilizer, avoid the brands that contain poultry waste. A database identifying some commercial fertilizers that contain poultry waste can be accessed through:
APPS.Ecy.WA.Gov/Fertilizer/Index.html.

"Modern factory farms raise animals in extremely unnatural conditions. Almost all 10 billion land animals who are slaughtered in the U.S. each year are forced to live in extremely crowded sheds. They are surrounded by their own filth and breathe ammonia-laden air that destroys their lungs and compromises their immune systems. It comes as no surprise that these facilities have become major sources for deadly disease outbreaks such as hoof-and-mouth disease, mad cow disease, Mycobacterium paratuberculosis (which is thought by most scientists to cause Crohn's disease in humans), and now the most dangerous of all: bird flu.

Avian influenza, or 'bird flu,' threatens humanity with the greatest public health crisis in recorded history. Experts warn that the disease could kill one in eight human beings, including 40 million Americans, and cause a collapse of the world economy. According to the Centers for Disease Control and Prevention (CDC) and the World Health Organization (WHO), while the virus is destroyed by thorough cooking, it can be caught simply by eating undercooked meat or eggs, by eating food prepared on the same cutting board as infected meat or eggs, or even by touching eggshells contaminated with the disease."
— GoVeg.Com/BirdFlu.asp, 2006

In 1918 the Spanish flu pandemic killed tens of millions of people, and sickened as much as half the world's human population. Now nearly 100 years later we are being warned by international organizations that we are on the edge of an epidemic that may lead to the deaths of hundreds of millions of people.

The Spanish flu was caused by a variant of H1N1, which is now a common form of influenza. It is believed to have originated as a bird flu. The current bird flu has a ripe breeding ground in the billions of chickens and turkeys that live in factory farms throughout the world. These warehouse bird farms have been built at an alarming rate to satisfy the global demand for bird flesh and eggs. The current bird flu has been around for thousands of years, but has existed as an intestinal infection in aquatic birds. Only now that there are billions of farm birds being bred and kept in crammed structures has the virus been able not only to spread, but also become resilient to the drugs given to the farm animals, which are the same drugs humans rely on to fight disease.

Because birds that carry the virus don't necessarily become sick, we have no idea how many birds have it, or where the virus exists. Because birds constantly fly hundreds, and some thousands, of miles it only takes months for an illness like this to be spread throughout the world. No need to punish the wild birds, it is the billions of birds kept on farms that are the real threat. And we may soon learn how big the threat is.

In November 2006 South Korea discovered bird flu on a chicken farm. As I write this they are slaughtering hundreds of thousands of birds that may have been exposed. They are also killing dogs and cats in the region, even though scientists say these animals don't harbor or transfer the disease to humans. South Korea is one country where dog meat is eaten.

Alzheimer's Disease and Type 2 Diabetes

"In the coming decades, science will probably be able to ascribe a cause to Alzheimer's with the same certainty that it can now ascribe a cause to heart disease. And I firmly believe that it will be the exact same cause: meat... Studies have shown that between five and 14 percent of those diagnosed with Alzheimer's actually suffered from CJD. The amyloid plaques – waxy clumps of protein called beta-amyloid – discovered at autopsy in the brains of Alzheimer's victims are not terribly unlike the plaques to be found in the brains of victims of CJD. In both cases, abnormal protein buildup in the brain is involved."
— Former Montana cattle rancher Howard Lyman, in his book *No More Bull: The Mad Cowboy Targets America's Worst Enemy: Our Diet*; MadCowboy.Com

Those who are concerned about mad cow disease may also want to concern themselves with Alzheimer's disease and Type 2 diabetes. And all those who consume any sort of animal protein, be it milk, cow, pig, fish, fowl, or eggs should also be concerned about all three.

In the U.S., Alzheimer's disease affects approximately one in ten people over age 65. Over 600,000 Americans under age 65 are living with the disease. For those over age 85 the chances of having Alzheimer's are nearly 50 percent. In 2006 approximately 4.5 million people had been diagnosed with the disease. As of 2005 the medical costs of supporting those with Alzheimer's was estimated to cost more than $100 billion.

From where did the protein misfolding disease called Alzheimer's originate? It appears that nobody knows for sure. It has only been a recognized disease since a German psychiatrist and neuropathologist, Aloysius Alois Alzheimer, first identified it as "presenile dementia." In 1901 Alzheimer noticed the curious behavior and short-term memory loss of a 51-year-old patient, August Deter, at the Frankfurt Asylum. After she died in April 1906, Alzheimer studied her brain and identified the amyloid plaques and neurofibrilary tangles that became the identifiable physical characteristics of the disease. On November 3, 1906, Alzheimer gave a speech identifying the pathology and clinical symptoms of presenile dementia. His colleague, Emil Kraepelin, later referred to the condition as "Alzheimer's disease." Back then it was considered rare. But now there are millions with it, and it is expected to become more prevalent and a huge burden to society. Over 100 times more Americans have it today than just 25 years ago.

Many studies have concluded that the more animal protein you consume, the more likely you are to experience Alzheimer's. It is interesting that the more animal protein you consume the more likely it is that you will develop Type 2 diabetes.

In Alzheimer's it is found that there is a buildup of amyloid protein in the brain. In Type 2 diabetes there is a buildup of amyloid protein in the pancreas. Like Alzheimer's disease, Type 2 diabetes is on the rise.

The heavier you are, the more likely you are to have Type 2 diabetes. People who consume animal protein are more likely to be obese than those who follow a vegetarian diet. Those who follow a vegan diet are even less likely to be overweight. Sunfoodists are even less likely to be overweight.

Currently the number of overweight children is increasing. The number of younger people becoming afflicted with Type 2 diabetes is increasing at the same rate.

Epidemiologists expect that about one in three U.S. babies born in the year 2000 will develop Type 2 diabetes. As those children become adults and continue to eat an unhealthful diet, it is likely that they increase their chances of having Alzheimer's.

As the consumption of meat and the number of people eating junk food is on the rise throughout the world, the number of children and young adults being diagnosed with Type 2 diabetes is on the rise. It is estimated that there were about 30 million people with Type 2 diabetes in the early 1980s. Today that figure has surpassed 225 million.

Not only the future, but also the present day holds the promise that the more animal protein you consume, the more likely you are to contract the human form of mad cow disease. As Howard Lyman points out in his book, *No More Bull*, the brains of those with the human form of mad cow disease are found to have a buildup of protein plaque in their brain in a similar manner to those with Alzheimer's disease.

When I first heard of mad cow disease and what it does to the human brain and body, I thought that perhaps there would be a link between mad cow and Alzheimer's disease. In 1995 I wrote about it in my book, *Surgery Electives*. I was hardly the first person to make the connection. In his book, *The Food Revolution*, John Robbins mentions studies concluding that many presumed U.S. Alzheimer's victims were actually victims of CJD. If those studies represent current statistics, then there are likely several hundred thousand Americans suffering from CJD.

More recently the book, *Dying for a Hamburger: Modern Meat Processing and the Epidemic of Alzheimer's Disease*, by Murray Waldman, the Toronto coroner, and Marjorie Lamb puts forth a convincing argument that Alzheimer's is related to infectious prions. The man who discovered prions, Stanley Prusiner, considered that prions might be causing Alzheimer's.

Another book that would likely be of interest to anyone wanting to know details about America's food supply is *Brain Trust: The Hidden Connection Between Mad Cow and Misdiagnosed Alzheimer's Disease*, by Colm A. Kelleher. Among the books that may be of interest on this matter is *How the Cows Turned Mad: Unlocking the Mysteries of Mad Cow Disease*, by Maxime Schwartz, a molecular biologist and former head of the Pasteur Institute in Paris, and Edward Schneider.

What will most certainly guard you from CJD? Not eating animal protein.

What will decrease your chances of becoming a member of both the Alzheimer's disease and the Type 2 diabetes clubs? It very clearly appears that avoiding animal protein while following a diet that is abundant in fruits and vegetables and other plant substances while staying physically fit are the most promising ways to avoid those dreaded diseases.

It is well documented that following a healthy, balanced vegetarian diet free from junk food while getting plenty of physical activity will greatly reduce your chances of experiencing diabetes.

In August 2006 *The American Journal of Medicine* published a study concluding that drinking fruit and vegetable juice reduces the likelihood that a person will develop Alzheimer's disease. The study concluded that those who drank fruit and vegetable juice more than three times a week were 76 percent less likely to develop Alzheimer's than those who had less than one serving of juice per week.

The study involved studying the diet and health of nearly 2,000 Japanese Americans in Washington State. They were chosen because it has been well known that Japanese people who live in Japan had a lower incidence of Alzheimer's disease than Japanese people who live in the U.S.

The study, which was supported by the National Institute on Aging, concluded that regularly drinking fruit and vegetable juice was particularly beneficial for those who have a so-called genetic marker linked to an increased risk of developing Alzheimer's disease.

Isn't it interesting that people in Japan are both less likely to eat meat and less likely to experience Alzheimer's disease than people living in the U.S.?

Researchers involved in the study of Japanese Americans living in Washington believe that polyphenols, a class of antioxidants in fruits and vegetables, seem to have a protective effect on the brain, reduce the likelihood of dementia, and prevent the development of Alzheimer's disease.

Where can you find polyphenols? They are in fruits and vegetables, and are more abundant in the skin and peels.

Polyphenols are also found in wine, which is considered to be a raw food, and even better if it is organic and vegan. If you have an issue with alcohol, or have a family history of alcoholism, you may find it beneficial to stick to fresh grapes, or grape juice.

Another study concluded that eating a diet that contained plentiful amounts of fruits, vegetables, nuts, whole grains, legumes, and quality oils also greatly reduced the risk of Alzheimer's disease. The study, which was sponsored by the National Institution of Health and conducted by Columbia University Medical Center, recognized this diet as that most often referred to as the "Mediterranean Diet." While that type of diet also contains some fish, the diet is low in red meat and cooked oils. The study concluded that those who follow a Mediterranean diet are 53 percent less likely to develop Alzheimer's disease.

A study conducted in Stockholm, Sweden concluded that quality raw oils, such as those from flax and hemp seeds, reduced the signs of Alzheimer's disease in patients with very mild symptoms.

Want to avoid Alzheimer's disease, Type 2 diabetes, and obesity? Eat fruits, vegetables, quality raw plant oils, and other plant substances. If you don't have a problem with alcohol, occasionally enjoy a glass of organic, vegan wine.

Avoid consuming animal protein.

Unhealthful Diet of Farm Animals

Grain-based diets for farm animals increased dramatically after WWII as the use of new and toxic chemical fertilizers led to a surplus of grain and soybeans. This in turn led to the mass use of antibiotics on factory farms.

Cattle are naturally grass eaters. But when they are fed a diet largely of grain, as they are on factory farms, they experience stomach ulcers and liver abscesses, which are then treated with, or prevented from happening, by giving the cattle mass doses of antibiotics.

Currently it is estimated that about 70 percent of antibiotics used in America are given to cattle, poultry, and hogs. And the majority of those drugs are used in factory farms. This is done even though hundreds of organizations, including the World Health Organization and the American Medical Association, have spoken out against it.

The overuse of antibiotics leads to drug-resistant strains of bacteria. An increasing number of these are playing a role in 60,000 deaths in America each year.

When considering the toxic ingredients of many pet foods, and the substances that are fed to farm animals, you can see that there are many things in those foods that are not natural for the animals to eat – and which are also very damaging to the animals. A good example of this is what factory farms are feeding to animals to make the animals grow as big as they can as fast as they can so that the farms can sell the animals at the best market price.

"Concentrating thousands of head of cattle from different origins in close quarters bred disease, so I added antibiotics to the feed like sugar to a breakfast cereal for kids. Since cattle were not designed by Nature to digest the grain that I was using to fatten them up, I fought a constant losing battle to control their digestive ailments. I injected steroids into my bovines to further stimulate their growth and to abort pregnant heifers."

— Former Montana cattle rancher Howard Lyman, in his book *No More Bull: The Mad Cowboy Targets America's Worst Enemy: Our Diet*; MadCowboy.Com

Many people don't know that a grain diet is not what cows naturally eat. But grain is what they are fed in the feed lots to fatten them. And they suffer for it. Cattle that are fed mass quantities of grain experience liver and stomach ailments that then are treated with massive doses of drugs. This is only a very small part of what is wrong with the way cattle are raised on factory farms.

Farms have been feeding the animals food that contains dead farm animals; blood meal made from the blood collected at slaughterhouses; animal dung sold to animal feed companies from farms; a variety of drugs; sawdust; cement; ground-up newspaper and cardboard; and ground-up road kill and the remains of dogs and cats from government pounds (yes, the dogs and cats and other pets that get killed at your city pound are often sold to companies that make products out of them – including ingredients that end up in cosmetics).

The result of all of this is that a very high majority of farm animals are sickly. They also get so heavy so fast that their bone structures cannot support the weight. One reason for this is that their muscles are so filled with growth hormones that they become like the freakish body builders who inject themselves with various chemical drugs to make their muscles ridiculously huge.

Among the body building drugs farmers feed to farm animals are sex hormones. These include 17 beta-oestradiol, progesterone, testosterone, trenbolone, and Zeronal. The drugs were banned by the European Union in 1995 because they are believed to cause cancer and damage to nerves, muscles, and bones. But farmers in other countries continue to use them. The animals suffer because of it, becoming sickly and with bodies so heavy that it strains their bones, legs, and feet.

If these animals were released back into the wild they would quickly go back to their natural diet of wild plants. Their digestive tract and physical form would transform to that which is much healthier.

Examples of this can be seen in animal sanctuaries that care for rescued farm animals. The people working in these animal sanctuaries have witnessed numerous cases of sickly farm animals being brought to them that were then fed natural diets, which brought back the health of the animals – or health the animals had never been able to experience because of the disgusting stuff they were fed on farms.

The Sad Lives of Today's Farm Animals

"Modern-day agriculture is all about profit. Animals aren't treated as emotional creatures. Animals are treated like widgets on a factory line."
— **Jenny Brown, Woodstock Farm Animal Sanctuary, August 2006; WoodstockFAS.Org**

"We prefer to numb ourselves physically to the fact of the slaughterhouse. We don't like to remember that a hamburger is a ground-up cow."
— **John Robbins, in his book** *Diet for a New America*

"Animals in agriculture:
In 2001, nearly ten billion land animals and fowl were slaughtered for food in the U.S., including:
- 9.3 billion chickens
- 309 million turkeys
- 27.7 million ducks
- 41.6 million cattle/calves
- 118 million pigs
- 4.2 million sheep/lambs"
— **A Voice for Animals, VoiceForAnimals.Net**

"Eight billion broiler chickens are killed for food in the United States each year, a number larger than the entire human population of the planet."
— **John Robbins,** *The Food Revolution*; **TheFoodRevolution.Org**

Most of the animals that are raised for human consumption in the U.S. today live sad lives and are treated horribly. The unnatural conditions prevent the animals from natural patterns of behavior and they are fed an unnatural diet. (Some countries, such as Sweden, have passed laws preventing farm animals from being treated as badly as the U.S. farm industry treats its animals.)

"U.S. society is extremely naïve about the nature of agricultural production.

If the public knew more about the way in which agricultural and animal production infringes on animal welfare, the outcry would be louder."
— **Bernard E. Rollin, PhD, Farm Animal Welfare, 2003**

The open-prairie type animal farming began disappearing in the U.S. after WWII. Factory farms where thousands of animals are kept in steel confinement buildings as long as football fields are corporate investors' way of making money by producing as much beef, pork, chicken, eggs, and milk in the quickest and cheapest way while using the least amount of land. Under factory farming arrangements, the corporations supply the animals, feed, drugs, and insecticides, and farmers working under contract provide the land, buildings, and labor. A few powerful companies now control the majority of animal farming in the U.S.

"Veal calves are a waste by-product of the dairy industry. A cow, like any other mammal, cannot give milk unless she has offspring. Her life is a constant round of pregnancies with her young wrenched from her when they are just a day or two old. Within a couple of weeks, the youngsters destined for the veal trade are taken to livestock markets where they are bartered like cheap jewelry before being loaded onto lorries for the Continent."
— **Animal Aid, Britain, 1996**

"Across the country, factory farms confine nearly 300 million egg-laying hens inside wire cages so small that each bird has less space than a sheet of typing paper. These social, intelligent animals cannot spread their wings, perch, dust, bathe, or even walk. There lives are filled with suffering."
— **Erin Williams, outreach coordinator for the Factory Farming Campaign of the Humane Society; Los Angeles Times editorial, Saturday, December 22, 2006, in response to the original "Egg City" factory farm in Ventura County burning to the ground**

Many people think that factory farming (where animals are kept indoors their entire lives) is used only to raise veal cattle. In 1980 Jim Mason and Peter Singer came out with their book titled *Animal Factories*. The book exposed conditions of the U.S. animal factories of the 1970s, revealing the number of cattle, chickens, turkeys, and hogs being kept in total confinement their entire lives. Since that book was published, factory farming continues to take over more and more of the U.S. livestock industry. Factory farming is now the most common way to raise millions of dairy cows as well as billions of other farm animals.

"Every year in Britain over 700 million animals, most of whom spend their brief lives confined in brutal factory farms, are slaughtered for human food."
— Animal Aid, Britain, 1996

As with veal cattle, many farm animals are taken from their mothers when they are only hours old, or as soon as possible. They then spend their entire lives in large warehouse-type structures – known as "total confinement housing" – where they are fed by computerized feed and water distribution systems.

"Every year 20 million sheep, cattle, and pigs are bartered in the U.K. livestock markets. Some go from market direct to slaughter. Others go to another farmer for further fattening.
Most British livestock markets are overcrowded and ramshackle. On stone floors, slick with urine and excrement, the animals spend hours awaiting their fate. All the while they are subjected to the clanking of metal gates and the slaps, kicks, and violent stick-work of often poorly trained drovers. Rarely will any of these animals be given water – even in the height of summer."
— Animal Aid, Britain, 1996

To prepare them for life on the factory farm, hundreds of millions of the animals are physically altered. The male chicks are not needed, so they are thrown into plastic bags where they suffocate, or are killed in other ways, such as by being tossed into a machine that grinds them up shortly after they hatch from their eggs. The chickens that are allowed to survive have the front half of their beaks cut off with a blade or hot wire to keep them from pecking at each other, some have their toes cut off, and, because of their sickening diet and farm restraints, the majority end up with leukemia. Pigs have their teeth cut so they can't bite each other; their tails sliced off (tail docking); their ears notched; many are castrated; and some have nose rings put in. Cattle are burned with red-hot branding irons, dehorned, castrated, and many have their tails cut off. All of this is extremely painful and done without the use of pain-killing medication.

If all the cutting and altering of body parts on animals isn't enough, consider what some companies were looking into doing:

> "Q: What caused you to become skeptical of your work [as someone involved in conducting surgical experiments on animals]?
>
> A: A moral twinge. Somehow it didn't feel right to be cutting off the wings of newly hatched birds [shown to save on feed costs]. Later some of them couldn't get up onto their feet when they fell over. It wasn't pleasant seeing them spin around on their side trying to get back onto their feet, without their wings."
>
> — Interview of Dr. Eldon Keinholz (1928-1993), former professor of poultry nutrition at Colorado State University's Department of Animal Science. By Karen Davis Ph.D., Founder & President of United Poultry Concerns, UPC-Online.Org

The wing-cutting plan didn't fly. But there are ongoing experiments to bring genetically altered featherless chickens into animal farming. That way the birds would eat less because their bodies wouldn't have to produce feathers, and the slaughterhouses wouldn't have to spend so much time on the defeathering process.

Once the animals have been physically altered, they then get to live a terrifying existence crammed into living quarters a tiny fraction of the size of what they would experience in the wild. It is animal hell.

> "Some of the birds' necks had been pecked at by other birds until the neck bone was visible. This was not an uncommon sight. We used to talk about how the cries of the birds started to sound as if they were screaming 'help.'"
>
> — Mitchell, a former egg farm worker, as quoted in Behind Closed Doors: Former Factory Farm & Slaughterhouse Workers Speak Out; Outrage: The Magazine of Mercy for Animals, Summer/Fall 2006; MercyForAnimals.Org

> "Every year in the United States, about 600 million chicks are hatched – half are females and half are unwanted males. The 300 million males are unceremoniously discarded upon hatching, since they cannot profitably be raised for meat. We don't have good statistics on methods, but it appears the vast majority are ground up while still alive or tossed alive into garbage bags, where they smother."
>
> — Erik Marcus, author of the books Vegan: The New Ethics of Eating, and Meat Market: Animals, Ethics, and Money, 2006

Often the factory farm structures are the size of one or two football fields. But there is no field. There is concrete and steel – just like prison and concentration camps. They may contain a several thousand dairy cows, tens of thousands of hogs, or more than 150,000 chickens or turkeys.

Other than egg hens, the animals on factory farms spend most of their lives in the dark, or in very dim lighting. Many are rarely, if ever, exposed to fresh air or Sun light – unless you consider their transport to the slaughterhouse. Most are confined to areas so small they cannot turn around or take a single step forward or backward. Those that are not confined to single small cages are kept in crowded cages. The smaller farm animals, such as chickens, turkeys, and hogs, are kept in cages two or three stories high – this is known as "vertical integration farming" – where the animals on the lower levels spend their days covered with excrement. Unlike prison, the animals are not allowed to exercise. They are bred to become as heavy as possible so that they will sell for the highest price. This unnatural weight creates more pain for their feet and legs. Some are chained at the neck or ankles, all have to stand on cement or grated steel flooring which affects the alignment of their bones, and injures their feet that are designed to stand on soil. Many of the millions of animals who are kept in these conditions get frustrated, are driven insane, and bite each other whenever possible – sometimes killing each other.

The noise of animal voices and of their bumping against the cages in large confinement barns is so loud that the workers often have to wear ear protection. If the noise in the buildings is not bothersome enough, there is the urine and poop of thousands of animals gathering day and night and creating an overwhelming stench.

While the manure from chicken factory farms may be sold off to companies that blend it into cattle feed, the manure and urine from cattle and hog factory farms are kept in enormous cesspool "reservoirs." These cesspools may be equal to the size of several Olympic-size swimming pools, and may contain millions of gallons of the putrid stuff.

Sometimes the earthen walls of these cesspools collapse. On August 10, 2005, this happened at the Marks Dairy Farm near Lowville, New York, sending millions of gallons of liquefied manure into the Black River, killing hundreds of thousands of fish. The river is a source for water for downstream towns, and eventually flows into Lake Ontario.

"Even without a manure spill, factory farm excrement can poison the water. The intensive confinement of thousands to hundreds of thousands of animals results in quantities of manure that often exceed the

soil's absorption rate. When the soil is saturated with higher levels of nutrients than can be absorbed, the result is runoff leading to potentially serious ground and water pollution.

Runoff that reaches the water can cause eutrophication, in which an increase in mineral and organic nutrients depletes the water of oxygen. The ensuing overgrowth of algae and other marine plants competes with fish for oxygen, creating an environment in which plant life thrives while animal life suffers.

Factory farm animal manure also threatens air quality. During decomposition, noxious levels of gases, such as hydrogen sulfide and ammonia, are emitted, putting workers and nearby residents at risk of developing a number of acute and chronic illnesses. Studies have shown that those who live near factory farms are more likely to suffer from a range of medical problems, including diarrhea, sore throat, cough, chest tightness, nasal congestion, heart palpitations, shortness of breath, sudden fatigue, headaches, nausea, sudden loss of consciousness, comas, seizures, and, ultimately, even death."
— **Marks Dairy Farm Manure Spill Threatens Environment and Public Health; Humane Society of the United States, August 24, 2005; HSUS.Org**

Large factory farms of all types continue to be built on every continent, increasing the animal suffering and the pollution of the land, water, and air.

"Every year up to two million baby and adult sheep are exported to foreign buyers, mostly in Europe. Increasingly, these animals are subject to the heavy burdens of intensive farming. Fattened on an unnatural, high-protein diet, they are forced to produce more lambs – twin births are common, triplets becoming more so – in punishing winter weather. Disease and lameness are rampant. The trade's own statistics show that between 10 and 15 percent of sheep die before they can be slaughtered."
— **Animal Aid, Britain, 1996**

There is more to eating meat than the taste of it. The piece of animal on the dinner plate is a tiny part of the livestock industry. People sitting at their dinner table are not exposed to the animals crammed in factory farming buildings, or the gory bloody hell of the livestock slaughterhouses where terrified animals screech, struggle, and fight as they watch each other getting killed.

As mentioned, because they are sold for their weight, farm animals are fed concoctions that contain anything that will fatten them in the fastest and cheapest way. Some ingredients found in cattle feed include shredded newspapers with all of its chemical dyes and processing residues; poultry feces; cement dust; cardboard scraps, and artificial flavors. Cow feed often contains ground-up parts of other farm animals as well as animals killed in city pounds, thus forcing the cattle to be meat eaters when they are naturally vegetarian. Some farm animals, particularly hogs, are fed their own urine to save on the cost of water.

Billions of farm animals are often given drugs by mouth or injection from their first day to nearly their last. These drugs include hormones, antibiotics, milk stimulants, tranquilizers, and chemicals that influence the birth rates. The animals are sprayed with toxic insecticides, fungicides, and pesticides. These drugs and chemicals along with the chemicals used to grow the feed accumulate in the fat cells of the animals. The chemical residues are transferred into the humans who consume the meats. This contributes to human illnesses, birth defects, and learning disabilities.

The conditions animals are exposed to in factory farms would be similar to a human spending his entire life in an area the size of a sleeping cot or a crowded elevator; urinating and defecating on a concrete or grated floor; being sprayed with chemical insecticides; injected with or fed antibiotics; and being fed a nauseating diet to fatten him up as soon as possible as cheaply as possible before he is finally hauled off to be killed in a room filled with his neighbors, then chopped and sawed into pieces sold to markets, restaurants, resorts, and cruise ships, and to prisons, schools, the military, and other institutions.

"The animals of the world exist for their own reasons. They were not made for humans, any more than black people were made for whites or women for men."
— Alice Walker

Slaughtering Farm Animals

"If slaughterhouses had glass walls everyone would be vegetarian."
— Paul McCartney

"On today's farms there is basically no such thing as a middle-aged hen or dairy cow. With each passing month, hens produce fewer eggs, and with each passing year, cows produce less milk. If there's one thing animal agriculture is great at, it's keeping track of the production of their animals and figuring out when yields have declined to the point that it's time to send the hen or cow to slaughter and bring in a new animal."

> — Erik Marcus, author of the books *Vegan: The New Ethics of Eating, and Meat Market: Animals, Ethics and Money*

"The animals who people eat are treated so abusively in this country that similar treatment of dogs or cats would be grounds for animal cruelty charges in all 50 states.

In the United States alone, more than 10 billion land animals (and billions more aquatic animals) are slaughtered for food every year – more than 1 million animals every hour. The overwhelming majority of them are kept on factory farms, where the goal is to raise as many animals as possible in the least amount of time and space."

> — VegAnswers.Com, 2006

As soon as the animals are large enough, or when the egg output of the chickens has decreased and the cows have slowed their milk production, they are sent off on the horrifying ride to the slaughterhouses. They often don't go easily. Electric shock prods are commonly used to make the larger animals get onto and off the trucks.

Anyone who has spent time with an animal knows how sensitive animals are to discomfort and to emotions, such as anger, fright, and danger. Animals are also intelligent, experience joy and sadness, and continue to amaze us by proving over and over that the level of their intelligence is much higher than we have considered. The compassion of animals is displayed when they care for their young. Many animals have saved the lives of humans. Keeping this knowledge in mind, consider the last days in the lives of farm animals.

What happens to farm animals when they are taken to the slaughterhouses is a far cry from the happy, "cute" commercials the meat industry uses to sell chicken, beef, pork, turkey, and lamb.

> "The meager regulations that do exist in Britain to limit journey times and to ensure proper feeding and watering of farm animals being transported are routinely ignored."
>
> — Animal Aid, Britain, AnimalAid.Org.UK; 1996

Farm animals spend their last days without sufficient food or water. They are crowded into hauling trucks and rail cars where they become covered with urine and feces. Many of the animals are injured and some die from injuries, illnesses, or suffocation during the long, bumpy, and exhausting trip to the slaughterhouse. The animals that are too sick to walk, are suffering from exposure to extreme temperatures, or have injuries that prevent them from walking off the hauling trucks and rail cars are often beaten, electrically shocked, or dragged by chains. Some of these sickly animals likely harbor illnesses, such as BSE, that can be transferred into the humans who eat the meat.

In the winter some animals become frozen to the inside walls of the hauling trucks. Because the trip may take more than a day the floor of the truck becomes covered in feces and urine. In the winter the feet of the animals can freeze to the floor. When they arrive at their destination, their skin that has frozen to the truck may be ripped off as they are forced off the truck. Those with frozen feet may have their legs broken to remove them. If they can't walk, a chain may be placed around them and they are dragged off the truck using a winch, a forklift, or by other means.

> "Have you ever stopped to ask yourself why we call some animals pets, and others food? Pigs, cows, and chickens feel happiness, fear, and pain just like dogs and cats. The only difference between the dogs and cats we consider beloved members of our families, and the pigs, cows, and chickens we eat, is our perception of them. Why?"
> — ChooseVeg.Com, 2006

In the slaughterhouses cows are often hung upside down by one leg, which fractures from the strain. While hanging, they twist in fright and anger next to one another before their necks are slit. Others are killed by having a mechanical rod shoved through their skulls. There is shouting. There are electric saws cutting the animals apart. It is loud. Workers wear ear plugs, but cannot escape the noise. It is bloody. Workers wear protective clothing, but cannot escape the slime of massive amounts of animal blood, vomit, urine, and feces. Chickens, turkeys, hogs, lambs, and other animals are treated with equal disdain, spending the last moments of their sad lives in the worst imaginable way. Hogs are stunned with 300-volt prods – which don't always work – before their throats are cut – which doesn't always work. Chickens taken out of crowded containers are hung by their feet on processing lines where their heads are cut off. All are terrified. All are slaughtered.

The slaughtering is done at rates often exceeding hundreds of animals per hour. As their bodies are cut into pieces they may still be alive because the killing mechanisms didn't work properly, or the animal's head or neck was at the wrong angle when their neck was to be slit or the rod jammed into their brain. Workers who have spoken against this practice of cutting apart animals that are still alive have been fired and/or found that nobody in authority seems to care.

In April 2001 the *Washington Post* published a series of articles about the business of slaughterhouses, *Modern Meat in America: A Brutal Harvest*. The series detailed the filthy conditions inside slaughterhouses. It also considered how it is that so many people get food poisoning from eating contaminated meat. The article covered the issue of animals being cut apart while they are still alive, and mentioned one Texas beef company that was "cited 22 times in 1998 for violations that included chopping hooves off live cattle." The article told of one incident where a live cow's leg got caught in machinery and workers simply cut off the leg. It mentioned one slaughterhouse worker who said he had witnessed thousands of cows getting slaughtered while they were still alive. Another worker said it was every day that cows were cut up while still alive. What usually happens when situations like this are exposed? Little, if anything. Closing the plant for a matter of hours or a day to retrain workers can cost many thousands of dollars. After that it is often back to business as usual.

You may know the pain you experience when you get a sliver, are scratched by a pin, or step on a sharp pebble. Take that pain to the severe extreme. Imagine having your body cut into pieces while you are fully conscious. This is what many defenseless, innocent animals experience in slaughterhouses.

"... It takes 25 minutes to turn a live steer into steak at the modern slaughterhouse where Ramon Moreno works. For 20 years, his post was 'second-legger,' a job that entails cutting hocks off carcasses as they whirl past at a rate of 309 an hour. The cattle were supposed to be dead before they got to Moreno. But too often they weren't.

'They blink. They make noises,' he said softly. 'The head moves, the eyes are wide and looking around.'

Still Moreno would cut. On bad days, he says, dozens of animals reached his station clearly alive and conscious. Some would survive as far as the tail cutter, the belly ripper, the hide puller.

'They die,' said Moreno, 'piece by piece.'"

— Modern Meat in America: A Brutal Harvest: In Overtaxed Plants, Humane Treatment of Cattle Is Often a Battle Lost, by Joby Warrick, *Washington Post*; April 10, 2001

"The 1,200 employees working at the Hudson Foods chicken slaugh-

terhouse in Noel, Missouri, kill and process 1.3 million chickens a day."
— **1,000 Miles of Hope, and Heartache, by Jesse Katz,** *Los Angeles Times,*
November 10, 1996

It is common practice in many slaughterhouses to dunk chickens, turkeys, ducks, geese, and hogs in scalding tanks of hot water to soften their flesh for skinning. The animals are supposed to be dead or stunned to the point of near death before they reach these scalding tanks. But, because their necks are not slit correctly, or the bolt gun or iron rod didn't hit their skulls at the right angle, or the stun gun was not working properly, many animals reach the scalding tanks fully aware and able to feel their skin being burned. They spend the last seconds of their tortured lives in extreme pain while drowning.

While slaughtering the larger animals, cows and pigs, the slaughterhouse workers sometimes wear protective gear, such as chest pads and head gear, while cutting up animals that are not yet dead. It hurts badly, and can break bones, when a cow kicks you.

"One of the most recent problems that I observed was the night-shift superintendent turning down the stunner and ordering the employees to leave it down. This machine is the device that is supposed to stun chickens before they are killed. Turning it down results in the chickens missing the killing machine and evading the killer behind the machine, so that they end up being scalded to death by water in the scalding tank. The scalding tank loosens the feathers so that they can be picked out. The chickens are supposed to be dead before they reach this point... they are scalded alive. When this happens the chickens flop, scream, kick, and their eyeballs pop out of their heads. Then they often come out of the other end with broken bones and disfigured and missing body parts because they've struggled so much in the tank."
— **Virgil Butler, former chicken slaughterhouse worker for Tyson, as quoted in
Behind Closed Doors: Former Factory Farm & Slaughterhouse Workers Speak
Out;** *Outrage: The Magazine of Mercy for Animals,* **Summer/Fall 2006;
MercyForAnimals.Org**

This slaughtering is done to feed the average Americans who, according to 1999 statistics from the American Meat Institute, ate 66 pounds of cow, 54 pounds of chicken, about 47 pounds of pork, and over 14 pounds of turkey.

Do you got milk? Do you eat meat? If so, you are supporting this abusive, horrifying, sickening, and massively environmentally destructive industry.

"You have just dined, and however scrupulously the slaughterhouse is concealed in the graceful distance of miles, there is complicity."
— **Ralph Waldo Emerson, Fate,** *The Conduct of Life;* **1860**

Slaughterhouse Workers

"Slaughterhouses are nothing less than hells on earth. Animals are stunned, bled, hung upside down, skinned, disemboweled, and chopped into pieces that will be wrapped in cellophane... The whole process is unspeakably filthy, as agricultural science, despite its best efforts, has yet to breed a cow or pig or chicken that can be chopped up without its blood, urine, feces and vomit inconsiderately spilling out all over and mucking up the whole proceedings...

Only a single industry in America has been cited by the group Human Rights Watch for violating human rights: the nation's meatpackers and slaughterhouses. In January 2005, the group issued a detailed, 175-page report calling meatpacking 'the most dangerous factory job in America.' "
— **Former Montana cattle rancher Howard Lyman, in his book** *No More Bull: The Mad Cowboy Targets America's Worst Enemy: Our Diet;* **MadCowboy.Com**

The injury rate of slaughterhouse workers is among the highest of any industry. In 1995, according to the U.S. Occupational Safety and Health Administration, 36 percent of meatpacking plant workers sustained serious injuries. Poultry slaughterhouse workers had a 22.7 percent injury rate.

A man I knew grew up in Mexico where he began working in a slaughterhouse at the age of 13. He eventually moved to the United States, where he continued to work in slaughterhouses. He spent a total of 14 years in that line of work. He often began his day by slitting the throat of a cow and drinking the fresh blood as it poured out of the wound. In the last slaughterhouse he worked in there would be about five additional workers kept on hand every day, in addition to the 30 who were scheduled to work. The extra five were there to take over for the workers who got injured that day. Every day there would be injuries that required a worker to take the rest of the day off, or to be taken to a hospital for stitches, or worse. He saw workers lose fingers, break bones, and get kicked in the face by cows, sometimes breaking facial bones. And he often saw cows being cut up before they were fully dead. He finally left the business after he suffered a stab wound on his arm that cut through tendons and nerves that controlled half of his left hand.

The injuries combined with the hellish visions the slaughterhouse workers are exposed to take a toll. Apparently killing and cutting up farm animals all day is not a very enjoyable job, and most workers do not hold onto their jobs for very long. Some animal-killing and meat-packing companies experience more than an 80 percent annual employee turnover rate. The low wages slaughterhouse workers are paid become even lower as companies may deduct charges for lunch meals, work clothes, and, when living on company property, rent.

"No one knows more about the suffering farmed animals endure than the workers in slaughterhouses and on factory farms, many of whom are desperate for employment and working for low wages in horrific conditions.

Although it seems easy to think of these workers as cold and uncaring individuals who abuse and torture animals for a living, there are many who took these jobs out of desperation – or were simply unaware of the conditions inside. In many ways they too are victims of a brutal industry."
– **Behind Closed Doors: Former Factory Farm & Slaughterhouse Workers Speak Out; *Outrage: The Magazine of Mercy for Animals*, Summer/Fall 2006; MercyForAnimals.Org**

The high turnover rate among workers in the $100-billion animal-killing and meatpacking industry has brought many U.S. slaughter-houses to rely on the cheapest and most uneducated labor they can find – often those labeled as "illegal immigrants," who may have been recruited by the meatpacking companies from their native towns in Mexico and Central America, from U.S. towns on the Mexican border, or from the Asian immigrant populations of larger U.S. cities.

During 2006 agents of the U.S. Immigration and Customs Enforcement office conducted a series of raids on slaughterhouses and meatpacking plants. The most recent as of this writing happened during the week of December 10. In this raid there were 1,282 "legal" and "illegal" immigrants arrested at Swift & Co. meatpacking plants in six states. The raids were part of a ten-month investigation into allegations that the immigrants were using fake or stolen identities of U.S. citizens. Swift & Co. executives say they relied on the government's own Basic Pilot system to check the identities of the employees, but that the system is flawed. The company operates nine plants in eight states, makes about $10 billion a year, and is the third largest beef and pork processor in the country. About 10 percent of its employees were taken away in the raids.

Many of the immigrants were taken to an immigration detention center in Atlanta, while others were taken to Camp Dodge, a National Guard base in Johnston, Iowa. They face deportation hearings. Even though some are married to Americans and have children here, they face a future far away from their families. Many other workers who have not been arrested in the towns where the raids took place have gone into hiding. Many of the households with children that are suddenly single-parent households will be relying on government assistance and charities to make up for lost income.

Hiring recent immigrants to work in the U.S. meatpacking plants is something that has been going on for decades. It has been mentioned in many books, and it was the subject of a special investigation, The New Jungle, that appeared in the September 23, 1996, edition of *U.S. News & World Report* magazine. That investigative report told of how meatpacking giant IBP advertises for workers on Spanish-language radio stations in southern Texas.

A report in the *Los Angeles Times* told of chicken slaughterhouses in Missouri, Mississippi, North Carolina, Arkansas, and Georgia recruiting workers from the Rio Grande Valley in southern Texas where unemployment is high and cheap laborers are easy to find. The recruiting was often done by placing English and Spanish help-wanted newspaper ads saying that no experience is necessary, transportation to Missouri is provided, and housing is available for those who want to work in the slaughterhouses (1,000 Miles of Hope, and Heartache, by Jesse Katz, *Los Angeles Times*, November 10, 1996).

Some slaughterhouse and meatpacking plants also use connections in Mexico to find workers to come to America. When officials working for the Immigration and Naturalization Service raided the Swift & Company meatpacking plant in Marshalltown, Iowa, in the mid-1990s they detained at least 125 suspected illegal workers out of the approximately 900 workers at the site. The raid took place after it was discovered that many of the employees had submitted false information to the company. This kind of raid where "illegal immigrants" are found working in U.S. meatpacking plants is not unusual. The New Jungle article told of a 1,000-an-hour hog-processing plant in Storm Lake, Iowa, owned by meatpacking industry giant IBP Inc, where 78 "illegal immigrants" were detained and sent back to Mexico.

Three companies control a majority of the beef and pork industry in

America: Cargill's Excel Corp., Con-Agra's Monfort, Inc., and Tyson.

The pay at the meatpacking plants is what entices the workers to come from Mexico and Central America. While workers in Mexico may make a few dollars a day, and unemployment is high, they can work for $6 to $10 or more per hour in the U.S. meatpacking plants. Towns in Mexico have long-term relations with certain meatpacking plants in the Midwest.

With more and more meatpacking plants being located in rural areas away from big cities, living quarters can be relatively cheap compared to city housing prices. The number of recent immigrants working at large meatpacking plants can transform surrounding towns into Spanish-speaking communities. It strains the towns to have to provide schooling for the large number of foreign-speaking immigrant children. It allows the meatpacking companies to keep expenses low by employing recent immigrants who work for the low pay without the medical benefits.

> "There are 220 packing plants in Iowa and Nebraska. Our estimate is that 25 percent of the workers in those plants are illegal."
> — Jerry Heinauer, district director of the INS, quoted in The New Jungle, by Stephen J. Hedges, Dana Hawkins, and Penny Loeb, *U.S. News & World Report*; September 23, 1996

Being an undocumented worker in America means that you do not get unemployment benefits if you lose your job, may not get proper medical care if you are injured on the job, and at any moment you can be deported if you are caught by agents working for the U.S. Federal Immigration and Naturalization Service, who may raid your place of work. If you do receive health insurance, you may not be able to afford the premium, and you may avoid going to the doctor altogether because you fear authority figures who may report you and have you deported. If you get deported before you get your weekly pay there is a strong likelihood that you will never receive it.

Finding work in a meatpacking plant is relatively easy for workers carrying fake immigration papers. While you may be able to get fake immigration papers, your employer doesn't have to prove the documents are legitimate — that is the job of the immigration agents who may show up at your workplace. It is also easy to find work in the meatpacking plants because many of them are no longer unionized. That presents another combination of problems because, as a nonunion and nonresident, if you have a grievance about your work conditions you have nobody to turn to, and little if any legal recourse.

For more information on this topic, read Eric Schlosser's book, *Fast Food Nation*. It is also now a theatrical film directed by Richard Linklater and featuring an excellent cast of actors.

Livestock by the Billions: A Global Environmental Disaster

"Of all agricultural land in the United States, 87 percent is used to raise animals for food. Twenty thousand pounds of potatoes can be grown on one acre of land, but only 165 pounds of beef can be produced in the same space.

[South and Central American] Rainforests are being destroyed at a rate of 125,000 square miles per year to create space to raise animals for food. Fifty-five square feet of land are consumed for every quarter-pound fast food burger made of rainforest beef."
  — PETA, VegNow.Com, 2005

"Nationwide, factory-farmed animals produce 130 times more manure than the human population – the equivalent of five tons of manure for every U.S. citizen. U.S. factory farms generate more than 350 million tons of manure each year."
  — Farm Sanctuary, VegForLife.Org, 2005

In addition to the incapacitating degenerative diseases, the food poisoning, and the suffering issues of raising, killing, and eating billions of animals, there are also the issues of the ecological damage to the planet caused by the livestock industry.

"Cattle and sheep grazing is ecologically destructive and an abomination against our national park system in areas as pristine as the Grand Canyon Park.

Grazing causes rapid depletion of wooded areas by clearing, cultivating and eroding the soil. Soil losses are as high as 44 tons per acre annually on steep slopes. Woodlands, waterways, and wildlife habitats have been significantly reduced or eradicated entirely due to overgrazing."
  — FarmSanctuary.Org, 2006

"Most wars are fought over control of natural resources: land, water, oil, and minerals. Yet, animal agriculture is by far the largest user and

despoiler of natural resources."
— **Citizens for Healthy Options in Children's Education, CHOICE.USA**

The livestock industry and companies that exist to service it use up more land and resources and create more pollution and ecological damage on the planet than any industry. There are tens of billions of chickens and turkeys, billions of pigs, over a billion cattle, and hundreds of millions of lambs and other farm animals being raised on millions of acres of land all over the world and this is ravaging the biodiversity (the full spectrum of living things including plants, insects, birds, and other land and water life) of the planet.

"Cattle are a chief source of organic pollution; cow dung is poisoning the freshwater lakes, rivers, and streams of the world. Growing herds of cattle are exerting unprecedented pressure on the carrying capacity of natural ecosystems, edging entire species of wildlife to the brink of extinction. Cattle are a growing source of global warming, and their increasing numbers now threaten the very dynamic of the biosphere."
— **Jeremy Rifkin, in his book *Beyond Beef: The Rise and Fall of the Cattle Culture***

"The less animal-based food you eat, and the more you replace those calories with plant-based food, the better off you are, in terms of your health as well as your contributions to the health of the planet."
— **Gidon Eshel, assistant professor of geophysics at the University of Chicago, co-author of a study concluding that becoming a vegan does more to reduce greenhouse gasses than the type of car you drive. (*Earth Interactions* journal, April 2006; It's better to green your diet than your car, *New Scientist Magazine*, December 17, 2005)**

Raising of livestock for human consumption and all of the ecologically destructive chemicals used by the animal-farming industry cause massive damage to the delicate ecosystems throughout the world. Livestock in the U.S. produces more than 130 times the amount of bodily waste of the nation's human population. As more people around the world are converting to an American diet style of meat and junk food, expansive stretches of virgin land and land that had been used to grow food for human consumption are being converted to provide space for cattle grazing and for growing feed for livestock.

"Rainforests cover less than two percent of the Earth's surface, yet they are home to nearly half of our planet's living creatures. Butterflies and birds fill the air, their colors are so intense, no artist could ever match them. Noble jaguars, howler monkeys, vines, fish, gorillas, orchids, lizards, and orangutans flourish there – and nowhere else on Earth.

A four-square mile area of rainforest teems with colorful variety: 750 types of trees, 1,500 different flowers, 125 mammal species, and 400 kinds of birds.

But rainforests are disappearing at the rate of a football field every second. The destruction of the Earth's most ancient complex ecosystem threatens the very survival of the human species.

Over 99 percent of the rainforest species have not yet been studied for possible medical use. A plant that holds the cure for AIDS – or a future epidemic – may be growing somewhere in the rainforest. Or a bulldozer may be crushing the last one right now as you read this.

Rice, potatoes, bananas, chocolate, coffee, oranges, tomatoes, yams and dozens of other food crops originated in the rainforests. The wild strains still found there provide genetic material necessary to keep world agriculture stocks hardy and healthy. Undiscovered rainforest species could provide new sources of food in the future.

Once the rainforest is gone, the vanished species won't return. And once the proud, ancient indigenous cultures are destroyed, the knowledge they possess – knowledge that could benefit all of humanity – will be lost forever."

– The Rainforest Action Network, RAN.Org; 2006

Anyone who studies the story of a Brazilian rubber tapper named Chico Mendez will begin to get an idea of how much corruption and damage the cattle industry has caused to the life-sustaining rainforests.

The main reason millions of acres of rainforests in South and Central America continue to be destroyed by cutting and burning is to clear new land for cattle grazing. This kills off many kinds of plants, insects, animals, amphibians, and birds, and also destroys natural water filtration systems within the rainforests that have existed for an unknown number of years. The cattle that are raised on the defiled rainforest land are used to supply beef to the Orient, to the Middle East, to North America, and to Europe – where millions of acres of land are already being ruined to raise, feed, and grow feed for hundreds of millions of cattle and billions of other farm animals.

"The livestock population of the United States today consumes enough grain and soybeans to feed over five times the entire human population of the country. We feed these animals over 80 percent of the

corn we grow, and over 95 percent of the oats... Less than half the harvested agricultural acreage in the United States is used to grow food for people. Most of it is used to grow livestock feed. This is a drastically inefficient use of our acreage. For every sixteen pounds of grain and soybeans fed to beef cattle, we get back only one pound as meat on our plates. The other fifteen are inaccessible to us. Most of it is turned into manure."
 — John Robbins, in his book *Diet for a New America*

In 1994 the U.S. Fish and Wildlife Service announced that California's state fish, the golden trout found in the waters in the High Sierras of California, was a candidate for the endangered species list. The declining population of the fish was blamed on cattle grazing in the U.S. government-owned Golden Trout Wilderness land adjacent to the streams where the fish spawn. The cattle the U.S. government allows ranchers to graze there have eroded the land and widened the river banks. As the cattle trample the soil it becomes compacted, making it unsuitable for new plant growth and prevents rainwater from being absorbed. Instead, the rainwater runoff carries soil into rivers and streams and the plants that do take up root are often invasive weeds. The vegetation degradation, soil erosion, and the manure from the cattle has affected the water temperature and clarity, smothered fish eggs, and has had a negative impact on the population of insects, which the fish and birds eat.

"In California, the number of gallons of water needed to produce one edible pound of: wheat: 25 gallons; beef: 5,214 gallons.
 Energy expended to produce one pound of grain-fed beef: equivalent to one gallon of gasoline."
 — EarthSave.Org

"McDonald's equals slavery and starvation."
 — Graffiti on a wall in Quito, Ecuador

"More than half of all the water and 33 percent of all the raw materials used for all purposes in the United States are used in meat production... the average chicken-processing plant may use 100 million gallons of water daily. More than 260 million acres of U.S. forest have been cleared to grow crops to feed to cattle. Cattle-grazing in the western United States has led to soil erosion and desertification."
 — *Take a Step Toward Compassionate Living,* by the People for the Ethical Treatment of Animals, PETA-Online.Org; 2004

Raising livestock and growing grains to feed livestock is not energy efficient. It takes significantly larger amounts of land, water, and other resources to produce cattle, poultry, and hog meat than it does to produce fruits, vegetables, herbs, legumes, and grains for human consumption. More than half of the water used in the U.S. goes to grow feed crop and to provide water for livestock. Those uses of water have been blamed for the droughts in California where water consumption by the livestock industry exceeds that of the state's human population. The beef industry in California is the state's third-largest agricultural sector. The number one reason California has had droughts where people were told not to use water and some people were fined for using more of their share of water is because so much water is going to raise grains and feed the livestock herds in California that it depletes the water supplies during the times where there is no rain. Water for farm animals, and to grow their food, is pumped out of the ground, draining aquifers; or is taken from streams, lakes, and rivers, damaging wildlife populations that depend on that water.

Enormous amounts of government money in the U.S. and other countries is spent to help irrigate livestock grain fields, and to build and manage water systems for the cattle industry. This water is then polluted by the chemicals used to grow the feed for the farm animals and by the farm animals themselves. This pollution and the soil erosion caused by livestock poison streams, rivers, ponds, lakes, and oceans.

"Livestock grazing on public lands accounts for less than one-tenth of one percent of employment in the eleven western states, including in Colorado (according to a study by Thomas Powers, chairman of the University of Montana's Department of Economics). However, this activity costs taxpayers anywhere from three to five hundred million dollars per year (according to the Cato Institute). More significantly, cows and sheep on public lands pollute streams and rivers, and jeopardize the continued survival of many rare wildlife species (according to the Congressional General Accounting Office)."
  — *Colorado Wolf Tracks*, **the newsletter of Sinapu.Org; 1996**

"The U.S. government spent $22 billion to build 133 water projects in the West. Every year the government spends $7 billion on these water projects. Farmers pay less than $1 billion per year to the government for water."
  — **NPR, 1997**

The farming of all the grains that are grown to feed farm animals takes up the majority of farmland on the planet, and has been and is causing a huge amount of damage and erosion to the land. It has led to and is leading to a huge amount of damage to streams, rivers, lakes, and oceans, as well as to underground water tables. Growing food for farm animals is a huge waste of resources in fuel, in water, in equipment, and in all of the resources used to manufacture and maintain the farm equipment used to grow all of that food for all of the billions of animals grown on this planet to feed the humans who choose to eat dead animals – the very same humans who would be a lot healthier if they did not eat animals and dairy products, but instead subsisted on a vegan diet.

> "You can use your food choices, your daily habit of eating, to say yes to life in a very profound way, and to say no to the corporate culture that is destroying the planet, and our communities. You can use your food choices, every meal, every bite, as an opportunity to take a stand for life, to take a stand for compassion."
> **– John Robbins, The Food Revolution; TheFoodRevolution.Org**

The California dairy industry is a billion-dollar industry that relies on the milk from of a population of 1.7 million dairy cows. These cattle create 65 billion pounds of manure each year, and this results in ammonia emissions that add significant amounts of pollution. Much of the manure is spread on farmland in the surrounding regions. Many dairies produce so much manure that it can't be used and it ends up poisoning the land, rivers, lakes, and ocean. A small fraction of California's 2,100 dairies have their manure taken away companies that bring it to "methane digester" plants that heat the slurry so that bacteria breaks it down to release methane gas to generate electricity.

Scientists at UC Davis have discovered that cows also emit a significant amount of gasses from their chewing and regurgitating. Combined with the nitrogen oxide emissions from vehicles and factories, the ammonia and methane from millions of cattle creates particulate-laden smog. This pollution is damaging to human lung tissue, and is especially a risk to babies, children, pregnant women, the elderly, people with weakened immune systems, and really everyone who breathes it. Smog also affects plant life in that it reduces growth and photosynthesis, and speeds aging within the leaves. This has an impact on crop farming as well as on forests, wildlands, and on wildlife of all varieties. The smog is the main reason that the dairy farming regions of California often have some of the worst air quality on the continent.

> "When emissions from land use and land use change are included, the livestock sector accounts for nine percent of CO_2 deriving from human-related activities, but produces a much larger share of even more harmful greenhouse gases."
> — Food and Agriculture Organisation, Rome, Italy; in a report on worldwide pollution caused by the cattle industry; 2006

According to a 1995 estimate by the San Joaquin Valley Air Pollution Control District, the average dairy cow releases 19.3 pounds of volatile organic compounds every year. California's vast San Joaquin Valley contains the most dairy cows of any region of the continent, and it also has the smoggiest air in North America. If you've bought California milk or cheese, you've supported that industry and have also played a part in that pollution.

The world would be healthier if people would stop eating animals as well as milk and eggs and foods made with them.

> "Raising animals for food causes more water pollution than any other industry in the U.S. because animals raised for food produce one hundred thirty times the excrement of the entire human population. It means 87,000 pounds per second. Much of the waste from factory farms and slaughterhouses flows into streams and rivers, contaminating water sources.
> Each vegetarian can save one acre of trees per year. More than 260 million acres of U.S. forests have been cleared to grow crops to feed animals raised for meat. And another acre of trees disappears every eight seconds. The tropical rainforests are also being destroyed to create grazing land for cattle."
> — Eating for Peace, by Buddhist teacher Thich Naht Hanh, on mindful consumption. From the FoodRevolution.Org Web site of John Robbins.

> "Raising animals for food consumes more than half of all the water used in the United States. It takes 2,500 gallons of water to produce a pound of meat, but only 25 gallons to produce a pound of wheat. The amount of water used in the production of the meat from an average steer could float a destroyer."
> — People for the Ethical Treatment of Animals, VegNow.Com

According to the United Nations, global meat production in 2001 was 229 million tons. It is expected to double by the year 2050. The milk industry produced an estimated 580 million tons of milk in 2001. It is expected to nearly double by 2050.

Pollution Caused by Farming Animals

Most pollution on this planet is caused by the meat, dairy, and egg industries – including the meat and dairy packaging, distribution, marketing, cooking, and consumption process. This is because of the misuse and abuse of resources such as fuel, metal, plastics, paper, electricity, and other items used to get meat on the plates of humans who choose to eat meat, dairy, and eggs. Consider the following:

1. The supplies and fuel used to manufacture the equipment that is used to farm the food for billions of farm animals.

2. The supplies and fuel used to run and maintain the equipment that grows the food for billions of farm animals.

3. The supplies and fuel used to transfer the food to feed billions of farm animals.

4. The supplies and fuel used to manufacture the equipment that is used to raise billions of farm animals.

5. The supplies and fuel used to run and maintain the equipment that is used to raise billions of farm animals.

6. The supplies and fuel used to transfer billions of farm animals to the slaughterhouses.

7. The supplies and fuel used to create and maintain the trucks and other equipment used to transport billions of farm animals to slaughterhouses.

8. The supplies and fuel used to manufacture the equipment that runs the slaughterhouses where billions of farm animals are killed.

9. The supplies and fuel used to run and maintain the slaughterhouses.

10. The supplies and fuel used to manufacture the equipment that transfers the dairy products to processing and storage facilities.

11. The supplies and fuel used to run and maintain those processing and storage facilities.

12. The supplies and fuel used to manufacture the equipment that transfers the meat and dairy products to the markets.

13. The supplies and fuel used to run and maintain the equipment that transfers trillions of pounds of meat and dairy products to the markets.

14. The supplies and fuel used to manufacture the equipment that is used in the markets – from the buildings to the shelving to the heating and air conditioning and refrigeration units.

15. The supplies and fuel used to run the markets that sell the meat and dairy products.

16. The supplies and fuel used to manufacture all the equipment used to advertise the meat and dairy products.

17. The supplies and fuel used to advertise the meat and dairy products – which take up millions of pages of newspaper and magazine pages, all sorts of outdoor advertising, and hordes of radio and TV commercial time.

18. The supplies and fuel used to keep and display the meat and dairy products in stores.

19. The supplies and fuel used to manufacture and maintain all the hundreds of millions of refrigerators, stoves, and microwaves used in the stores, restaurants, hotels, homes, cruise ships, schools, hospitals, prisons, military bases, and other places where meat and dairy products are kept and prepared for consumption.

20. The supplies and fuel used to fuel all the hundreds of millions of refrigerators, stoves, and microwaves.

21. The massive amounts of water, soaps, and other cleansers used to clean the farms, slaughterhouses, equipment, markets, and kitchens of all sorts where all of that meat and dairy are produced, killed, sold, prepared, cooked, and eaten.

22. All the pollution left from the manufacture, marketing, packaging, and shipping of the meat and dairy products.

23. All the supplies and fuel used to deal with all of that pollution.

When a person considers the environmental destruction caused by the meat, dairy, and egg industries, they should take into account the litter from fast-food and junk food that is strewn among the roads and highways of the cities, towns, and country. These are the main source of litter. The other two main sources of litter are products that also lead to health problems: cigarettes and unhealthful drinks, beer and soda bottles and cans, and coffee cups by the billions.

Then there are all the resources used to run the allopathic medical industry, which largely exists to treat the results of unhealthful living. It does this by utilizing toxic drugs and risky, invasive surgery.

The entire obesity industry – from liposuction to stomach stapling and intestinal bypass to "diet" pills and programs – is the result of unhealthful living. The large majority of heart surgery is the result of people eating unhealthful food (especially dairy, meat, eggs, and processed foods), and not exercising.

All of this pollution, all of the animal farming, and all of the products associated with it, are not good for human health, or the health of Earth.

Humans do not need to drink soda or eat meat or dairy, fried foods, grilled or barbecued foods, or anything containing artificial dyes, preservatives, flavors, scents, emulsifiers, or sweeteners. The world would be a much healthier place without any of these toxic concoctions.

> "This is a global business, and it's not only that we need to add to supply, but we need to reduce demand... In the United States alone, we have about two percent of world oil reserves, five percent of the population and yet we use about 25 percent of the world's consumption of oil."
> — James J. Mulva, chairman of ConocoPhillips Co., speaking on NBC TV's *Meet the Press*, June 18, 2006. On the same show, Shell Oil Co. President John Hofmeister explained that oil companies are holding "discussions with the White House quite frequently" with the goal of gaining greater access to U.S. federal lands (such as Nature preserves and national parks), as well as local waters to explore and drill for oil. That is truly deplorable.

Again I ask, what industries use up the most amount of petroleum in North America?

The large majority of the food we grow on the continent is fed to farm animals. Raising, slaughtering, packaging, marketing, refrigerating, and cooking billions of farm animals every year use up tremendous amounts of fuel.

> "The typical U.S. diet, about 28 per cent of which comes from animal

sources, generates the equivalent of nearly 1.5 tons more carbon dioxide per person per year than a vegan diet with the same number of calories... By comparison, the difference in annual emissions between driving a typical saloon [sedan] car and a hybrid car, which runs off a rechargeable battery and gasoline, is just over one ton."
   — **According to study done at the University of Chicago; It's better to green your diet than your car,** *New Scientist* **magazine, December 17, 2005**

"Raising animals for food requires more than one-third of all raw materials and fossil fuels used in the United States. Producing a single hamburger patty uses enough fossil fuel to drive a small car 20 miles and enough water for 17 showers."
   — **PETA, VegNow.Com, 2004**

If you want to help save the world, stop eating meat, dairy, eggs, and processed foods.

Becoming vegan is the single most effective way you can improve the environment and the health of the world.

"If anyone wants to save the planet, all they have to do is just stop eating meat. That's the single most important thing you could do. It's staggering when you think about it. Vegetarianism takes care of so many things in one shot: ecology, famine, cruelty."
   — **Paul McCartney, vegetarian, animal rights proponent, and music maker**

If you are a meat eater and think that eating meat, dairy, and eggs is your business, and none of mine, think again. Similarly to how Howard Lyman and others have stated it, I repeat the defense to the stance of vegans: If your diet style is relying on the mass breeding of animals, then it is my business, and it is the business of everyone on the planet. It affects us environmentally, socially, physically, and financially. Your diet style pollutes the air I breathe, the water I drink, and the food I eat. It has led to, and is leading to the extinction of species, and the entire animal farming industry is the main cause of global warming.

A vegetarian diet uses substantially fewer resources than a wasteful and unhealthful meat-based diet. A plant-based diet is not only healthier for humans, but also for farm workers, for the land, for plant life, for the water, for the air, for the animals, and for Earth.

Hog Farm Pollution

When pigs live in a natural, wild environment they walk and explore many miles a day, and sleep with other pigs in a bed of twigs and/or grass. They are clean, smart, and social animals.

Today most pigs that are grown for human consumption are raised indoors in smelly, filthy, noisy conditions with cement floors that deform their feet. They are kept in cramped pens and fed horrible diets that are a far cry from what they would naturally eat. Pregnant pigs are kept in narrow cages that restrict their movement to the point that they can't turn or lie or stretch. Often the pregnant pigs are kept with a chain or leash around their neck that is tied to the floor or pen.

When the babies are born the piglet's teeth are cut, their tails are sliced off, and their ears are clipped off. Then they are placed in a pen where they will spend their entire lives with hundreds and often thousands of pigs living a similar grim fate of confinement. They are limited to eating a poisonous diet that will make them as fat as possible as fast at possible. Most U.S. pigs have respiratory infections at time of slaughter. Several hundred thousand of them are slaughtered every day in the U.S., and more than that are being born.

"Basically, pork producers figured out some years ago that if they packed the maximum number of pigs into the minimum amount of space, if they pinned the creatures down into fit-to-size iron crates above slatted floors and carved out giant 'lagoons' to contain the manure – if they turned the 'farm,' in short, into a sunless hell of metal and concrete – it made everything so much more efficient. An obvious cost-saver, and from the industry's standpoint, that should settle the matter.

... It turns out that when you trap intelligent, 400- to 500-pound mammals in gestation crates 22 inches wide and seven feet long, when their limbs are broken from trying to turn or escape and they are covered in sores, blood, tumors, 'pus pockets,' and their own urine and excrement, they tend to act up a bit.

Indeed, the most notable thing is how the appearance of any human being causes a violent panic. A mere opening of the door brings on a horrific wave of roars, squeals and cage-rattling from the sows. Another memorable sight is the 'cull pen,' wherein each and every day, the dead or dying bodies of the weak are placed, the ones who expired from the sheer, unrelenting agony of it.

– **Matthew Scully, author of *Dominion: The Power of Man, the Suffering of***

Animals, and the Call to Mercy; **in an article published in the** *Arizona Republic,* **February 9, 2006**

"A typical pig factory farm generates raw waste equivalent to that of a city of 12,000 people."
— PETA, VegNow.Com, 2004

Raleigh, North Carolina, *News and Observer* newspaper reporters Joby Warrick and Pat Stith, along with editor Melanie Sill, worked for several months on a series of articles that exposed the environmental disasters and health risks of hog farming in factory farms in North Carolina. In April 1996 the newspaper won the Pulitzer Prize gold medal for meritorious public service.

The articles, known as the *Boss Hog Series,* told how politicians involved in hog farming helped pave the way for a billion dollar hog farming expansion where corporations are taking over the industry and elbowing out the small farmers. The politicians did so by influencing state agencies, introducing bills, helping to pass laws, and forming policies that provide weaker environmental regulations and zoning protection for corporate hog farming. Many legislatures in North Carolina have a history of receiving money from the hog industry, and some are investors in hog farming.

The expansion of big business hog farming in North Carolina was done in spite of complaints and concerns voiced by long-time residents, local leaders, and environmental groups. But key to the rapid expansion is the way self-serving politicians, along with contributors to political campaigns, make millions from the hog industry. The issues detailed in the *News and Observer* are not confined to North Carolina; they are issues being faced by farming and business communities all over the world. Corporate pig farm interests spent $1 million in 1998 to defeat legislators who were working to clean up the environmental hazards of factory hog farm cesspools.

The massive amounts of pollution from the hog farms in eastern North Carolina come from housing several million hogs in large steel barns (factory farms). The combination of the hogs, barns, flies, and pollution has changed the landscape, real estate value, smell, and water quality of the region. The odors from the hog farms have invaded the homes, schools, churches, and businesses of residents angered that their communities are being spoiled by the rapidly expanding hog industry.

The hog population in North Carolina resulted in the state jumping from the seventh to the second largest hog-farming state in the U.S.

Since the 1990s there are more hogs than humans in North Carolina. Each hog produces two to four times as much waste as the average human.

By the year 2000 it was estimated that hog farms in North Carolina were producing more than ten million tons of waste every year. With millions of hogs in such a small area producing that much waste, North Carolina hog farms are turning out more raw sewage than both New York City *and* the suburbs that surround it.

The pollution produced by the hog farms in North Carolina is overwhelming the land and the people who live there. By 2005 the state had over 16 million hogs producing raw waste equal to at least 32 million people. The situation has been able to magnify so fast because North Carolina has weaker and imposes fewer environmental regulations for hog farms than any major hog-producing state.

> "Animals raised for human consumption in the U.S. generate 2.2 trillion pounds of waste each year."
> — A Voice for Animals, VoiceForAnimals.Net; 2002

The putrid waste from the hog farms is stored in thousands of cesspools that the hog industry likes to charmingly refer to as "lagoons." Those in the hog industry say the hog waste safely decomposes in the cesspools before it is sprayed onto crop land. The problem is that the land cannot absorb that much waste. The waste stored in the cesspools also leaks into ground water.

The *60 Minutes* TV show reported in December 1996 that over 30 percent of water wells near hog farms were contaminated by hog waste. The cesspools also overflow into streams and rivers during heavy rains. Millions of gallons of hog farm sludge, hog feces, hog afterbirths and blood, as well as cropland fertilizer have leaked into surrounding waterways where it has been killing aquatic life and causing algae overgrowth that chokes waterways. In one incident an estimated 25 million tons of hog waste flowed out of an eight-acre cesspool when a levee broke. Many farms have been caught dumping hog waste directly into surrounding streams, rivers, and lakes. The pollution has killed millions of fish and many other types of waterlife and caused rivers and lakes to be closed off to swimming and water sports.

In 1995 a 120,000-square-foot hog cesspool lagoon released over 25 million gallons of crap into the headwaters of North Carolina's New River. It took months to reach the ocean and killed millions of fish and unknown numbers of water mammals unfortunate enough to be in the contaminated river. In 1999 Hurricane Floyd caused so much flooding in Eastern North Carolina that it is estimated that well over 120 million gallons of hog waste made its way into the rivers, and out to the sea. It carried with it tens of thousands of drowned pigs, and killed unknown millions of fish. There were too many dead fish for birds to eat, and too many pigs in the ocean for sharks to feast on.

Nitrate-nitrogen from the hog cesspools continues to leak into ground water. This is a major problem because the chemical causes methemoglobinemia, a disease that hampers the ability of the blood to absorb oxygen. It can be particularly lethal to infants who drink contaminated water.

Other ingredients of hog waste that may threaten human and animal health include bacteria, viruses, and parasites. Pfiesteria piscicidia is one of the microbes. It results in massive fish kills. When humans are exposed to this microbe they can experience skin sores, nausea, vomiting, headache, blurred vision, breathing difficulties, liver and kidney problems, memory loss, and cognitive impairment. The putrid smell from the hog farms can saturate everything in the community, including well water, food, laundry, and the structures of the homes.

In addition to the hog waste that is polluting the air, water, and land of North Carolina, the people regularly find dead hogs dumped in the countryside. The corporation may own the pigs, but the farmers who are under contract with the corporation are supposed to take care of the pigs that die and the hog waste. When the farmers are under contract raise thousands of pigs they can quickly get overwhelmed with the waste and carcasses.

What is a growing problem in North Carolina is not limited to that state. The corporate players in the hog industry have expanded in several states as well as to other countries, including Eastern Europe. The hog pollution experienced in North Carolina and Iowa is a growing problem in Poland.

Some factory hog farm facilities are designed to hold several hundred thousand hogs with adjoining cesspools holding millions of gallons of urine mixed with feces containing all the drugs the animals were given, all of the toxic sprays they were treated with, all of the farming chemicals used on the foods the pigs ate, and a wide variety of bacteria. I addition, the lagoons contain the afterbirth of hogs, as well as stillborn pigs and piglets that died soon after birth.

One hog factory in Utah has about 500,000 pigs. Since hogs produce about three times as much excrement as humans, those 500,000 hogs produce more waste than 1.5 million people. It is a subsidiary of Smithfield Foods, a company responsible for the slaughter of about 27 million hogs in 2005. An article that appeared in *Rolling Stone* compared this Smithfield Foods slaughter in body weight to killing all of the human population of America's 32 largest cities (Boss Hog, by Jeff Tietz, *Rolling Stone*, December 14, 2006). That same article estimated that the excrement from Smithfield Foods hog farms for one year would fill four Yankee Stadiums. The article tells of factory hog farm workers who have died in these cesspools of hog waste, including five members of one family.

"The animal-rights people want to impose a vegetarian's society on the U.S. Most vegetarians I know are neurotic."
 — Joseph Luter III, Chairman of Smithfield Foods, which is the world's largest pig farming company. It produces several billions of pounds of hog meat every year. As quoted in Boss Hog, by Jeff Tietz, *Rolling Stone*, December 14, 2006. The Environmental Protection Agency has cited Smithfield Foods for thousands of violations of the Clean Water Act.

If you eat ham or bacon, you are supporting this horrible hog industry.

"When nonvegetarians say that 'human problems come first' I cannot help wondering what exactly it is that they are doing for human beings that compels them to continue to support the wasteful, ruthless exploitation of farm animals."
 — Peter Singer, *Animal Liberation*, 1990

War on Wildlife: Killing Millions of Wild Animals to Protect Farm Animals

"Every year, tens of thousands of bison, coyotes, wolves, and other wildlife are maimed, shot, poisoned, and even burned alive because the meat industry claims these animals interfere with raising animals for food. This war on wildlife is carried out with the full support of state and federal agencies, which fund so-called predator control programs."
 — FarmSancturary.Org

"Animal agriculture directly kills annually nearly 50 billion animals worldwide, after subjecting them to the cruelties of factory farming. It

also kills uncounted numbers of wildlife on land and in the seas."
— Citizens for Healthy Options in Children's Education, CHOICE.USA

"In reality, ranchers are the most pervasively destructive force on our public land, with logging as a distant second. Via outlandish subsidies, you, I, and Uncle Sam support the cattle industry with drought and fire relief, fencing, water tanks, windmills, and bargain-basement grazing fees. Our government kills hundreds of thousands of wild creatures each year to protect ranchers' herds against predators such as wolves, mountain lions, and coyotes.

In return we get erosion, endangered species, habitat destruction, flash floods, exotic weeds, desertification, and some of the most degraded landscape on Earth."
— Tim Lenerich, *Dispelling the Cowboy Myth*, Earthsave.Org/News/03Summer/ Cowboy_Myth .htm; 2004

"But it [cattle ranching] is anything but benign. It is the number one source of water pollution in the West. It's the number one source of soil erosion in the West. It's the number one cause of species endangerment in the West. It's the reason we don't have wolves throughout the West. It's one of the major reasons that more than four-fifths of all native fish west of the Continental Divide are endangered or threatened."
— George Wuerthner of Eugene, Oregon, is one of the most outspoken leaders against public-lands ranching. From *Dispelling the Cowboy Myth*, by Tim Lenerich, Earthsave.Org/ News/03Summer/Cowboy_Myth.htm; 2004

"Nearly 20 million taxpayer dollars fund the trapping, poisoning, and shooting of native predators deemed a threat to agriculture by the USDA Wildlife Services agency, which each year kills approximately 100,000 coyotes, bobcats, foxes, bears, wolves, and other predators. In 2001 the program also killed 1.6 million other 'nuisance' animals.

Almost two-thirds of all large mammal species are threatened or endangered in the lower 48 states. Less than 10 percent of all endangered and threatened species in the U.S. is improving.

About 20 percent of all endangered and threatened species are harmed by grazing."
— A Voice for Animals, VoiceForAnimals.Net; 2004

"In response to ranchers' complaints of coyotes attacking cattle in southern Arizona, the federal government took to the air this past January, killing 200 coyotes. The hunt was conducted by Wildlife Services, a division of the U.S. Department of Agriculture, and took place on both public and private land."
— Earth First! Journal, May-June 2006; EarthFirstJournal.Org

Some people would like the public to believe that pollution is the only and worst offender to wildlife in the U.S. While pollution does take an enormous toll, the reason populations of native animals in the U.S. have dwindled is that the animals have been killed to provide grazing land for livestock, and to protect grazing livestock.

To make it possible for cattle and other livestock to graze in open fields there has to be a safe haven created for them. This means that native animals have to be killed off. These animals include wolves, coyotes, foxes, lynx, mountain lions, bobcats, bears, elk, bighorn sheep, deer, porcupine, beaver, badgers, skunks, possums, prairie dogs, and antelope.

"In 1914, Congress first appropriated money for the U.S. Biological Survey (now known as Animal Damage Control) to exterminate wolves from the face of the continent. Though the agency failed to eradicate the species entirely, by 1945 it had killed every wolf in Colorado."
— *Colorado Wolf Tracks*, **the newsletter of Sinapu.Org; 1996**

Eliminating the native animals is done with poisons, with steel jaw leghold traps, by shooting them from helicopters, and by damaging their food supplies. The government offices involved in these activities include the Bureau of Land Management (BLM) and the Animal Damage Control (ADC) program of the Department of Agriculture. According to *Wildlife Damage Review*, in 1994 the government spent over $56 million of federal, state, and cooperative funds to kill 783,585 wild animals.

The land that has been cleared of native wildlife is then used as pasture for grazing livestock such as cattle, sheep, and goats. The ranchers lease the land from the government, and they do so at very low rates that do not make up for the money spent by the government to manage the land for the ranchers. The balance is made up from tax dollars – thus providing government welfare programs for ranchers.

In addition to killing wild animals for pastureland, the U.S. Department of Agriculture also is involved in killing millions of birds. They regularly use poisoned rice laced with DRC-1339 to kill grain-eating birds, such as grackles, red-winged blackbirds, ravens, magpies, vultures, and yellow-headed blackbirds. The killing doesn't stop there. That's because predator birds, such as Cooper's hawks and prairie falcons that eat the poisoned birds, also die.

Killing predator animals damages the natural cycle of native animal life. When the predator animals are killed off, the animals they feed on are able to reproduce in massive numbers. This has resulted in large populations of animals such as mice, rats, gophers, squirrels, badgers, prairie dogs, skunks, possum, rabbits, chipmunks, deer, and raccoons.

The ADC programs attempt to control the populations of the smaller animals by sending out trappers to eliminate them. They eliminate the smaller animals by burning them, by bludgeoning them, and by poisoning their young. Many smaller native animals are also killed to prevent them from eating the crops that are being grown to feed livestock, and to prevent them from creating nesting and dwelling holes in the ground, which may result in livestock injuring their legs.

To help control the population of some animals, such as deer, hunters are allowed to enter into controlled areas to kill a certain number of animals every year. When bows are used to hunt deer, about half of the deer escape with the bow stuck in them, and then the deer suffer slow, agonizing deaths.

"Trapping and/or hunting are allowed on more than half of the 540 U.S. National Wildlife Refuges. According to the U.S. Fish & Wildlife Service, of 27 million people who visited refuges, 22 million came for wildlife observation, while only 1.2 million visited to hunt or trap animals."
— A Voice for Animals, VoiceForAnimals.Net, 2005

The techniques used to kill off smaller animals, and to eliminate brush and other native plants used by larger animals, also harm the bird populations. Not only do birds die when they get caught in traps and when they eat poison meant for other animals, large birds die after eating animals that have been poisoned. A decrease in the bird population allows more insects to populate the land. To kill off the insects, the government and farmers use more chemical poisons. The pesticides then do even more damage to the bird population, create insects that are resistant to pesticides, destroy beneficial insects, and pollute the land and water, and so forth, in a cycle that would naturally take care of itself if man would not interfere.

"The ADC program, created by the Animal Damage Control Act of 1931, is greatly responsible for the virtual extinction of the grizzly and wolf in the lower 48 states as well as for putting the black-footed ferret, jaguar, black-tailed prairie dog, bald eagle, and other wild animals in, or

close to, the endangered category. ADC reported it poisoned 1.8 million animals in 1991 and distributed thousands of pounds of restricted-use pesticides to private individuals who poisoned untold numbers more. The U.S. Agency for International Development works with ADC to export ADC pest control practices and chemicals, including those banned in the U.S., to developing countries."
    — *Wildlife Damage Review*, the newsletter of Sinapu.Org;1997

Ranchers and BLM workers eliminate shrubs that are used for food and shelter by native animals, and then plant grasses to feed grazing cattle. By eliminating native plants that provide food and shelter for wild animals, by eliminating small animals that provide food for predator animals, and by killing all kinds of native animals, the government has had an enormous negative impact on the populations, life cycles, migrating patterns, and social structures of native animals of North and Central America. This is done at great cost to taxpayers to provide grazing land for livestock ranchers. It is welfare farming and it is destroying the biodiversity and ecosystems of the continent. Sadly, because more and more cattle are being raised on other continents, these practices are becoming the standard in other countries.

Predator animals not only manage populations of large animals in the natural circle of life, they also improve conditions for small animals, fish, insects, and plants.

When wolves were reintroduced to Yellowstone National Park, willow trees, cottonwoods, and aspen trees began to grow more abundantly there. This was the result of elk seeking the safety of higher ground away from the wolves. The new vegetation has attracted other wildlife. The banks of the rivers and creeks, which had been damaged by elk, began to show more vegetation growth, which in turn improved the health of the rivers and creeks. This improved conditions for fish populations. And the new trees have also attracted native birds to nest there and provide shade for certain varieties of plants to grow.

"Next to an all-out nuclear war, today's intensive animal agriculture represents the greatest threat to human welfare in the history of mankind."
    — Farm Animal Reform Movement, FarmUSA.Org; 2005

"The love for all living creatures is the most noble attribute of man."
    — Charles Darwin

Fish and Waterlife

"It is estimated that in the past thirty years, the human species alone
has used up 1/3 of the entire planet's natural resources... over-fishing,
in all parts of the world, is just one example."
— ZeroImpactProductions.Com

Many people think that vegetarians eat fish. Some people who
consider themselves to be vegetarians do eat fish. A true vegetarian does not eat fish of any sort.

While many people are aware of the damage to water life that is
caused by pollution, most people are not aware of the damage to the
oceans, lakes, rivers, and streams that is caused by fishing. It is because
of fishing that many types of sea life have disappeared and others are
being seriously threatened with extinction. Many populations of sea
life the fishing industry seeks are at dangerously low levels.

- The term seafood includes hundreds of species of water-dwelling
  creatures, from fresh and saltwater fish, to crustaceans (lobster,
  prawns, etc.) and mollusks (clams, squid, etc.) to cetaceans (water
  mammals: whales, dolphins, porpoises, seals, etc.).

- The average international per-person consumption of seafood has
  nearly doubled in the last half of the 20th century.

- According to the National Oceanic and Atmospheric Administration of the U.S. Department of Commerce, in 2004 the average
  American ate 16.6 pounds of seafood. That indicates a 1.4-pound
  increase in four years.

- In 2005 the consumption of land animals (cows, pigs, chickens,
  turkey, lamb, etc.) was 2.5 times greater than that of seafood.

- In 2004 the average American consumed 4.2 pounds of shrimp.

- In 2005 there were over 1.2 billion cans of tuna sold in the U.S.

- Seafood taken from the world's waters, including fish farms, has
  gone from about 20 million tons in 1950 to about 130 million tons
  in 2000.

- About a fourth of the sea creatures taken from the oceans aren't used
  for human consumption, but are instead turned into pet food, into
  feed for farm animals (mostly fed to pigs, chickens, and turkeys), and

into feed pellets for fish farms.

• China, with only four percent of the world's coastlines, is the world's number one consumer of fish, and produces over 28 million tons of farmed fish yearly.

• Advances in refrigeration combined with the building of airports around the world have made it possible for people in virtually any region to eat sea food from any other region.

• Commercial fishing continues to be one of the most dangerous professions in the U.S. According to the U.S. Coast Guard more than 630 fishermen died between 1992 and 2002.

> **"Researchers say the global fish harvest will have to increase by near-ly 50 percent by 2020 just to meet new demand in China and other developing countries."**
> — **The Great Open Ocean Sell-off: A Glut of New Offshore Factory Fish Farms May Be Just Over the Horizon, by Craig Cox; *Utne* magazine, November-December 2004**

In 1940 a sardine fishing boat named *The Western Flyer* left the Monterey, California, waters and traveled down past the Baja California coast and up to the top of the Sea of Cortez. The boat carried a group of people – including *The Grapes of Wrath* author John Steinbeck and his marine biologist friend, Edward F. Ricketts, who wrote the landmark book *Between Pacific Tides*, a study of intertidal marine biology. The 4,000-mile six-week trip was recorded in Steinbeck's nonfiction 1951 book, *The Log from the Sea of Cortez*. The book stands as a survey of the sea life he encountered on the trip.

Steinbeck wrote about a sea filled with life, where sea turtles were common; where massive schools of groupers appeared, some weighing 500 pounds; where giant manta rays leaped from the water; where schools of yellowfish chased schools of sardines; where hammerhead sharks fed; where tuna jumped from the sea; where leaping swordfish cut through the water; where dolphin swam alongside the boat; and where pelicans dove to pick fish from the aquamarine waters. His descriptions of the coast of Baja portray a quiet and unspoiled land with random villages of Native people. The coastal waters had plentiful amounts of a variety of vertebrates and invertebrates. Pearl oysters were common, as were starfish, sea cucumbers, jellyfish, crabs, stingrays, snails, barnacles, anemones, and urchins.

Even as late as 1986 internationally renowned oceanographer

Jacques Cousteau declared the Sea of Cortez to be the "aquarium of the world."

> "The web of life in our oceans is being pulled apart as top predators like tuna have crashed from overfishing; trawling for groundfish and scallops has scraped some areas of the ocean bottom clean like a parking lot; and pollution and nutrient-rich runoff have fed algae blooms and jellyfish population explosions, resulting in what one scientist calls 'the sliming of the oceans.'"
> — Jon Christensen, Steinbeck Fellow, San Jose State University, *Back to the Sea of Cortez: Sailing with the Spirits of John Steinbeck and Ed Ricketts on a New Journey of Discovery Around Baja California*, SeaOfCortez.Org

In 2004, Chuck Baxter, a retired Stanford University marine biology professor; Jon Christensen, a freelance writer (and keeper of the blog SeaOfCortez.Org); William F. Gilly, a neurobiologist; and Nancy Packard Burnett, who, with Baxter, is a cofounder of the Monterey Bay Aquarium, gathered a group of people together and retraced the 1940 voyage taken by Steinbeck and Ricketts. They used the writings of Steinbeck and Ricketts as a guide while making the trip on a shrimp trawler named *Gus D.*

What Baxter's group found was vastly different from what Steinbeck recorded in his book, and what Ricketts wrote about in his field notes. Not only were many types of sea life described by Steinbeck and Ricketts not seen, but even many of the creatures in the tide pools were missing, or in obvious steep decline.

Baxter, Christensen, and the others did not see turtles, sharks, schools of tuna, leaping swordfish, or giant manta rays. Over the decades, those and many other forms of life once common in the Sea of Cortez, such as tuna, shrimp, and yellowtail, have vanished, or have been brought to the edge of extinction in those areas because of over-fishing and pollution. In addition, much of the shellfish, including the pearl oysters, have been hunted to death. The sea life ended up in grocery stores and restaurants, as pet food, and feed for farmed animals. As time passed much of the coast of Baja has been built into tourist traps, retirement communities, college student party zones, and harbors for yachts and cruise ships.

Steinbeck had written about the fishing industry, which he called "a large destructive machine," and which was involved in "committing true crimes against Nature." What the group traveling in 2004 saw was the result of those crimes: a sea with relatively few forms of life left compared to just 64 years in the past.

What has happened to the Sea of Cortez has happened and is happening to oceans and seas, lakes and streams all over Earth. Pollution from urban runoff, from the oil industry, from the burning of fossil fuels, from the shipping industry, and from such things as cruise ships, the military, golf courses, and the chemicals used in the farming industry has resulted in poisoned waters and "carbon sink-holes" where oxygen is so depleted that natural sea life cannot exist.

Chesapeake Bay, which, like the Sea of Cortez, was once compared to a giant aquarium, is also void of many forms of sea life that once flourished there. Instead, Chesapeake Bay is highly polluted from the runoff of cities, animal farms, and chemicals used on farms, lawns, and golf courses. The sea life in the bay is being strangled by water-clogging algae that feed off the nitrogen in the fertilizers and farm runoff. The bay is the world's main spawning ground for striped bass, which are now often found to be starving and with bacterial infections eating away at their flesh. The natural water-filtering sea creatures, such as oysters and menhaden fish, are on the steep decline caused by pollution and fishing, adding to pollution.

There are vast areas of dead water covering several thousand miles of water in the Gulf of Mexico where sea life has died off and is unable to exist. Throughout the world's seas there are similar dead zones consisting of mass quantities of pollution.

In 1995 the United Nations Environment Program identified at least 146 dead zones in the world's seas. Some exist near the surface of the water, and some are deep down. Because of this, great numbers of marine species are at risk from the increasing acidification of the water. It is one reason why sea life, such as sharks, and schools of fish, are found swimming where they don't normally swim, and a main reason why some forms of sea fish and vegetation are vanishing from the oceans.

"It is estimated that nine out of ten organisms on the entire planet live in the ocean. Some of these are tiny unicellular algae which make up part of the plankton that produce four times the amount of oxygen than terrestrial plants do."
— ZeroImpactProductions.Com

"Basic chemistry leaves us in little doubt that our burning of fossil fuels is changing the acidity of our oceans. And the rate of change we are seeing to the ocean's chemistry is a hundred times faster than has

happened for millions of years.
     ... Failure to (cut carbon dioxide emissions) may mean there is no place in the oceans of the future for many species and ecosystems that we know today."
       — John Raven, oceanic expert with Britain's Royal Society, which reported that the oceans were absorbing one ton of carbon dioxide (the primary greenhouse gas) per person per year, and are running out of the capacity to absorb it; June 2005

As I write this I sit on the end of a pier overlooking Santa Monica Bay. It is an interesting vantage point to write about the health of the oceans. This is one of the many areas of the oceans directly affected by a city built on the edge of it. Just over a hundred years ago this bay was a pristine oasis for a variety of wildlife. But for the past several decades it has been the focus of environmental groups working to halt toxins from flowing into it. The city of Santa Monica has built a $12 million urban storm drain runoff treatment facility that treats an estimated 350,000 gallons of street runoff every day, intercepting pollution that would otherwise go directly into the ocean. Plastics and other solid waste are removed and taken to a landfill. Some of the treated water goes to the local police department's plumbing, where it flushes the toilets. Other treated water is used to irrigate city parks and the cemetery.

Despite the efforts to protect the bay, the water quality here often gets a very low grade. While other coastal cities are considering ways to treat urban-runoff, the Santa Monica Urban Runoff Recycling Facility remains the only urban runoff treatment plant in the country. During heavy rains the facility backs up and the polluted water is released directly into the ocean. Because of high bacterial levels the beaches on this bay often get posted with signs warning swimmers and surfers that the water is unsafe. The bay water has been used as a dump for the military and various companies looking to unload various junk. When it rains in Southern California the trash and grime from the thousands of miles of the region's streets flow into storm drains that empty into the ocean, contaminating everything that lives here. When that happens, Santa Monica Bay is often the dirtiest ocean area of western North America.

     "The U.N. Environment Program estimates that 46,000 pieces of plastic litter are floating on every square mile of the oceans...
     An estimated one million seabirds choke or get tangled in plastic

nets or other debris every year. About 100,000 seals, sea lions, whales, dolphins, other marine mammals, and sea turtles suffer the same fate."
— Altered Oceans: A Chemical Imbalance, Usha Lee McFarland, *Los Angeles Times*, August 3, 2006; LATimes.Com/Oceans

As I look at the murky water I can see lots of bits of trash floating in it. I wonder what the people who are fishing off the end of the pier think of all the pollution here. If I were someone who ate sea creatures, I would certainly lose my appetite looking at this water. Unfortunately, the pollution here does not stay in one area.

Because the oceans of the planet are really just one big body of water with merging currents, what we toss into this ocean in the form of toxic chemicals and garbage often shows up thousands of miles away in another part of another ocean. As fish migrate to various parts of the oceans just as birds migrate across continents, the pollutants that fish pick up in one part of the ocean is spread to another part of the ocean.

As I look across the water I see a brown pelican skimming the surface. This is a very good thing to see.

By 1992 the brown pelican species around the coast of Los Angeles County was one generation away from extinction. That was the year the pesticide DDT was outlawed. The pesticide caused the birds to lay eggs with shells that were so thin they would break in the nest. In 2006 it is estimated that there are 7,000 breeding pairs of brown pelicans in California.

The white croaker caught in Santa Monica Bay are still unsafe to eat because of the DDT in their systems, and this is happening over twenty years after DDT was outlawed.

Unfortunately the pollution issues of Santa Monica Bay are nothing compared to what other regions of the world's oceans are facing.

In March 2004 the U.S. Department of Health and Human Services as well as the U.S. Environmental Protection Agency released information detailing the levels of mercury and other heavy metals in the tissues of fish that are commonly eaten by humans, such as tuna, shark, swordfish, king mackerel, and tilefish, as well as shellfish. Mercury occurs naturally in the environment, but the increase in mercury in the tissues of waterlife is largely the result of industrial pollution, and much of that consists of pollution from coal-burning power plants and from concrete processing kilns. While the press release mentioned how pregnant women, nursing mothers, and small children should avoid some types of fish, it stupidly also said that people should continue eating fish and shellfish – likely a way to appease the multibillion dollar fishing, seafood, and restaurant industries.

> "Unfortunately, what fish does contain is enough mercury to help you take your temperature."
> — Former Montana cattle rancher Howard Lyman, in his book *No More Bull: The Mad Cowboy Targets America's Worst Enemy: Our Diet*; MadCowboy.Com

The high levels of mercury and other heavy metals are among of the many reasons why it is unhealthful to eat fish. Small sea creatures are exposed to all sorts of toxins in the water that are the result of poisoned rivers emptying into the oceans; of pollution directly flowing into the oceans from coastal cities, military operations, and industries; from toxic chemical fertilizers and pest controls spread on the greens of golf courses, lawns, farms, schools, and corporate campuses; from the shipping and oil industries; from cruise ships; and from air pollution.

When larger forms of sea creatures eat the smaller sea creatures, the toxins from the smaller creatures accumulate in the tissues of the larger fish. When a person consumes tuna, shark, red snapper, and other large fish, they are exposing themselves to all of the toxins that have accumulated in the tissues of those larger fish. As the U.S. government has reported, this exposure can lead to nerve damage, miscarriages, learning disabilities, birth deformities, and cancers in humans.

Mercury concentrates more in the blood of fetuses than in pregnant mothers; this is why women who are planning on becoming pregnant and those who are pregnant are advised to avoid eating tuna, king mackerel, shark, swordfish, and tilefish. Babies whose mothers consume fish are at greater risk. Those whose mothers consume a plant-based diet are at a lower risk. According to the Centers for Disease Control and Prevention statistics released in 1995, based on blood surveys of women of childbearing age, about 5.7 percent of infants in the U.S. could be at risk of mercury poisoning absorbed from their mothers during pregnancy.

Solid white albacore tuna has been found to be especially high in mercury contamination. One single tuna sandwich may contain enough mercury to interfere with a child's learning, concentration, behavior, coordination, and language. Because their bodies are smaller and are developing, children should also abstain from eating these fish.

The food companies that package and sell the fish you see in supermarkets have been pressuring the Food and Drug Administration to refrain from any actions that may interfere with the profits of the fishing industry. In meetings held between FDA officials and fish industry executives in the fall of 2000, the executives expressed concerns that FDA advisories against the consumption of eating tuna may result in class action lawsuits from consumers.

[An advisory released by government agencies telling people not to eat certain types of seafood] "could have an irreversible impact on American dietary habits, profoundly affecting consumers and producers of seafood and resulting in significant segments of the population turning away from the proven health benefits of fish consumption."
— The National Food Processors Association, the National Fisheries Institute, and the U.S. Tuna Foundation, in a letter to an FDA commissioner, 2000; as quoted in Balancing Interests, Agencies Issue Guidance at Odds with EPA Risk Assessment: A Schoolboy's Sudden Setback, by Peter Waldman, *The Wall Street Journal*, August 1, 2005

In 2001 the FDA released a revised fish advisory in 2001 that didn't mention tuna but did mention king mackerel, shark, swordfish, and tilefish. Americans are more likely to eat tuna, and to accumulate mercury in their bodies from tuna than from the fish mentioned in the mercury advisory.

"In order to keep the market share at a reasonable level, we felt like we had to keep light tuna in the low-mercury group."
— Clark Carrington of the FDA in an FDA Food Advisory Committee meeting with officials from the Environmental Protection Agency, 2003; as quoted in "Balancing Interests, Agencies Issue Guidance at Odds with EPA Risk Assessment: A Schoolboy's Sudden Setback," by Peter Waldman; *The Wall Street Journal*, August 1, 2005

When the FDA may be taking actions to protect the profits of the fish industry rather than protecting the health of people, one has to wonder how reliable the information is that is being released by government agencies in relation to the safety of eating fish.

It would be wise for adults to consider the findings on mercury contamination of both fresh and saltwater fish and the health problems related to this poison, and to act accordingly.

"Animals accumulate and concentrate toxicity from the environment. This is especially true with fish, as they live in and constantly filter impure water, which leaves residues of toxins in their tissues. Because toxicity is channeled to the liver of animals, fish liver oil is likely to con-

tain large doses of poisons.
    We must keep in mind that either we filter out what we are allowing into our bodies, or we ourselves will become a filter."
    — **David Wolfe**

Those who believe that there are health benefits to be had by consuming fish liver oil are only fooling themselves. The oil from the body tissues of seafood contains all of the toxins that the creature was exposed to. Cod liver oil is also so rich in vitamin A that regular consumption of that oil can contribute to osteoporosis.

Much healthier and safer oils are those that have been extracted from raw and organically grown olives, flax seeds, grape seeds, pumpkin seeds, walnuts, and especially from raw hempseeds. Hempseed oil contains a most excellent balance of quality nutritional oils. Oil from seafood should be avoided.

Nobody needs to be eating seafood for the purpose of getting essential fatty acids. There are no health benefits from eating seafood that can't be obtained in better quality by eating a variety of raw plant substances.

Pollution is only a part of the major problems facing the world's waters.

"Longline fishing, used to catch swordfish, tuna, and other species, may be 80 miles long and carry several thousand baited hooks at a time. Each year longlines catch and kill hundreds of thousands of other animals, including sharks and birds."
    — **A Voice for Animals, VoiceForAnimals.Org**

"A longline is a fishing line usually made of monofilament. The length of the line generally ranges from 1.6 km (one mile) to as long as 100 km (62 miles). The line is buoyed by Styrofoam or plastic floats. Every hundred or so feet, there is a secondary line attached extending down about 5 m (16 feet). This secondary line is hooked and baited with squid, fish, or in cases we have discovered, with fresh dolphin meat. The baited hooks can be seen by albatross from the air and when they dive on the hooks, they are caught and they drown. The lines are set adrift from vessels for a period of 12 to 24 hours.

The use of longlines in international waters is not illegal in itself. However, if the lines take an endangered or threatened species [which they often do], they become illegal because the taking of an endangered species is a violation of the Convention on the Trade in Endangered Species of Flora and Fauna. International maritime law dic-

tates that a longline that does not bear an identifying flag is in effect legally salvageable, i.e., free for the taking because it is not attached to the ship or boat that deploys it."
— **Sea Shepherd Conservation Society, SeaShepherd.Org; 2006**

Fishing boats place billions of hooks in the oceans every year. Additionally, diesel fuel-spewing fishing trawlers drag nets across the ocean waters, with some nets reaching to the oceans' floors. Over the years the nets have become larger and are being dragged by larger and larger boats. And there are drift nets, set out like some sort of game play to see what shows up. Some boats can carry a couple hundred thousand pounds of fish kept on ice. Many of these fishing fleets, especially from Asian and European countries, receive money from their governments in the form of subsidies to help pay for boats, fuel, and supplies. All of this goes to supply the world markets with seafood. While Asian countries capture an estimated 2/3 of the world's seafood supply (much of it exported to other countries), the fast-food restaurant industry uses hundreds of millions of pounds of fried fish every year.

As this trend continues, fishing is taking place deeper and deeper in the seas, and resulting in more damage, not only to the types of sea life that people eat, but to sea life that people do not eat, and sea life that other forms of sea life depend on for their existence in the circle of life. Fishing companies are constantly killing all sorts of sea life that get tangled or caught in their nets or on their hooks.

More and more the fish that are being caught are smaller and younger. They often don't get the chance to grow to their full adult size because they are caught before they reach adulthood. Fish stocks are depleted the world over. Fishing fleets ignore quotas. And fish markets and restaurants are selling varieties of sea life that are at risk of vanishing from the oceans.

With trawlers removing all varieties of sea life from an area of the ocean, generations of populations of sea life are swept away, including the young and unborn of the fish that the fishing trawlers seek, as well as those they don't. Some of the sea creatures unwanted by the fishing companies survive by being thrown back into the water. Many don't. Many that are caught are smaller fish on which the larger fish survive. So not only are the large fish being removed, but the food for the remaining larger fish is depleted as well.

One or two boats pull trawler nets, which may reach as far as 4,600 feet below the surface, often scraping the bottom. The World Conservation Union estimates that between 500,000 and 100 million species inhabit the bottoms of the seas, known as the benthic regions.

In November 2006, when United Nations negotiators tried to get a measure approving strict regulations on high-seas bottom trawling, Iceland led other nations to oppose the measure. Companies in Denmark, Estonia, Iceland, Japan, Latvia, Lithuania, New Zealand, Norway, Portugal, Russia, and Spain own fleets of bottom trawling boats. Countries that supported the measure to strictly limit bottom trawling fleets included Brazil, Britain, Canada, Chile, Germany, India, New Zealand, Norway, Palau, South Africa, and the U.S.

The trawling will continue without limits by the United Nations and will remain a tragically destructive practice on the high seas, where every season is open season.

Furthering the problem in the oceans is that the food for the smaller fish is in trouble. Phytoplankton is the food for a variety of sea life. One of the main sources of food for larger fish is the foot-long menhaden, and the chief source of food for the menhaden fish is phytoplankton. When there is too much phytoplankton, which occurs when menhaden populations are overfished, as they currently are, the phytoplankton block Sun light from reaching aquatic plants that support a variety of other sea creatures, such as oysters that help filter the water.

Because of pollution flowing into rivers, and eventually into the oceans from farms, golf courses, and lawns, the coastal waters are out of balance with an overgrowth of algae. Much of this is the result of fertilizers. As the populations of phytoplankton-eating sea life are on the decrease, and algae on the increase, the coastal waters, and increasingly large areas of water away from the coasts, are being devastated by algae overgrowth. The overgrowth robs the water of oxygen, causing massive fish kills. The rotting vegetation sinks to the bottom where it kills even more sea life. The dead and dying at the bottom include oysters, which have already been overfished, killed off by pollution, and are extinct in areas where they flourished just a few decades ago.

With the oceans absorbing more and more pollution, the fish are becoming toxic to themselves, and to the humans that eat them. Some nursing sea mammals have such high levels of pollution in their bodies that their nursing young are being poisoned from pollutants that concentrate in mother's milk. Unfortunately this is not the only threat to sea mammals.

It isn't only haddock, tuna, snapper, salmon, rockfish, cod, whiting, bass, herring, sardines, pollack, halibut, grouper, orange roughy, mackerel, anchovies, marlin, tilefish, swordfish, squid, and other commonly eaten sea life that are being killed by fishing.

Many people are unaware that whales, dolphin, and porpoises are still being killed and sold for food in many regions. Whales continue to be hunted by commercial fishermen from Japan, Norway, Iceland, and by indigenous people in Denmark, Korea, Russia, and the U.S.

> "It is unbelievably brutal and inhumane to slaughter such intelligent animals like this. Boats surround the animals and the hunters bang long metal poles under-water to create a wall of sound that disturbs their sonar and confuses them.
>
> The boats push the dolphins into a small lagoon where they are trapped by nets. They are then left for a night or two – they're strong animals and the hunters want to tire them out.
>
> They are harpooned from boats while some men jump into the bloody water with big knives to cut their throats. Sometimes they're hooked and lifted out of the water while still alive."
>
> — Clare Perry of the Environment Investigation Agency describing the slaughter of dolphin by Japanese fleets, quoted in the article Slaughtered: They're Friendly, Intelligent and Our Kid's Dream of Swimming with Them. So Why Are Thousands of Dolphins Still Being Slaughtered?, by Gary Anderson, *Sunday Mirror*, September 17, 2006 (SundayMirror.Co.UK). The article mentioned that it was expected the Japanese fishermen would kill about 20,000 dolphins over the following sixth months. (See: EIA-International.Org; MarineConnection.Org; and EarthIsland.Org/SaveTaijiDolphins/JapanDolphinDay06.html)

Japan is often held up as the worst offender when it comes to killing sea mammals, including dolphin, and minke and fin whales, who all struggle and scream as they are mercilessly killed in ways that may take hours as the water around them turns red with their blood.

Japanese fishermen have caused great harm to populations of Dall's porpoises. In January 2002 it was reported that because the population of Dall's porpoises has plummeted, the fishermen have resorted to killing female porpoises that are pregnant or are still nursing, which often results in the death of the calves through starvation or by shark attack. When the fishing boats surround the dolphin pods and use large nets to drive them into coves, the adult dolphins surround the females and young to protect them. After the boat crews gather some of the dolphins to sell them to aquariums and tourist parks, the remaining dolphins are stabbed.

> "The U.S. is currently not importing live dolphins, but many of the marine mammals currently on display in the U.S. were caught in the

wild. We reward the industry described above when we pay for tickets to see them. When we swim with captive dolphins while on vacation in other countries we are directly supporting the slaughter."
   — Karen Dawn, October 2006; DawnWatch.Com

The meat of one adult dolphin can be sold for about $600. It doesn't seem to matter to consumers that dolphin meat is contaminated with high levels of methyl mercury, a particularly toxic form of the toxin. Whale meat, which is also consumed in Japan, has also been found to contain levels of the toxin.

"The Japanese drive hunts are an astonishingly cruel violation of any reasonable animal welfare standards."
   — Lori Marino, Ph.D., Emory University and Diana Reiss, Ph.D., New York Aquarium and Columbia University. These two scientists proved that dolphins can recognize their reflection in a mirror, a cognitive complexity that elephants and chimpanzees can also do.

"During drive hunts, migrating pods of dolphins and other small whales are first panicked and confused by loud banging, then herded, by the hundreds, into shallow coves and butchered, one by one, by fishermen. Every year, some 20,000 small cetaceans of several species, some of which are endangered, including bottlenose dolphins, striped dolphins, spotted dolphins, Risso's dolphins, short-finned pilot whales, white-sided dolphins, and false killer whales, are killed or taken in the drives, sometimes illegally.
   This cruel and inhumane practice is sanctioned and controlled by the government of Japan, which claims that these animals compete with the fishermen and slaughtering them is a means of pest control, but no evidence for this claim exists. The dolphins are processed and used as pet food or fertilizer, and the government is encouraging the consumption of dolphin meat. In fact, the hunts would be economically unviable without the sale of live dolphins captured during the drives to dolphinariums in Asia and elsewhere."
   — TheOceanProject.Org/ActForDolphins

"Scientific research shows that dolphins are highly intelligent, self-aware and emotional animals with strong family ties and complex social lives."
   — from the Scientist Statement Against the Japanese Dolphin Drive Hunts, to the Government of Japan. The statement was signed by hundreds of scientists from around the world. TheOceanProject.Org/ActForDolphins; November 2006

"You cannot ignore any longer the fact that these animals have very

large brains, highly developed societies, social relationships, and sophisticated cognitive abilities."
— **Richard Connor, Ph.D., University of Massachusetts, Dartmouth**

It is a travesty that about 300,000 dolphins, porpoises, and whales are being killed by fishing teams every year; it is so much worse that so many other forms of sea life are being killed for no reason other than they just happened to be in the wrong place at the wrong time. In so many areas these large sea animals, including endangered sea turtles, are being killed because they get caught in gillnets that stretch from the surface of the water to the ocean floor. The dolphins and porpoises cannot detect the nets, get tangled in them, and drown.

There are simple, low-cost modifications that can be made to gill-nets that would greatly reduce the number of dolphins and porpoises that are killed, but the fishing companies have not made the changes. (Dolphins, Porpoises Require Immediate Action on Baycatch; WorldWildlife.Org; June 2005.)

In June 2005 Japan announced to the International Whaling Commission in Ulsan, South Korea, that it was increasing the number of mink whales it will kill annually from 440 to 935. Japan claims that it kills the whales to study them, but ends up selling the meat for food, which clearly appears to be the main reason they are killed. The commission had banned commercial whaling in 1986.

"According to the Marine Fish Conservation Network, north Atlantic swordfish caught today are only a third the size caught in the 1960s when I was out spotting for snappers – and well below that [weight] which females must be to reproduce. Sea Web reports that of the 157 fish species tracked in U.S. waters, 36 percent are overexploited and 44 percent are fished to the max. Populations of cod, haddock, halibut, red drum, and yellowtail flounder are at record lows. Chilean sea bass is so overfished that many scientists predict commercial extinction within five years."
— **Will the Real "Slob" Fishermen Please Stand Up?, by Doug Moss, founder, E magazine, July/August 2005**

The big fish have been and are being killed off by overfishing to such an extent that currently there may be only ten percent of them left from what existed just 50 years ago. This is leading to a dangerously small gene pool. At the same time, the small fish are killed because of net fishing; dynamite fishing; damage to mangrove forests, coral reefs, and sea grass terrain; and from pollution. The creatures at the bottom are being killed off by overfishing, pollution, and overgrowth of algae. The water plants are overgrowing because of pollution and this causes the death of fish and bottom feeders. Oysters and menhaden and other sea life that work as natural water filters are being overfished, are dying because of pollution, and are suffocating because of radical algae blooms. In other words, every form of sea life is suffering.

Some may argue that the nondesirable sea creatures that are killed by fishing companies are not a total waste as much of the kill ends up being sold to companies that turn it into feed for farm animals and for fish farms (such as those shrimp farms on the rims of the Indian Ocean that have caused vast amounts of damage to the mangrove forests, and helped contribute to the tragedy of the tsunami that devastated that region of the planet in December of 2004). In addition, much of the sea life that is caught that can be fed to humans *also* end up being turned into feed for farm animals and farmed fish.

> "It takes three to five kilograms of other fish, such as herring and anchovy, to make the feed necessary to produce one kilogram of farmed salmon resulting in a loss of edible animal protein worldwide.
> In Canada it is illegal to make animal feed out of proteins otherwise suitable for human consumption. As a result most of the feed for British Columbian (farmed) salmon is obtained from South America. This reduces the amount of food energy available to people there."
> — FarmedAndDangerous.Org; 2006

Today's massive fishing operations are devastating to the ecosystems of the oceans, seas, lakes, and rivers.

Who owns some of the largest fishing companies? Some of the largest animal farming companies, such as Tyson Foods, the Arkansas company that produces millions of chickens every year. Tyson Foods is truly one of the most environmentally destructive companies.

Many types of sea life are not killed for their meat. Oysters are killed for pearls. Many sea animals are killed for their pretty shells.

Some types of coral are killed for use in calcium supplements and use in bone surgery. Many types of coral are killed to supply pet stores with aquarium supplies.

Many sharks are killed for their fins, which are used in Chinese medicine, and in shark fin soup. Whale sharks, which are considered to be harmless to humans, are being killed off for their fins. Hammerhead and great white shark populations have been reduced by about three-fourths in the past two decades. The Caribbean is basically empty of silky white-tip sharks. Very often the sharks are hauled onto fishing boats, their fins are sliced off, and the sharks are thrown back into the ocean where they struggle to swim until they die.

In addition to the fishing industry that kills untold millions of wild fish, there is another threat to sea life.

No story about the health of the oceans would be complete without mentioning the growing threat of fish farms.

> "Shrimp farms are the primary cause of the destruction of the world's mangrove forests."
> — A Voice for Animals, VoiceForAnimals.Org; 2005

> "Imagine the raw sewage that half a million people would create in one day. It is probably too much to imagine. Now imagine if it were pumped directly into the ocean without having been treated. There are presently over 85 open net cage fish farms currently operating in the coastal waters of British Columbia producing waste that is equivalent in volume to the raw sewage released from a city of 500,000 inhabitants."
> — FarmedAndDangerous.Org; 2006

> "Though funded with public money, the process of developing open-ocean aquaculture has been conducted with an astonishingly arrogant degree of secrecy."
> — Ben Belton, *The Ecologist* magazine, July-August 2004

Farmed fishing is a new, quickly growing, and serious problem for the seas. It destroys coastal mangrove forests, water ecosystems, wild fish populations, and results in the deaths of many thousands of sea mammal and waterfowl. Farmed fish colonies create enormous amounts of pollution. Not only from the fish waste, but from the chemicals used in the fish farming industry. The water is treated with herbicides to prevent water plant growth. Even the nets used to surround the fish farms are damaging to the environment as the nets are often treated with toxic chemicals to prevent the growth of sea organisms, such as barnacles and mussels, which encrust the nets. The pellets fed to farmed salmon contain dyes to make the flesh of the salmon take on the color that wild salmon get from eating their natural food, krill.

Issues of concern for fish farming:

- Pollution from the fish farms altering nearby waterlife, and killing it.

- Chemicals used to treat the fish farms damaging surrounding waterlife.

- The governments selling off parts of their Exclusive Economic Zones (EEZs) in the oceans to companies and private investors and allowing the "ocean ranches" the right to commercially exploit the water, waterlife, and minerals within those zones. This is especially common among poorer countries.

- Disease developing in the fish farms, and spreading to nearby wild fish populations.

- Genetically modified fish in fish farms escaping into the wild and contaminating wild fish.

- Fish farmers killing sea mammals and marine birds that show up to feed from the farmed fish.

Farmed fish are more likely to carry increased levels of toxic chemicals and heavy metals that are known to cause such conditions as birth defects, miscarriages, immune disorders, learning disabilities, and various types of cancer.

> "The groundbreaking study, 'A Global Assessment of Organic Contaminants in Farmed vs. Wild Salmon: Geographical Differences and Health Risks,' was released January 2004 in the respected journal *Science*. The study, which is being considered the most thorough analysis of farmed and wild salmon to date, found in most cases that consuming more than one serving of farmed salmon per month could pose unacceptable cancer risks, according to U.S. Environmental Protection Agency (EPA) standards for determining safe fish consumption levels. Farmed salmon were found to have up to ten times higher levels of PCBs and dioxins than wild salmon."
> — FarmedAndDangerous.Org; 2005

The meat of the farmed fish is less healthful than fish that is wild. Farmed fish meat is higher in saturated fat, which is one reason it is also higher in toxic chemicals as environmental pollutants gather in fat cells. The antibiotics that are given to the farmed fish contribute to human health problems, especially through the increased likelihood of drug-resistant bacteria.

Farmed fish are more likely to become diseased through bacteria, through sea lice and other parasites, and through viruses, such as the highly contagious virus, infectious haematopeoietic necrosis, that contaminates salmon farms. This creates a serious risk factor for the wild fish that swim or feed near the fish farms.

It has become increasingly common for fish farms to be growing types of fish that are not native to the region of the farms. When these non-native fish escape into the wild, they compete with native fish, and in some cases kill or otherwise damage the populations of wild fish, as well as surrounding ecosystems.

Fish farmers also kill predator sea life, such as seals and sea lions, to stop them from eating the farmed fish. Fish farmers along the coast of British Columbia have reportedly killed hundreds of thousands of seals and sea lions in the past decade. The farmers are also known to use underwater noisemakers to deter whales and other marine mammals from entering into the surrounding waters. This interrupts the migration patterns of the sea mammals.

Some fish farmers use bright lights to keep the fish eating all night so they become fatter faster. This confuses wild fish, and contributes to the damage of the surrounding ecosystem.

The entire fishing industry has wreaked havoc on populations of all sea life – from the lobsters, shrimp, and shellfish to sea birds and sea mammals, such as dolphin, porpoise, and whales. The populations of most types of creatures of the sea have been decimated, and some have become regionally extinct as the direct result of the fishing industry.

Across the board you can look at all types of water creatures that humans consume and see that not only are every one of them "overfished," but also their populations are continuing to decline. Not only are populations of sardines, mackerel, and herring being fished to regional extinction, all forms of sea life have been reduced, and many have become extinct in the past 100 years. Others are endangered, or are on the edge of becoming extinct, such as beluga sturgeon, which are killed for their eggs, which are sold as caviar.

"We thought the ocean was an inexhaustible source of food, and that it would always regenerate more creatures to replace those we remove. But today's ocean is failing to produce fish as it did in the past, and the reason increasingly appears to be an overall decline in marine nutrient

cycling. Simple starvation now increasingly limits the growth of fish and other marine life. 'Overfishing' appears to have affected not only the targeted species, but also the ecosystem in general... and ramifications of this disturbance may extend as far as the ocean-atmosphere CO2 balance."
— **The Starving Ocean, FisheryCrisis.Com; 2005**

When waterlife is damaged, all life is damaged. John Robbins explains this very well in his book *The Food Revolution*. Fish of all size play a critical role in the existence of all other sea life. When one type of fish is overfished, or becomes extinct, it disrupts the entire ecosystem. This includes both saltwater and freshwater fish. And it impacts not only life within the water, but also the lives and population of birds, animals, and insects. It also affects the plants and trees in the forests; this is because as the animals that feed on waterlife defecate, they nourish the plants, and when the animals die, their bodies further feed the plant life. Marine carbon and nitrogen isotopes are two beneficial atomic nutrients brought into the forests by animals and birds eating fish.

A global study authored by 14 marine biologists that was published in the November 3, 2006, issue of the journal *Science* concluded that unless humanity makes enormous changes in the way they live and in what they eat, the entire populations of the world's fished species will collapse by about 2048. The study considered evidence from all of the world's 64 large marine ecosystems. They found that 91 percent of native species suffered from a 50 percent decrease, and 7 percent were extinct. Continued overfishing as well as coastal land development, habitat destruction, and world pollution are to blame. The study pointed out that nearly 29 percent of species that are fished have collapsed (defined by being below 10 percent of historic highs). The study said that the fish populations were rapidly decreasing and losing entire functional groups. The study says that the oceans will not be able to recover from the decline of so many species. The study authors wrote, "Our analyses suggest that business as usual would foreshadow serious threats to global food security, coastal water quality, and ecosystem stability, affecting current and future generations." Many scientists throughout the world voiced their opinions in agreement with the study.

"There's no question if we close our eyes and pretend it's all OK, it will continue along the same trajectory. Eventually, we're going to run out of species."

— Dalhousie University marine biologist Boris Worm, leader of the global research team that authored the study titled Impacts of Biodiversity Loss on Ocean Ecosystem Services, November 2006

There are efforts being made to make seafood eaters more aware of where and how their meal was caught. The Marine Stewardship Council works to certify some types of seafood as sustainable by allowing packaging to feature a blue and white certification label. The MSC also encourages people to avoid eating large fish, and instead to eat low on the food chain by eating oysters, scallops, crabs, and squid, which reproduce more quickly than large fish. However, when it is taken into consideration that the smaller forms of sea life play a part in the health of the seas, it should be clear to see why these forms of waterlife need to be protected from harm.

People do not need to eat seafood. Fish should not be taken from the waters of the world to make pet food, and especially not for food to feed massively overbred farm animals, which also is so unnecessary and damaging to the planet. The creatures of the seas should be left alone and protected from harm.

Animals and Humans

When I was ten, walking alone on my way home from school one early spring day, I stepped on the last bits of ice that were undermined by water running in the street gutter. As I stepped on these little shelves of ice they collapsed into the thin stream of water. Those that wouldn't easily break got stomped on. As they collapsed, they splashed water onto me – which was part of the fun of it.

As I walked along I noticed that the water was turning pink. Looking ahead I saw a thin stream of red that had slowed alongside the street gutter. I wondered why someone had spilled a bunch of red paint. With my eyes I followed the streak of red and saw that it was running in a very thin line down the middle of a driveway of a neighbor's house. Walking up to the driveway, I stopped. My breath left me.

The only time I had seen large animals was at the zoo and on my relatives' dairy farm. But I had never seen a deer up close.

That day I did.

My absent neighbors had returned from a hunting trip. Maybe they were inside taking showers.

I stood alone trying to understand what my eyes were seeing.

Hanging by its hind legs from the backyard tree next to the driveway was a large deer. Its limp body had given up the ghost. Someone had slit through its neck so deeply that its head looked to be hanging from a bit of flesh. Its face on the nearly decapitated head looked to be painted red. Its snout dripped with blood into a puddle on the lawn.

With my eyes, I followed the blood from the puddle, down the driveway, past my feet, and into the street gutter, where it turned the water from the melting ice a bloody pink.

I walked away with a memory I knew I would never forget.

Where I grew up there were wild berry bushes and cherry and other fruit trees. I often saw birds eating the berries and cherries, and they seemed to do so with great pleasure. When you see animals enjoying themselves by doing such things as feasting on wild berries, or playing with their young, you realize that they are beings that feel pleasure, establish relationships, and care for each other. Observing these behaviors displayed in wild animals has helped to make me want to protect them from harm.

Animals are not simple stimulus response mechanisms. It has been proved that the brains of animals release hormones in relation to the thoughts they are displaying; this is similar to how human brains function.

Ethologists are scientists who study animal behavior. Throughout the years those working in this field have conducted numerous studies concluding that animals have memories, show affection, romance their lovers, establish community standards, and role play among themselves; are aware of their behavior as compared to others; experience moods and express emotions of eagerness, jealousy, excitement, compassion, distress, guilt, sadness, depression, and joy; mourn for their dead; have preferences; understand reasoning; are able to remember where they buried things; can experience post-traumatic stress; show favoritism, socialize, teach their young, form intention, practice intimidation tactics, anticipate needs, are cautious, display an understanding of cause and effect, gather observations and make conclusions from them, are able to do simple math; cooperate with the agreements of others; communicate desires; plan strategies, and sometimes hide things from others. They not only form friendships, but their health deteriorates if they do not experience physical and mental stimulation.

From ants that cultivate fungus farms, to animals that protect and care for the young of other species, and to dolphin that guard humans from sharks, to New Caledonian crows that fashion hooks to forage for bugs, to bee birds in Africa that know how to lead badgers and humans to beehives, wildlife is made up of active thinkers who display individual personalities and various levels of understanding, and clearly show that they each have a consciousness.

Koko, a gorilla living at the Gorilla Foundation in Northern California, has learned sign language to the point of recognizing over 1,000 signs, as well as thousands of English words. She displays an IQ that may be higher than a certain U.S. president.

Animals deserve to live freely on this planet we share. Free from animal farming and free from being experimented on in laboratories. Their habitat needs to be protected, and large parts of it need to be restored so they can survive and prosper.

Witnessing the damage humans have done to wildlife sickens me. Vast areas of Earth and wildlife have been violated by humans in the pursuit of making money, conducting warfare, and simply selfishly disrespecting the treasures of Earth and Nature. All throughout the world humans have violated the wild animal kingdom. Within human society many more billions of animals are violated by animal farming, by the exotic animal trade, and in scientific experimentation. All of these activities create bad energy and damage all forms of life on Earth.

"The factory-farming techniques of present-day civilization have created a frightening karmic debt and health danger for anyone consuming animals. Factory-farmed animals are injected with, sprayed with, and fed antibiotics, artificial hormones, and toxic chemicals of many kinds. These toxins are present in the flesh when the animals are slaughtered, and pass directly into the body of the people who eat the meat. Factory-farmed animals are kept in darkness, and squeezed together in inhospitable cages. They are fed the most outrageous and unnatural diet imaginable."
— David Wolfe

"Suffering is suffering, whether experienced by animals or humans. The physiological process is identical."
— Professor Mirko Bagaric, Head of Deakin Law School

The way farm animals are treated, the drugs they are given, the unnatural foods they are fed, the toxic chemicals they are treated with, and the conditions they live in make them stressed, depressed, confused, angry, frightened, and diseased. It is no wonder why the rates of degenerative diseases are so high in countries where the most amount of meat is consumed. People who are eating meat are eating stress, confinement, depression, frustration, confusion, repression, anger, fright, poison, and disease.

> "When a person eats the flesh of tortured animals, or the milk of dairy cows, or eggs from factory chickens, one also ingests the fear, pain, exhaustion, and sorrow of those innocent beings. These energies manifest within the consumer in the form of negative attitudes and illness."
> — David Wolfe

By consuming a diet that consists of plants in the form of a vegan diet, a human can release the energies and illness they have absorbed into their system through their previous consumption of meat, eggs, and dairy products. The longer people consume a diet that is free of meat, eggs, and dairy, the more they will improve not only their own life, but those of the people and animals around them. As their body absorbs a higher quality of nutrients it spins a new fabric of molecules and they resonate with a new level of energy that is attuned to and that will attract vibrant health.

> "Just as you cannot make others happy while being unhappy, one cannot heal while inflicting hurt. Hurting animals to try and find a way to heal only inflicts pain, and never heals anything. This exposes the fraud of animal experimentation (vivisection)."
> — David Wolfe

The book, *Old MacDonald's Factory Farm*, by C. David Coats contains a preface about the absurdity of man. It tells of how it is an odd world where humans inflict so much pain on animals; then kill and eat the animals, which makes humans ill, then, in an attempt to "cure" themselves of the diseases formed by eating the animals, they turn to toxic chemical drugs produced by the pharmaceutical industry, which spends hundreds of millions of dollars developing the drugs and testing them on tortured animals in outrageous laboratory experiments. Many of the drugs people take also contain ingredients that are derived from animals killed in slaughterhouses. (See *Naked Empress*, by Hans Ruesch; PETA.Org; and the books *Mad Cowboy* and *No More Bull*, by

Howard Lyman, MadCowboy.Com.)

> "Once we know that we thrive on a raw vegan or raw vegetarian diet,
> then there no longer remains any reason to exploit animals."
> — **David Wolfe**

Not only does following a raw vegan diet protect animals from exploitation, it also protects wildlife, wildlands, the oceans, lakes and rivers, and Earth. This is because a raw vegan diet has a much lower impact on Earth than that of the standard American diet (SAD) that consists of meat, dairy, eggs, and highly-polluting junk food. It starts with the fact that most food grown on the planet is being fed to farm animals. This may come as a surprise to those who thought that there is a food shortage on the planet. As I stated earlier, humans could not possibly consume all of the food that is growing on Earth. There is more than enough food to feed every human on the planet. The largest part of the problem is that most food grown on the planet is used to feed farm animals so that the rich countries can have their meat and dairy products.

When we refuse to eat animals, dairy products, and junk food, and instead subsist on a plant-based diet, we are agreeing to live in tune with Nature. We are not participating in the animal-killing industries of factory farms and slaughterhouses. We are not part of the farming industry that grows more than 60 percent of its products to feed to animals on meat farms. We are not a part of the fishing industry that kills millions of fish and hundreds of thousands of sea mammals and birds every year. We are not part of the ranching industry that kills many millions of wolves, bear, lions, raccoons, predator birds, and other wild animals every year. We are not part of an industry that is cutting down the rainforests to provide cattle-grazing land. When we follow a vegan diet we are protecting wildlife, wildlands, forests, the oceans, lakes and rivers, and Earth.

Nature and animals can teach us things simply by being part of our existence.

> "There are some barbarians who will take this dog, that so greatly
> excels man in capacity for friendship, who will nail him to a table, and
> dissect him alive. And what you discover in him are the same organs of
> sensation you have in yourself."
> — **Voltaire, Philosophical Dictionary**

Centuries of writing from all areas of the planet, among the people who didn't know that others existed, and who had no way of communicating with people on other continents, have recorded events where humans have communicated with animals. Native people from various continents even include their communicative thoughts with animals and Nature as part of their spiritual practices. An example is that of the Native Americans who include in their prayers an acknowledgment of a spiritual connection to animals such as deer, bears, wolves, serpents, fish, and birds. Writers of novels and songs often include references of communicating with animals and Nature in their works.

Animals are tuned into an energy that humans ignore, don't seem to consider, think of as impossible, or don't believe they can tune into. Where hope falters, possibilities fail.

Migratory birds often fly away at the same time of year, returning to the same spots year after year. Fish, such as salmon, do the same thing. Whales, sea turtles, and even butterflies do the same. Animals seem to know where they are and where they are going. Dogs and cats removed from their owners often find their owners, even when the owners move to new homes miles away. Farm animals have escaped from their confinement only to be found later at distant farms where their babies had been sold off.

A magnetic field that wraps the earth, the alignment of the stars, the angle of Sun and the moon, the smells of different regions of Earth, polarized ultraviolet light patterns, and other factors may play a part in migration. But there are also factors that guide living things that seem to be tuned into a resonance or energy – an invisible power.

Is this energy field, or a connection to instinct and Nature, something humans are missing out on by eating such unhealthful foods and living in a way that is disconnected from Nature? I believe so.

> "Would Nature have placed our very means of survival – food – in mobile animals, another mammal's skin, and under a hen, or in 260,000 varieties of plants spread over Earth?"
> — **Rex Bowlby, author of *Plant Roots: 101 reasons why the human diet is rooted exclusively in plants***

Eating Meat and Junk Food

> "The beef industry has contributed to more deaths than all the wars of this century, all natural disasters, and all automobile accidents com-

bined. If beef is your idea of 'real food for real people,' you'd better live real close to a real good hospital."
    — **Neal Barnard, M.D., President, Physicians Committee for Responsible Medicine, PCRM.Org**

Those who say that we need meat to survive, and that the human body is meant to eat meat, often point out that even chimpanzees are known to occasionally kill and eat other animals. But this is a faulty argument because the chimps rarely eat meat, and basically subsist on a raw vegan diet. The fact that apes and ape-like creatures, including the gorillas, eat a raw vegan diet invalidates the opinion of those humans who say you need to eat meat to become strong. As David Wolfe points out in his book, gorillas are known to even remove insects from vegetation before eating.

"I never saw gorillas eat animal matter in the wild – no birds, eggs, insects, mice, or other creatures – even though they had the opportunity to do so on occasion. Once a group passed over a dead duiker without handling the fresh remains, and another time a group nested beneath an olive pigeon nest without disturbing a single egg."
    — **Dr. George Schaller, *The Year of the Gorilla***

When you observe all of the varieties of life, you notice that each has its own specific way of obtaining what it needs. These activities that provide for sustenance come naturally. Bees get what they need from blossoms. Bears get fish from the rivers. Birds eat seeds and fruit, some eat worms, and others (such as vultures) eat dead animals. Various wild animals hunt and kill their food. Many animals eat leaves and fruit. Some dig for and eat roots.

To me seeing humans eating meat appears as unnatural as it would appear for chickens to hunt and kill bears, or for fish to climb trees and eat bird eggs. Sometimes when I pass fancy restaurants it seems absurd to see the so-called high society fashionable people using their fancy forks and knives to cut through platters of expensive meals that consist of some sort of bits of slaughtered and cooked animal.

"At its inception, each new genus form is associated with a definitive energy and a specific physiological design. Its functioning environment, physical form, social life, physical life (i.e., how to spin a web), and food/fuel choice are pre-determined within a narrow variable range. These are not subject to change and do not (actually cannot) adapt

beyond a certain threshold."
— **David Wolfe**

Among meat products sold in markets, processed meat is the worst. According to a study by the University of Hawaii, people who consume processed meats containing sodium nitrite greatly increase their risk of pancreatic cancer, leukemia, and brain tumors. Sodium nitrite was nearly banned in the U.S. in the 1970s, but the meat industry prevented the USDA from doing so because the meat industry relies on the chemical to give meat a more appealing color.

The diseases of societies that eat unnatural diets are evidence that it is not good for the body to subsist on anything but real whole foods provided by Nature. The elements in Earth, water, and sunshine are transformed by plants into a wide variety of fruits and vegetables that consist of all of the nutrients a person needs, and this is what humans should be eating. Humans should not be eating things consisting of toxic chemical dyes, preservatives, flavorings, scents, and other food chemicals, or things that have been grown using toxic chemical growth hormones, pesticides, herbicides, fungicides, insecticides, and so forth.

It is when we drift from what Nature provides that we risk damaging the delicate balance of life that exists throughout the plants, animals and world around us, and within ourselves.

Your body is a living mechanism. Eating foods that have had their life force killed through the process of cooking only deadens the body. There may be nutrients derived from low-quality food; but there is also a lot of other stuff in cooked and processed foods that clog the system, and this stays in the body in the forms of plaque and residues that detract from all areas of health, and weave a fabric of disease and lameness into the tissues.

One of the ways the human body tries to cope with all of the unnatural forms of food being put into it can be found in the way the body produces stronger digestive juices to try to digest the unhealthful concoctions of junk food people eat. But these stronger digestive juices — enzymatic mutations — take more energy and nutrients for the body to produce than those that are produced by the body when a healthful diet is eaten. The mutations also work against the system in the long term, leading to a damaged digestive tract, and a system out of balance.

As humans have changed their diets from that which is natural to that of modern day junk food, the human body has not changed. The lips, teeth, throat, stomach and the rest of the digestive structures have not changed. There has been no "evolution" in the way the human body grows. It is the same as it has been throughout human existence.

All forms of cooked food, and foods that contain animal protein (meat, milk, and eggs) require the body to produce stronger enzymes than those which would normally exist in the body of someone who follows a more healthful vegan diet. While the enzymes produced to digest animal protein in its various forms exist in those who eat such things, the enzymes needed to digest plant foods exist in everyone, and are natural.

Simply because the body can work to digest unnatural and unhealthful food does not mean that garbage is the natural diet of the human. You can shove any number of crazy concoctions down your throat and your body can work it through your digestive tract, but this does not mean you are eating that which is natural or good for you. It does not mean that you have progressed to that sort of diet in an evolutionary manner. It simply means that the body has the capability of tolerating certain combinations of foods and nonfoods. But the longer the body is fed unhealthful food the more that fact is evident in the existence of obesity, organ diseases, a weakened immune system, premature aging, and mental and physical lethargy.

There are those who promote a raw food diet that includes raw eggs, raw meat, and raw milk. Some refer to this type of diet of raw meat as "instinctive eating," which is a philosophy of the man Wolfe refers to as the "staunch evolutionist Frenchman, Guy Claude-Burger." This type of eating is possibly more unhealthful than eating cooked animal protein. This is because of the parasites, bacteria, and other elements of raw animal protein, and especially in raw meat products. Meat also includes the saturated fat, cholesterol, uric acids, hormones, and environmental pollutants that are so damaging to human health.

For these reasons the raw meat diet is what we refer to as the DUM diet (dead uncooked meat diet).

Some people claim that they need to eat meat to get protein. This is nonsense. The human body creates protein from amino acids. There are plenty of utilizable amino acids in edible plants. This topic is covered very well in John Robbins's book, *The Food Revolution*. I encourage everyone who desires to understand the relationship between humans and their food choices to read that enlightening book.

Some people say that they need to eat animal protein to build their muscles and maintain their strength. Would they consider horses to be muscular and strong? How about gorillas, giraffes, kangaroos, elephants, deer, and other large wild animals? Those animals maintain strong, muscular bodies by eating nothing but plant matter. They are all vegetarians. In fact, because they don't eat eggs or dairy products, and don't cook their food, they can be considered to be raw vegans. And their muscles are amazingly strong and defined.

Meat (from any of the creatures of the air, land, and water) does not fit into the classification of healthful food. But a diet that includes meat does resonate with the energies of environmental destruction, selfishness, greed, abuse, suppression, confinement, anger, violence, death, and murder.

> "As bees sip nectar from many flowers and make a hive of honey, so that not one drop can claim, 'I am from this flower or that,' all creatures, though one, do not realize that they are one."
> — Upanishads

Milk and Growth Hormones

A farming drug that has been the target of much concern is the milk-production stimulant known as recombinant bovine growth hormone (rBGH, also called bovine somatotropin, or BST). The drug is injected into cows to increase their production of milk by inducing a marked and sustained increase in levels of insulin-like growth factor-1 (IGF-1). It is IGF-1 that stimulates milk production. While cows not treated with the stimulant may produce a couple of gallons of milk at each milking, a cow given the drug may produce five gallons of milk at each milking.

Organic Pastures Dairy in California's San Joaquin Valley does not treat their dairy cows with milk stimulants or the typical antibiotics used on factory farms. The farm also allows its cows to graze in an open field, and feeds the cows alfalfa instead of grain. The dairy has found that its cows live an average of eight years. Cows treated with BST and antibiotics may live less than three years, and are likely to have lived a life of stress from intensive milk production induced by drugs while eating an unnatural diet of grain, which increases the acidity of the intestinal tract and allows for the growth of E. coli O157:H7.

IGF-1 is normally found in both humans and cows and plays a part in cell division. The rBGH-treated cows produce milk that has a higher than normal amount of IGF-1. The controversy in the use of rBGH is that it is likely that an unnatural amount of IGF-1 in the diet will promote tumors by causing cells to divide at an abnormally fast rate. Many people believe that high levels of IGF-1 may transform normal breast tissue to breast cancer and stimulates and maintains malignancy of cancer cells, including their ability to spread to distant organs in an aggressive manner.

The chemical drug company Monsanto, the producer of such chemicals as PCBs and Agent Orange with its toxic dioxin components, began marketing rBGH in February of 1994 after reportedly spending hundreds of millions of dollars to develop the drug. Many countries have banned the use of rBGH. But not the U.S., Mexico, or Brazil.

The U.S. Food and Drug Administration has said they have found no unusual problems with cows that have been injected with the bovine growth hormone. The FDA has also said that they believe there are no risks involved with the ingestion of the milk from cows that have been treated with the hormone.

Oh, really?

Perhaps the FDA spends too much time listening to the financial concerns of the dairy industry. Perhaps the people who work for the FDA also are financially connected to the dairy industry, and to the company that produces the hormones. Perhaps the FDA is also looking out for how much money is made by exporting American dairy and beef. Perhaps the FDA is ignoring many scientific studies regarding growth hormones. Perhaps the FDA simply and blatantly lies to the American consumers to appease the dairy industry.

One manufacturer's list details 21 side effects that cows may experience from rBGH treatments. Cows that have been treated with the hormone have a higher incidence of painful udder infections, and this results in pus-contaminated milk. The antibiotics used to treat these infections also end up in the milk products that are sold for human consumption.

In a letter written to the FDA, Dr. Samuel Epstein, a professor of occupational and environmental medicine at the School of Public Health at the University of Illinois, warned that the effects of IGF-1 could include premature growth stimulation in infants, breast enlargement in young children, and breast cancer in adult females. He says that IGF-1 survives digestion, stimulates cell growth of the intestinal wall, and may promote colon polyps and other abnormal growths. He also believes that the hormone makes its way to other areas of the body by being absorbed into the bloodstream and may then promote or stimulate abnormal cell growth, resulting in tumors.

In an article written for the *Los Angeles Times*, Epstein noted that the Council on Scientific Affairs of the American Medical Association stated, "Further studies will be required to determine whether the ingestion of higher than normal concentrations of bovine insulin-like growth factor is safe for children, adolescents, and adults."

On December 14, 1994, the unresolved human health issues related to rBGH caused the European Council of Ministers to impose a ban through the year 2000 on the commercial use of the drug (Citizens for Health Report, Volume 3:1, 1995). Because of the hormones in U.S. cattle, in 1988 the European Union placed a ban on importing beef from the U.S. In January 1996, U.S. Trade Representative Mickey Kantor, working in the interests of the cattle industry, conducted talks to try and reverse the 14-nation EU ban, but talks failed to resolve the matter. The EU has claimed that rBGH makes the beef unsafe for human consumption. The ban prevents the export of from $100 million to $200 million in beef products to Europe (1996 figures). Under World Trade Organization rules, countries are supposed to justify trade policy restrictions by using scientific evidence. The U.S. trade representatives claimed that there is no strong scientific evidence to support the EU ban on hormone-treated beef. The EU did not budge.

Meanwhile, in the U.S., dairy farms keep using hormones on dairy cattle and keep putting forth the message that we should be drinking lots of milk. The dairy industry works for dairy farmers by promoting the products of the dairy farmers. Could their advertising and PR campaigns be biased to the point of being not exactly the truth?

The dairy industry often bases its claim that milk is good on the fact that dairy products have a lot of calcium. So drink lots of milk and you will get lots of calcium – and the dairy industry will make lots of money. But your blood will keep pulling calcium out of the bones to neutralize the acidic level of the blood that is put off balance by the acid forming dairy products. The more animal protein you take in, the more calcium that is excreted by your kidneys and the more likely you are to have kidney stones.

The blood uses the calcium that is stored in the bones as a bank. When you eat things that raise the acid level of the blood – such as meat, fish, and eggs – the blood pulls calcium out of the bones to balance the pH level of the blood. Most fruits and vegetables have an alkaline ash, and do not make the blood take calcium out of the bones. The calcium in fruits and vegetables is more available to the body because of the calcium/phosphorous ratio found in fruits and vegetables.

A study by researchers at Washington University School of Medicine in St. Louis found that raw vegans have surprisingly robust bones. How could this be when vegans don't do what the dairy industry wants by drinking lots of milk? Raw vegans have strong bones and they have a plentiful amount of vitamin D. The raw vegans in the study even had "markedly higher" vitamin D levels than those who follow an average diet. The raw vegans also had low levels of C-reactive protein, an inflammatory molecule linked with susceptibility to heart disease, diabetes, and other chronic degenerative diseases. They also were found to have lower levels of IGF-1, which is a growth factor associated with the risk of cancers of the prostate and breasts. Those were the finding of the study that was published in the March 25, 2006 issue of the *Archives of Internal Medicine*. The study also found that raw vegans have an average body mass index of 20.5, which is clearly in the range of a healthy BMI, which is considered to be 18.5 to 24 (BMI is a measurement of height to weight).

If a person stays a vegetarian, and stays away from milk, eggs, and cheese, they lower their chances of experiencing osteoporosis. Vegetarians have stronger bones and when their bones break they heal faster than the bones of people who eat animals and dairy products

Meat, dairy, and eggs contain cholesterol. Other than non-fat milk, all of these products also have saturated fat. Some people say that you need cholesterol in your diet. You don't need cholesterol in your diet and this is because every cell in the human body makes the cholesterol that you need. No one ever died of a cholesterol deficiency, only of cholesterol overload — heart attacks and strokes. Gallstones are made up largely of cholesterol. Plants do not contain cholesterol. Vegetarians have lower rates of gall stone problems.

The less fiber you have in your diet, the better your chances are of getting colon cancer. Dead animals, dairy products, and eggs do not have any fiber in them — at all. Fruits, vegetables, grains, and legumes have lots of fiber. All countries that consume the most dead animals, dairy products, and eggs also have the highest rates of colon cancer.

Dairy is not a good source of iron. You would have to drink 50 gallons of cow milk to get the iron available in a single bowl of spinach.

You need vitamin C to be able to use iron. Fruits and vegetables contain vitamin C. Vegetables such as broccoli, peas, cucumbers, tomatoes, spinach, and some others are good sources of iron.

Like human milk that is specific to the needs of human babies, cow milk is specific to the needs of baby cows.

Got Sunfood cuisine?

Chemicals and Drugs in Milk, Meat, and Eggs

Most farm animals are given drugs by mouth or injection from their first day to nearly their last. These drugs may include hormones, antibiotics, milk stimulants, tranquilizers, and chemicals that influence the birth rates. The animals are also sprayed with toxic insecticides, fungicides, and pesticides.

The insecticides that are used on and around the animals not only kill flies but also kill needed insects such as bees that pollinate plants; preying mantises and ladybugs that help control damaging insects; and other helpful bugs and insects. The chemicals also poison the air, water, and land.

The drugs farm animals are given along with the pesticides and insecticides used on and around them as well as the chemicals used to grow their feed accumulate in the fat cells of the animals and these residues are transferred into the humans who consume the meats, milk products, and eggs.

The fats in farm animals contain residues of all the chemicals used to grow their food. Because the feed given to animals raised in factory farms often contains portions of ground-up farm animals that died prematurely, the amount of drug and chemical residue found in meats from these animals contains a larger dose of the residues.

As if giving the naturally vegetarian animals a cannibalistic diet were not bad enough, some farm animals are also fed their own excrement. Some pigs are fed their own urine. Poultry waste and feathers are mixed in with feed that is fed to other farm animals. Other farm animal feed contains the leftovers of slaughterhouses, road kill, and the bodies of animals from county and city animal control shelters. Not only does this magnify the amount of chemical and drug residues in the fat of the animals, it also increases the likelihood that the animals are harboring infectious diseases. The farm animals that die are not tested for diseases. Using ground-up animals to increase the protein content of animal feed increases the likelihood that contagious diseases, such as mad cow disease, are becoming rampant within farm animals.

Leonardo da Vinci considered the bodies of humans who eat animals to be the tombs of the animals. A modern-day Leonardo might consider the bodies of humans who consume farm animals, eggs, and dairy to be toxic waste dumps of all the farming chemicals and drugs found in the animals.

Cooked Food

Nobody knows where or when the first cooked meal was made. On every continent there is evidence that ancient humans used fire to cook food, including meals consisting of both plant matter and animal flesh. But like the belief that Sun revolves around Earth, or that air causes infections in wounds, the idea that cooked plant substances are better for you should go the way of the other two beliefs.

The way Nature provides food is already in its best form. You can't improve fruits, vegetables, herbs, berries, nuts, seeds, flowers, or sea vegetables by cooking them.

Heating plant substances alters their molecular structures, placing them outside of the way Nature formed them. When you consume those altered molecules, they become part of your body tissues. In this way eating cooked food changes your body in the most basic way. This sets the stage for other unnatural things to take place within your body, such as disease and illness of all sorts.

You are what you eat. Either you can be eating living, vibrant foods as Nature grows them, or you can be eating cooked food that has been degraded by heat.

Cooked foods are no longer alive. Cooking kills their enzymes, eliminates their life energy, and damages nutrients. Cooked food is dead. Just as a cooked seed will not sprout into a plant, a cooked food diet will not provide for vibrant health. Eating deadened food deadens your life force, your spirituality, and your thought processes.

Cooking foods at high temperatures creates chemicals that do not naturally exist in plants. The substances also have no place in the human body. When you are eating cooked food you are eating elements that your body would not naturally have to deal with. They are foreign, useless, and damaging.

Eating cooked food triggers an immune response in the body called leukocytosis. When someone eats food cooked at high temperatures, the body responds as if it is being invaded, and there is an increase in the white blood cells. This confuses the immune system, is wearing on the system, and results in fatigue.

Eating a diet of cooked and processed foods leaves residues in the tissues that inflame and damage the tissues, decrease vitality, cause mood swings and grogginess, clog the system, and make each cell work harder to maintain health. Ultimately this leads to a body that is overweight, discolored, filled with residues the body has trouble getting rid of, and that is not functioning at the level it would be if the person would simply eat a diet consisting of a variety of vibrant, living foods.

When you consider that an addiction is a craving for something that is void of the true needs of the person, and that satisfying the craving takes time and energy, and that the craving is often related to substances that are liable to have damaging effects on the person, then cooked food is addictive in every sense of the word. Cooked food causes a chemical change within the body. The consumption of cooked food leads to a physio-chemical pattern that alters the body and limits the ability of the body and mind to function at their best level, leading to diseased organs and to traumatic health events like heart attacks, strokes, organ failure, and cancers.

Pollution from Cooked Food Diets

Governments around the planet constantly spend tremendous amounts of money to manage the trash their citizens produce from eating processed foods. Typical packaged foods cause more solid pollution by bulk than any other product. At least one-fourth of the plastic used in the U.S. is used for toss-away packaging, and much of this is used for packaged food. Most of this packaging is from foods that are cooked or otherwise processed, and especially those that contain animal products, such as meat, eggs, and milk. These forms of pollution are spreading around the world as more countries adopt the "American way" of food processing, marketing, and consumption.

The U.S. has only about 5 percent of the world's population, but uses an estimated 30 percent of the world's resources, emits over 28 percent of the world's greenhouse gasses, and consumes 20 percent of the world's beef. Taking that into account, it is clear to see why it is important to change our ways.

Besides requiring the use of millions of ovens the world over, which use enormous amounts of fuel, cooked food is wasteful in another way.

Cooking food destroys or damages many nutrients in the food. If a large amount of the nutrients are destroyed, then so is a large amount of the time, energy, and resources used to grow and handle the food before it is cooked (see *Survival into the 21st Century*, by Viktoras Kulvinskas).

The cooking of food causes a lot of damage to the forested areas of the planets. Some areas of the world (where there are few trees) are that way because people have cut down the trees to cook food. Much of Haiti has been deforested not because the trees were used for building houses, but because people used the trees to create fire for cooking. This sort of thing continues to happen on all of the continents and islands of the world, especially in areas that are not using electricity or gas to cook food.

According to a study conducted by a team of researchers from around the world and that was published in the March 2005 issue of the journal *Science*, the number one source of climate-changing black carbon pollution in the air of south Asia is from cooking fires. In addition to wood, the people of that region also use agricultural waste and animal manure to cook their food. The study concluded that 42 percent of black soot was the result of cooking fires, and 25 percent was the result of burning fossil fuels. The result is that pollution in the air collects the heat of Sun light, warming the atmosphere and altering weather patterns.

In addition to the pollution caused by burning wood to cook food, a tremendous amount of air pollution is caused by people using other types of fuel to cook. From restaurants to delis, schools, prisons, military bases, and hospitals, hotels and homes, enormous amounts of fuel are used to cook food. This is done in the form of natural gas, coal, and in the use of electric stoves and ovens and microwaves. A mile from my home there is a restaurant that is famous for its cheap (and very unhealthful) lunch menu consisting of large hamburgers, barbecued meat, and beef chili. The place is usually packed, and the chimney pumps out so much smoke from its cooking that the surrounding area sometimes smells of hamburgers. If you magnify this one restaurant by millions of restaurants around the world that are spewing cooking fumes into Earth's atmosphere, you begin to get an idea of how much pollution is the result of cooking food.

Food cooking is a major source of air pollution, and in many regions of the planet ovens and stoves cause more pollution than that caused by engines.

In Los Angeles the number-one cause of air pollution is not automobiles, but is the result of cooking food with gas, electricity, barbeque, wood, and microwaves. Not everyone drives a car, but nearly everyone in Southern California eats cooked food.

Cooks working in busy restaurants are more likely to experience asthma attacks. This is because they are exposed to gasses being emitted by the ovens and stoves. Cooking food creates pollution that causes lung damage, global warming, and harms all life forms on Earth.

On the other hand, eating a diet that consists of eating raw plants saves all of the resources used to cook food.

The Sunfood diet results in less pollution and trash. While you may have been subsisting on an unhealthful diet that consisted of a lot of processed foods that were in all sorts of plastics, boxes, and other type of packaging, on the Sunfood diet you will basically be eating fruits and vegetables, nuts, seeds, and things made of them. These can be grown by you, purchased at a farmers' market, or bought in the bulk or produce sections of your local natural foods market. Thus you will be causing less pollution. If you shop with a cloth bag that you bring to the store every time you shop, you will also eliminate your need for "paper or plastic" bags.

Poisons in Cooked Foods: Glycotoxins and Acrylamides

Cooked food is simply not good for the tissues of the body – from the surface of the teeth to the innermost areas of every cell.

Chemicals (glycotoxins) that form during cooking, and especially in the browning of cooked food, are damaging to the kidneys, ignite inflammation, weaken the immune system, and lead to tissue damage. This is because when cooked food enters the body, it is treated as a foreign substance.

Cooked food is foreign in that the cooking process chemically changes the substances from those that occurred naturally in Nature to those that do not exist in Nature, unless things have been burned. When you put the cooked food substance in the body, which was designed to consume and digest natural substances, an adverse reaction takes place as the body works to recognize it, to create the digestive juices necessary to digest it, and to deal with the cooked food chemicals as they travel through the body.

The toxic glycotoxin compound is formed when sugars, proteins, and fat are exposed to high temperatures. This compound damages blood vessels and results in tissue damage throughout the body. This is one reason why people who eat an unhealthful diet consisting of cooked and fried foods end up looking older than their actual age.

Interestingly, the "proinflammatory" substance (glycotoxin) that is formed in cooked food has been given the name "heat-generated advanced glycation end products." The abbreviation for the name of this substance is "AGEs." So you see, AGEs, which are created in cooked food, damage and *age* the body.

"AGEs attack virtually every part of the body. It is as if we have a low-grade infection. They tend to aggravate the immune cells."
— Dr. Helen Vlassara, of the Division of Endocrinology, Department of Medicine, Mount Sinai School of Medicine, New York; first author of a study on AGEs: Inflammatory mediators are induced by dietary glycotoxins, a major risk factor for diabetic angiopathy, *The Proceedings of the National Academy of Sciences*; November, 12, 2002; PNAS.Org.

The study concluded that AGEs damage body tissues. Switching to a diet that consists of raw plant substances can aid in reversing the damage done by AGEs. In the Mt. Sinai study, those diabetic patients who didn't cook their foods at high temperatures, preventing their foods from browning, experienced a 30 percent decrease in AGEs in their body within two weeks.

Age-related macular degeneration (age-related blindness), which is much more common in countries where meat consumption is high (diets containing large amounts of animal protein), and less common in countries where meat consumption is low (vegetarian-based diets), may also have a connection to the AGEs factor. Earlier studies have established a connection between the occurrence of age-related macular degeneration and those following a diet high in cholesterol and saturated fat.

Furthermore, another substance in cooked foods, acrylamide, which is in all fried and baked starches, is a known carcinogen (cancer-causing agent). There have been studies done on this substance at such institutions as the Food and Drug Administration, Harvard, the Center for Science in the Public Interest, and Sweden's Karolinska Institute. Scientists working for the British, Swiss, and Norwegian governments have confirmed the presence of the substance in foods. And the health ramifications of acrylamide have been discussed at meetings of the World Health Organization.

> "The FDA has been strangely silent about acrylamide. It should be advising consumers to avoid or cut back on the most contaminated and least nutritious foods while more testing is done across the food supply. The FDA also should be intensively investigating ways of preventing the formation of this carcinogen."
> — **Michael F. Jacobson, Center for Science in the Public Interest, 2002**

Acrylamide is found in everything from cooked cereal to coffee, cookies, fries, chips, bread, crackers, rice, taco shells, tofu, and cake. The more that starchy foods are cooked, the more acrylamide forms within them. According to scientists who studied this at the FDA, soft bread has very little acrylamide, but when you toast bread, it greatly increases the substance in the bread.

Acrylamide is formed when an amino acid in foods, asparagine, is heated. But it is unknown what the exact chemical reactions are that lead to the formation of the chemical. It occurs at varying levels in different foods. But some foods that have lower acrylamide levels may be a main source for them in the diet. This is because those foods may be eaten more often than foods that have higher levels.

According to the FDA's Office of Food Additive Safety, the foods containing acrylamide that are most common in American diets include bread, breakfast cereals, cookies, French fries, potato chips, and toast.

Tests conducted by the CSPI conclude that, among foods tested, French fries showed the highest levels of acrylamide. A study involving the lifelong eating habits of thousands of female nurses concluded that children who eat French fries have a much higher risk of breast cancer as adults (Nurses' Mothers' Study, *International Journal of Cancer*, August 2005).

> "I estimate that acrylamide causes several thousand cancers per year in Americans."
> — **Dale Hattis, Clark University research professor**

As an industrial chemical, acrylamide is used in some water treatment facilities, which is a good reason to avoid tap water and to seek natural water sources. According to the CSPI, a large order of fast-food French fries contains at least 300 times more acrylamide than the U.S. Environmental Protection Agency allows in a glass of water.

Raw plant substances, even uncooked potatoes, test negative for acrylamide.

An Italian study compared the diets of 767 kidney cancer (renal cell carcinoma) patients with the diets followed by 1,534 people without the disease. The study researchers found that those with the cancer ate diets that were heavy in bread. Those who consumed the most bread were at nearly two times the risk of the cancer than those who ate the least amount of bread. The study also identified increased risk factors for kidney cancer among those who consumed the most milk, yogurt, rice, and pasta, but the risk was greater for those who ate bread. I speculate that the reason for this is that bread is baked while rice and pasta are boiled. The study authors speculated that the incidence of cancer in the test subjects might also have something to do with the blood sugar-raising effects of cooked starches influencing the level of insulin-like growth factors, which have been linked to cancer. The study, which suggested eating more vegetables, was done at the Mario Negri Institute for Pharmacological Research in Milan and published in the October 20, 2006, online edition of the *International Journal of Cancer*. According to the American Cancer Institute, about 39,000 Americans are diagnosed with kidney cancer every year.

"Some vegetables have a large proportion of cellulose (an indigestible fiber) and are also difficult to properly digest. The Brassica genus, including cabbage, broccoli, cauliflower, Brussels sprouts, and kale, tends to be tough to suitably digest. Blending, fermenting, and lightly steaming 'tough' vegetables are good solutions for easier digestion.

Blending tougher vegetables into a soup or chopping them finely and marinating them in lemon juice helps for easier digestion.

... Lightly steaming 'tough' vegetables and sprouted beans and grains is very helpful for delicate or transitioning digestive systems. Light steaming is not a crime in raw foods preparation. Although some nutrients and enzymes are lost, the steaming also breaks down the cellulose, the main constituent of cell walls, allowing the nutrients inside

those cells to be accessed and assimilated. Good deal."
— **Renée Loux,** *Living Cuisine: The Art and Spirit of Raw Foods;*
EuphoricOrganics.Com

As Renée points out, steaming or fermenting certain vegetables may help to make their nutrients more bioavailable. Fermenting foods for lengthy periods, such as with sauerkraut or kimchi, partially digests the plant substances through bacterial and enzymatic activity. This works in the same way that trillions of bacteria in the digestive tract help us to digest food. Soaking finely chopped vegetables in lemon juice and a little salt for half a day, or overnight, also helps to make some plants easier to digest.

For those who desire heated foods, I suggest steamed vegetables; steamed wild or whole grain rice that has been partially sprouted for several hours before steaming; and low-temperature-simmered vegetable soup that has been made without salt and oil, but adding the salt and oil only after the soup has been made.

Avoid eating heating salt because heat can change the chemistry of the salt, making it rough on the system. Also, avoid heating oils because the heat will damage the essential fatty acids and create a lower-quality oil that slows the electrical charge within the cells of the body.

Low-temperature heated foods

For those who desire heated food, here is a recipe for a low-heat simmered vegetable soup that will not create the harmful chemicals that form in foods heated at high heat:

Simmered Iron Soup

Place a steamer basket in the bottom of the pot. Fill with water to above the top of the basket. Heat the water to almost the boiling point. Add a selection of vegetables that may include one or more of a variety of chopped organically grown greens (consider: chard, spinach, collards, kale, dandelion, and celery), diced ginger root, diced garlic, chopped onion; herbs (oregano and thyme); freshly ground black or white pepper; and a good splash of organic vinegar.

Cover and simmer at the lowest heat possible until the vegetables are slightly soft, but not mushy. Turn off the heat. Use a long serving fork or other kitchen tool to pull out the basket, allowing the vegetables to gently slide off into the water.

After the soup has been made, just before serving, add lemon juice; salt to taste, and add raw olive oil and/or grapeseed oil. Shoyu, a fermented, raw soy sauce may also be used to add flavor. Some chopped raw bell pepper and/or summer squash can also be added just before eating. You might also sprinkle a little nutritional yeast on top just before serving.

Steamed whole grain or wild rice on the side also goes well with the soup.

If you steam vegetables:

Use a double boiler. This is a pot that has a second pot that fits inside. If you don't have one of these, use a steamer basket or other utensil that keeps the vegetables from sitting in the water. Fill the bottom pot of the double boiler with water to the point where it meets the inside pot, or set a basket into the pot and fill the pot with water only to the bottom of the basket. This way you will keep more nutrients in the vegetables, and not in the water. It also prevents the vegetables from touching the bottom of the pot, where they would be exposed to higher heat.

Vegetables that can be steamed at low heat include artichokes; asparagus; slightly sprouted beans; sliced beets; burdock root; celery root; green beans; parsnips; sliced fresh pumpkin and other hard squash; stinging nettles; radish; sliced sweet potatoes or yams; and turnips.

If you choose to eat bread:

Take into consideration that the study indicates there is very little acrylamide in soft bread. Hard breads, such as bagels, have more acrylamides. You can reduce your exposure to acrylamides by not toasting your bread, and by removing the crust.

I advise people to refrain from eating white breads, and to choose breads that are made using whole, organic grains.

Just because a label on bread says that it is "seven-grain bread" does not mean that it is made using whole grains. Food labels are misleading.

Seek organic breads. Look for unusual breads, such as those made without wheat, or those made using hemp.

Avoid any bread containing margarine, butter, corn syrup, molasses, rice syrup, fructose, sugar, preservatives, whey, eggs, white potatoes, cheese, colorings, flavorings, and other artificial ingredients and additives.

While there are some health benefits to eating quality, whole grain, organic breads, eating a lot of bread is clearly not in your best interest. Whole grain bread can help reduce your desire for sweets while providing carbohydrates that your muscles and brain rely on for energy. The fiber in whole grain bread can aid digestion, and improve colon and heart health.

Bread making is very easy. If you choose to eat bread, consider making your own bread from organic, locally grown ingredients.

Remember that it is better to eat fresh, raw foods. Accompany your bread with quality raw nut spreads; raw berry spreads; thin slices of raw vegetables; or raw vegan pesto sauces and herbal raw oil dips.

Those who do choose to eat foods cooked at high temperatures should see that the majority of their diet consists of unheated vegetables, herbs, berries, fruits, nuts, seeds, sea vegetables, and the occasional small portion of edible flowers. The largest influence should be on eating unheated, raw, organically grown green vegetables to keep the body alkaline and the lymph system and muscle structures free from the constriction that occurs on an acidic diet. Locally grown organic produce is ideal, especially if it is home grown.

People who are truly interested in improving their health should refrain from eating cooked foods; food containing heated oils; and food containing trans fats. They would also benefit by avoiding foods containing animal protein, especially from animals that were raised on factory farms. The protein, hormones, uric acids, and blood sugars, and the farming chemical residues in meat, dairy, and eggs are damaging to the human system, and result in degenerative diseases such as diabetes, heart disease, arthritis, kidney disease, gall stones, some types of cancer, some types of blindness, and weak bones.

A person who follows a lifelong diet that consisted mostly of cooked foods, animal protein, processed foods, and trans fats is left with an unbalanced and weakened immune system, and has likely damaged the blood system, including the heart.

A diet chiefly consisting of cooked food, animal protein, bleached foods, and processed foods is particularly unhealthful for those with diabetes and viral infections.

Eating Naturally

While it is true that some pesticides have been made illegal for use in the U.S., there are still companies in the U.S. manufacturing the pesticides and selling them to other countries, such as Mexico and Chile. U.S.-owned companies also manufacture banned farming chemicals in other countries, and sell them wherever there is a market for them. Many fruits and vegetables that have been sprayed with the illegal pesticides are then imported into the U.S. and are sold in U.S. markets.

The more fruits and vegetables that are grown using fertilizers, the more pesticides will be used. Plants that grow with the aid of fertilizers are nutritionally weak and are chemically out of balance, which provides nesting grounds for more insects. Plants grown using chemical fertilizers grow faster, and their root systems grow shallower than plants grown without chemical fertilizers. The result is the plant does not accumulate the full spectrum of nutrients that deeper roots would naturally mine.

Chemically grown plants tend to have higher concentrations of free amino acids and sugars, and are weak in the nutrients needed for the plant to convert these into lignans, proteins, starches and other plant substances. This provides food for insects that feed off the sugars and free amino acids in the plants. As bugs go about searching for plants that provide them with food, they land more often, and lay more eggs on and around plants that are grown using chemical fertilizers. This results in the use of sprays that kill bugs and poison food. You can think of chemically grown plants as addictive sugary junk food for bugs. And because chemically grown fruits and vegetables are nutritionally weak, they aren't as good for us either.

The most ecologically responsible and most healthful way to grow food is to use organic methods. Some farms also use the low-input sustainable agriculture (LISA) and the integrated pest management (IPM) techniques. Healthier farming techniques rotate their crops to help maintain a healthy soil and do composting to build the soil base. Some farmers use natural soil bacteria and fungi to improve their harvests. These forms of farming are safer for the soil, for wildlife, for native plants, for the health of humans, and for farm workers.

People can reduce exposure to farming chemicals on imported

produce by purchasing fruits and vegetables in season. Other ways to avoid exposure to food-processing and farming chemicals are to purchase produce from local farmers' markets; purchase unpackaged items from the bulk bins at the local natural foods store; choose organic produce at the market; buy foods with labels indicating they are certified organic; make your own food from scratch; and especially by growing an organic home food garden.

The larger farming corporations have mostly stayed out of the organic farming movement. By choosing organic produce you are supporting smaller farmers and their families. You are also supporting food distributors that concentrate on the organic market.

By choosing to eat organic foods, you are saying "no" to the chemical companies that make pesticides, insecticides, fungicides, herbicides, waxes, and other chemicals used on farms and that pollute the land and water, damage wildlife, risk human health, and contribute to global warming.

To absorb the most high-quality energy available from plants, seek out organically grown, nongenetically modified food. Organically grown food should be the first choice above any chemically "conventionally" grown produce. Naturally grown local foods will provide the best nutrients, ground you, integrate and adapt you with the environment, and tune your energy to be more in alignment with Nature.

Many types of produce found in grocery stores are of plants that have been genetically modified. These are energetically and nutritionally weaker plants that have been changed from their natural state, and cannot grow as easily in the wild as plants that are in their natural state. To further understand the dangers of genetically modified foods, please use the references in the Genetic Engineering and Food Safety Section of this book.

Those who desire to eat the highest quality produce while also protecting the planet should seek organically grown, nongenetically modified produce.

It is better to eat your food as close as possible to its unprocessed form in Nature. It is better to eat raw food than cooked food. While low-heat dehydrated food is okay, and is commonly eaten by many raw vegans, it is better to eat fresh food than food that has been dehydrated or dried. It is better to eat organically grown food than chemically grown food. It is better to eat nongenetically modified food than food from genetically altered plants. It is better to eat locally grown food than it is to eat food that was grown thousands of miles away. It is better to grow some of your own food than to eat only store-bought and restaurant food.

Some people believe that fruits and vegetables that are harvested without killing the entire plant are better karmically than those that have been harvested in a way that kills the entire plant. But if I held this belief I would not be using foods such as ginger, garlic, and onions. I love making salad dressings that include blending some combination of garlic, onions, peppers, mustard, and lemon with olive oil or hemp seed oil, grape seed oil, or flax seed oil; tomato, avocado, olives, sea salt, vinegar, and fresh herbs (or dried herbs when fresh are not available). The blenders, food processors, and juicers here have been presented with about every mix of raw fruits, vegetables, nuts and seeds that we can possibly think up – sometimes to disastrous effect.

Naturally grown produce carries strong positive Nature energy, which is truly something that plants bring to us when we eat them, and they often grow in sizes that are perfect for eating. They have a powerful way of beautifying and bringing a vibrant health frequency into the body. They grow in all parts of the world, and in amazing varieties.

When fruits are in season in the region where you live, you should take advantage of that. Your body will thank you in the form of increased health and energy. Berries are particularly vibrant; these should be sought out when they are in season. Even the wild animals are attracted to berries.

One way to keep quality raw greens in your diet is to grow your own culinary herbs, such as oregano, thyme, basil, sage, mint, green onions, chives, curry, dill, and others. Those who don't have land to grow herbs may be able to grow them in pots. Fresh herbs are of a much higher quality nutritionally than dried herbs. Several pots of herbs grown in a small space and that are well tended can provide herbs for everything from salads and soups to Sun teas. Even though fresh herbs are best, if you find that you have more than you can use, they are easy to dry by hanging them from a string. Then you can store the dried herbs in glass jars for use when they are out of season.

Genetically Altered and Overly Hybridized Foods

Certain plants are out of balance with what Nature originally created. Some have been altered through many years of hybridization. And others have been altered through the very unwise and growing practice of genetically altering plants.

Overly hybridized plants are those that have been bred to alter their appearance, and often their shape and/or ability to survive shipping. I'm not talking about some of the basic produce that has been selectively bred. I'm talking about fruits and vegetables that have been crossbred to the point that they are genetically weak, do not contain viable seeds, and cannot survive in the wild. They mostly only exist on farms or gardens, where they need to be protected from the elements and wildlife to survive – which often means using toxic chemicals to grow and protect them. Some have been bred to the point that their sugar content is very high. Their mineral content is also out of balance to the point of being nutritionally deficient, especially if they were grown using chemicals.

Genetically engineered foods are far more detrimental than those that have been overly bred to be seedless. Genetically engineered foods are those that have genes from another plant or animal installed into their gene structure. This includes creating plants that contain the genes of animals, fish, bacteria, bugs and other life forms. The companies involved in this are truly and dangerously screwing with the structure of life. Their products have been given the name of "Frankenfoods." Their experiments are no longer in their labs, but are growing on many farms around the world. Most cotton, corn, and soybeans in the U.S. are grown from genetically engineered seed stocks. These genetically engineered crops are also grown using mass quantities of toxic farming chemicals.

Genetically engineered foods are so new that we have no real idea of the dangers they may pose, not only to our immediate health, but also to the long-term health and stability of humans, plants, and wildlife as well.

Educate yourself about the latest information about genetically engineered foods to keep updated on what has been done, and what you can do about it. It is likely that genetically engineered foods will result in a new profile of food allergies, as well as other health issues. Many people believe they already have.

Because large food companies often combine ingredients from many different sources, most food products that contain milk, such as butter, cake, candy, cheese, cookies, ice cream, and yogurt also contain milk treated with genetically engineered hormones. So, if you got milk, you also likely got genetically altered substances streaming through your body.

Likewise, because GE corn products, canola oil, cotton seed oil, soy products, potato products, and wheat products, as well as GE papaya and GE squash, are becoming so widely used, most people living in the U.S. are likely to be eating GE foods, wearing GE cotton, using paper made from GE trees, and using body-care products containing ingredients derived from GE plants.

In addition, some animals are used in the experiments conducted to create new forms of farm animals. These animals are also sent to the slaughterhouses and sold to the unsuspecting public. If you eat meat or meat products from U.S. grocery stores or restaurants, you likely have eaten some amount of GE animal. Some of these animals have had human DNA engineered into their genes. Got human?

Eating overly hybridized and genetically altered produce may create imbalances in the human system, especially if they are eaten often, or make up most if not all a person eats.

To counter this overhybridization and genetic engineering of food plants there is a growing movement of an increasing number of people involved with creating seed banks of open-pollinated heirloom plant seeds. If you plant a home garden, or are involved with farming, you would do yourself a favor by learning more about heirloom food plants, as well as organic gardening.

Because hybridized foods are more likely to contain higher levels of sugar, they are especially prone to molds that feed off sugar. Fruits that give you a "sugar high" are not the best things to eat in large quantity. Those who have experienced blood sugar problems and/or candida should especially avoid eating overly sweet fruit.

Eating too many sweets creates a situation within the body that makes the body pull minerals out of the bones and other tissues in an attempt to balance the sugar rush. The liver and pancreas also don't deal well with too many sweet foods, even if the foods consist of something like apples or dates. The effects of eating unnaturally sweet fruits and/or vegetables can be softened by eating foods that counteract the effect, such as green vegetables, nuts, olives, herbs, and especially sea vegetables.

> "People become addicted to bread made from hybridized grains; corn chips made from hybridized corn; French fries and potato chips made from hybridized potatoes; and even such things as carrot juice made from hybridized carrots. These hybridized foods contain an addictive quantity of sugar and low levels of minerals."
> — **David Wolfe**

While many of the hybrid fruits and vegetables sold today are nutritious and fine to eat because they are still rather close to their original state, as mentioned earlier, some have been altered to the point that they don't even bear seeds – such as seedless watermelon, seedless grapes, and seedless citrus. These are of the weakest produce, and should be eaten in limited quantities, if at all. Their genetic makeup no longer carries the balance that would exist in Nature. It is better to choose seeded fruits than those that are so out of tune with Nature that they don't produce seeds, or that have seeds that are not viable. As Wolfe points out, even the Bible advises (in Genesis 1:29) to eat fruits "bearing seed."

Organic Living

While many people know of the adverse effects that a tiny mosquito bite or bee sting may have on the health of a person, even to the point where a bee sting can cause death, they do not take into consideration what illnesses may be related to the hundreds of millions of pounds of various chemicals used to farm and process food. Toxic chemicals in foods cause distress in humans similar to the allergic responses humans have to tiny bits of dust or pollen. Repeat exposure to the chemicals can result in serious health problems.

Beside the toxins found in today's supermarket foods, there are many hazardous materials found in today's homes, businesses, schools, churches, and sport facilities. On a long-term basis, chemicals used in food, around the household, and in the atmosphere assault human health and cause and contribute to disease.

Where are the toxins in your surroundings?

• Pesticides, fungicides, insecticides, weed killers, and chemical fertilizers in your food.

- Growth hormones, antibiotics, and other drugs and chemicals used on the animals and dairy products you eat if you are not a vegan.

- Paints, stains, varnishes, adhesives, and caulkings used around your home, business, school, club, church, sporting facility, stores, and other buildings.

- Gasoline, motor oil, antifreeze, windshield fluid, cleaners, waxes, battery fluids, transmission fluid, brake fluid, dust from tire wear and break pad wear of your car and all the cars in your city or town and the surrounding communities

- Weed killer, gardening chemicals, pesticides, pet sprays, flea collars, bug repellents, disinfectants, and other chemicals used on the plants and animals in your neighborhood and home.

- Cleaning chemicals used in the homes, businesses, stores, schools, clubs, sporting facilities, and other places you spend time in and around

- Cosmetics and body care products that contain various substances and chemicals derived from fossil fuels and the animal farming industry.

As billions of dollars are poured into research to try to find a cure for human diseases, much of the money could be spent more wisely on finding what man-made chemicals in the food and water supply may be causing the very same diseases researchers are seeking to cure, and then banning the manufacture of those chemicals that poison the food supply and damage the ecosystems and seasonal rhythms of Earth.

Chemical companies started funding research at agricultural colleges several decades ago. Since then there has been a huge increase in the amount of chemicals used on farms, and a strong relationship between industrial farming, chemical companies, and college programs.

There are now over 400 pesticides licensed for use on foods in the U.S. alone. Other countries do not ban the same assortment of farming chemicals that are banned in America. So when you eat food that is not organically grown in other countries you really have no idea what type of farming chemicals you are also eating. If you cook food that was grown with the use of chemicals, the heating process is likely to be creating new chemicals out of the combination of those chemicals that were used to grow the food.

"In our country over two billion pounds of pesticides – in 21,000 different pesticide products – invade our lives every year through the air we breathe, food we eat, and water we drink.

Every day that pesticides are used, we allow the poisoning of our children and families. Sometimes the effects are vivid and dramatic, as captured by studies linking brain cancer to home pesticide use. Or, the effects may be more subtle and take the form of learning disabilities or problems with physiological development. The effect of low-level exposure to pesticides on the central nervous system can be devastating to normal productive lives."
— **National Coalition Against the Misuse of Pesticides, BeyondPesticides.Org; 2004**

It is known that pesticides and insecticides are toxic, many can cause cancer, birth defects, neural disorders, and other health problems. They are not only a risk to the health of humans, but also to all wildlife, including helpful bugs and ground organisms. One study found a fourfold increase in the risk of soft tissue sarcomas in children exposed to household pesticides in the first fourteen years of life (*Journal of Public Health*, February 1995). In the last forty years the incidence of cancer in the U.S. has increased at a rate of about one percent per year. This corresponds with the growing use of chemicals for growing foods, killing household bugs, spraying lawns and yard plants, preserving wood, and to the rise of fossil fuel culture.

Because of their exposure to farming chemicals, farm workers have higher rates of cancer than the general population. For instance, non-Hodgkin's lymphoma is one type of cancer that is more common among those who work on farms where chemicals are used. Farming chemicals are also suspected of causing an increase in cancers of the breasts and testicles; in reproductive organ disorders, such as endometriosis; and in birth defects of the reproductive organs.

The farming community is aware of the problems the farming chemicals may cause. In 1994 midwestern farmers were urged to wash their clothes separately from other family members to avoid exposing their families to the toxic farming chemicals. But that is clearly not enough. Luckily people are starting to understand the dangers of pesticides. There are changes being made. However, they aren't happening fast enough.

Methyl bromide was the world's most popular fumigant. During the 1980s in California, approximately 16 million pounds of methyl bromide were used every year in soil where dozens of crops including carrots, peaches, cherries, cotton, grapes, and strawberries were grown. It was also used to fumigate crops exported from California and to fumigate homes to kill termites. Only the state of Florida used more of the chemical.

Overexposure to methyl bromide gas can cause dizziness, blurred vision, headaches, nausea, vomiting, loss of muscle control, and permanent damage to the kidneys, brain, and liver. When liquid methyl bromide comes in contact with the skin it causes severe burns. The chemical also damages the ozone layer that protects us from Sun's ultraviolet rays. The California Department of Pesticide Regulation reported 454 illnesses caused by exposure to methyl bromide between 1982 and 1993.

When horrible laboratory tests were conducted on dogs to determine the toxicity of methyl bromide, the dogs went into convulsions and slammed themselves against the sides of their cages. The tests were supposed to last for four days but were stopped after two days to save the lives of the dogs so that federal animal protection laws would not be broken. As is the case with many laboratory tests conducted on animals, the results were ignored when the California governor signed papers allowing extended use of the pesticide.

The Environmental Protection Agency classifies methyl bromide in the category of the most deadly substances. Under EPA guidelines, use of the chemical was to be stopped nationally by 2001. Under international agreement as specified under the United Nations 1987 Montreal Protocol the pesticide was to be out of use by 2005.

Banning methyl bromide is a very good thing. But it is still being used. Under the international pact that has been ratified, the U.S. and other countries can be granted annual exemptions to continue manufacturing, stockpiling, and using the chemical. Shamefully the U.S. has stockpiled millions of pounds of the chemical and continues to allow it to be used on certain crops, including tomatoes grown in Florida, strawberries grown in California, and on bell peppers. The branch of the government that authorizes new production of the chemical is named the Environmental Protection Agency. Seems the only things they are protecting in this case are the profits of the chemical company that makes it, Chemtura Corp. of Middlebury, Connecticut. In 2005 over 21 million pounds of methyl bromide was used on U.S. crops.

Unfortunately there are hundreds of other very toxic pesticides still being used, and more being developed by these companies that apparently have no concern for the damage they are doing to the planet.

Research is showing evidence that some widely used pesticides, fungicides, manufacturing chemicals, and other chlorine-based substances imitate estrogen and others block testosterone. The chemicals, known as endocrine disrupters or "hormone modulating pollutants" are suspected of depleting human sperm counts, feminizing animals, and causing hormonally related cancers. Pesticides and industrial chemicals are believed to be the cause of wild animals being found with half-female, half-male sex organs. The animals also have abnormal testosterone and estrogen levels. Animals with those deformities include otters in the Pacific Northwest, trout in British rivers, alligators in Florida, and birds found in the Great Lakes area and on the coast of California. One study conducted by scientists at Tulane University found evidence that some pesticides may become hundreds of times more powerful when combined with other pesticides (*Science*, June 7, 1996).

"Possible synergistic reactions in which chemicals from different pesticides combine to form other possible more toxic compounds are often not considered (in Environmental Protection Agency review processes).
Insufficient data on the health effects of inert ingredients in pesticides represent another flaw in the evaluation process. Disclosure of these chemicals is not required by the EPA as they are considered 'trade secrets' by the pesticide industry... Although these 'secret' ingredients aren't actively involved in pest control, the EPA has determined that as many as 50 of these inert ingredients pose serious health hazards."
— *Greater Los Angeles Green Pages*, A Project of Environment Now & Green Media Group, 1993

Many people have recognized the dangers that man-made chemicals in the food and water supply pose to health. This knowledge is motivating a growing number of people to turn to whole organic foods in what some are calling a "clean-food diet." This way of eating includes water that is free from additives, and foods that have been grown or farmed organically. To satisfy the demand for these types of foods, the organic food market has taken off. It nearly doubled in the five years from 1989 to 1994. According to the Natural Marketing Institute, organic food and beverage sales increased 18 percent from 2003 to 2004. And the market keeps growing as more people become aware of the importance of organic foods and the problems caused by toxic farming chemicals.

Clean foods are vegetables, fruits, grains, legumes (beans, peas, lentils, etc.) that are free from refined carbohydrates, unnatural food dyes, flavorings, sweeteners, pesticides, herbicides, insecticides, ripening agents, growth-promoting chemicals, preservatives, waxes and shellacs, and other synthetic and unnatural food additives and farming chemicals.

Some people also consider clean foods to be dairy products and food from animals that have been farmed without the use of growth hormones, antibiotics, steroids, and other drugs, and that have been fed a free-range, natural, organic diet.

Under the Organic Foods Production Act of 1990, producers of organic foods must be certified by independent agents registered with state government agencies. The act established what is now a 15-member volunteer board, the National Organics Standards Board, to set standards for how organic foods must be grown. Under the NOSB standards, if a product contains at least 95 percent organic ingredients by weight, then it can be labeled "organic." Organic foods must be grown on land that has not had nonorganic farming substances applied to it for at least three years. The act allows for foods made with at least 50 percent organic ingredients to be labeled "made with organic ingredients."

"The prime source of toxic pesticides and other chemicals for most Americans is in the consumption of food high in fat content, such as meat and dairy products. A vegetarian diet, or one that minimizes animal products, can substantially reduce one's exposure to most of these cancer-causing chemicals."
— Lewis Regenstein, in his book *How to Survive in America the Poisoned*; 1982

Organically Grown Foods

"Before we go back to an organic agriculture in this country, somebody must decide which fifty million Americans we are going to let starve or go hungry."
— Earl Butz, farming chemical industry suck-up and U.S. secretary of agriculture during the Nixon administration

As mentioned, in the last several decades farms have been using more and more poisonous chemicals to grow food. There are chemicals to kill bugs and molds, and chemicals to make the food grow faster and to a certain color or ripeness. Foods grown using these toxic herbicides, pesticides, fungicides, and fertilizers are not natural, and can lead to diseases in the humans who eat the foods grown or treated with them.

When it is taken into consideration that chemical pesticides are made using cancer-causing elements that are designed to kill living organisms, it should be pretty obvious why these are not something a person seeking vibrant health would want on or near their food — or even on the same planet.

Organically grown food may cost a bit extra, but it is worth the extra expense to support farmers who are working to change the world for the better. The more people purchase organically grown foods, the lower the price will be.

There are many benefits to growing and/or purchasing and eating organically grown foods.

One 12-year study of organic produce, known as *The Schuphan Study*, found that organically grown foods are nutritionally superior to chemically grown foods. The study concluded that organic produce has a greater content of minerals than chemically grown foods. Organic foods were also found to have greater concentrations of vitamins. With this in mind, remember that you are getting more nutrition in the same size plant material when you are buying organically grown food.

Some fruits and vegetables are grown using more chemicals than other types of produce. This makes it more important to look for the organically grown versions of these to avoid the toxins that are used to grow them on nonorganic "conventional" farms.

It is always good to purchase organically grown produce, but especially important that you purchase the following as organically grown, as they are the most contaminated by pesticides and farming chemicals when they are not grown organically:

- Apples
- Asparagus
- Avocadoes
- Bananas
- Bell peppers
- Blueberries
- Broccoli
- Cabbage
- Carrots
- Cauliflower
- Celery
- Cherries
- Corn
- Cucumbers
- Dates
- Grapefruit
- Grapes
- Green beans
- Hot peppers
- Lemons
- Lettuce

- Mangoes
- Melons
- Mushrooms
- Nectarines
- Nuts
- Onions
- Oranges
- Papayas

- Peaches
- Peanuts
- Pears
- Peas
- Pineapples
- Plums
- Radishes
- Raspberries

- Spinach
- Squash
- Strawberries
- Sweet potatoes
- Tangerines
- Tomatoes

"There is growing consensus in the scientific community that small doses of pesticides and other chemicals can adversely affect people, especially during vulnerable periods of fetal development and childhood when exposures can have long-lasting effects. Because the toxic effects of pesticides are worrisome, not well understood, or in some cases completely unstudied, shoppers are wise to minimize exposure to pesticides whenever possible."
— **Environmental Working Group, EWG.Org**

The better quality of food you put into your system, the better your body can function. Whenever you have the opportunity to purchase organically grown food, choose it rather than "conventionally grown" food. You can also connect with organic farmers in your area. Ideally you will also be able to grow some of your own food.

As mentioned earlier in the book, one group working to provide information to people interested in growing food gardens is Food Not Lawns (FoodNotLawns.Com).

For a more in-depth experience in organic gardening, there are work exchange and volunteer opportunities on organic farms around the world. An organization called World Wide Opportunities on Organic Farms (WWOOF) is part of an effort to link volunteers with organic farmers, promote educational exchange, and build global community consciousness of ecological farming practices. For more information, access WWOOFUSA.Org. (If volunteering on an organic farm is something you are interested in, you can always simply ask your local organic farmers if you can volunteer to work on their farm. Or access OrganicVolunteers.Org)

Seasonal and Seeded Produce

Not that I am one who eats only what is in season, but it is good to at least make an effort to eat things that are in season in your region. That way you will be more grounded, in tune with your atmosphere, and connected to the season you are living in.

Here in California we have a situation where many fruits and vegetables — even those that are grown organically — are available year-round. This is because of the ability to grow a wide variety of fruits and vegetables in the mild climate, and because some are grown in enormous greenhouses. It is also because California is also home to several ports of entry, including shipping docks and international airports, where produce arrives from throughout the world, and then is shipped all over the continent.

It can be an odd feeling to know that a piece of fruit you are eating may have traveled several thousand miles. One reason is that you don't know how it was grown. Another is that even though the label says organic, you don't know what kind of fumes it was exposed to. You also may be wondering if there are waxing agents on it, and if these contain substances that are not good for health. You also may be wondering if it was grown in ways that aren't good for wildlife, for the environment, or for farmer health. These are issues that should be considered. They are questions that are easier to answer if you purchased the produce from local farmers, grew them yourself, or harvested them from wildland.

In addition to taking some effort to eat what is in season and to what is grown locally, pay attention to those fruits that contain growable seeds. If you have the choice, avoid fruits that are "seedless" when you know they would naturally have seeds. A seedless fruit or vegetable is not in its natural state, and has a weaker energy than a natural fruit or vegetable. Look for or grow fruits and vegetables that contain seeds. If you buy your produce at a natural foods store, ask the produce manager if they could please order some seeded fruits and vegetables. Local farmers are often a good source for organically grown heirloom produce that contains seeds.

Those new to Sunfood may discover that there are many varieties of fruits and vegetables that they have never heard of, including those that are grown locally, or that are wild to their area. Looking through raw vegan recipe books may introduce you to some foods that are unfamiliar to you. You can also seek out information on foods that grow in the wild, and then take a wild food foraging hike to gather some of these.

As you adopt a healthful diet, you will likely also naturally tune into the seasonal fruits and vegetables, and recognize how they can benefit you. Nature is a very wise angel, and she provides for us in many whimsical and mysterious ways. Help her along by planting your own garden, and by planting and tending to native edible plants in nearby wildlands.

The Plight of the Family Farmers

"Family farms are an important part of the American tradition of self-sufficiency, forming the bedrock for communities across the U.S.

Since 1935, the U.S. has lost 4.7 million farms. Fewer than one million Americans now claim farming as a primary occupation.

Farmers in 2002 earned their lowest real net cash income since 1940. Meanwhile, corporate agribusiness profits have nearly doubled (increased 98 percent) since 1990.

Large corporations increasingly dominate U.S. food production.

... Encourage your local grocery store and area restaurants to purchase more of their products from local farmers."
— FoodRoutes.Org, 2006

There was once a time when families ran the farms. They would work the land, grow a variety of fruits and vegetables, rotate the crops to manage a healthy soil, maintain seed supplies, and sell their produce to the markets.

More recently, farms in the U.S., as well as an increasing number of farms in other parts of the world, are being taken over by large multinational companies worth billions of dollars and that control many different levels of the food manufacturing and distribution process. These monolithic companies buy up land and turn what were once many farms into one large complex involved in intensive monocropping (massive single-crop farms). They also contract with land-owning farmers and dictate what the farmers grow and how the farmers grow it. They use tons of chemical fertilizers, pesticides, fungicides, insecticides, and other toxic chemicals to grow, protect and process the grains, fruits, and vegetables.

This has created a nightmare for family farmers, some of whom find themselves dealing with depression, life-threatening stress-related illnesses, and suicidal tendencies as they witness multigenerational farm life come to an abrupt halt. The family farm may have been all they and generations before them have ever known. The farmer can experience deep anguish when the farm is taken away instead of handed on to the next generation.

In the U.S., this change in the farm community has taken place because the government has been foreclosing on loans and because corporations are taking over the farming industry. Several multinational corporations, such as Cargil, Continental Grain, and Archer Daniels Midland, control much of the U.S. food supply.

Mental depression related to economic stress among farmers is such a problem that one of the leading causes of death among farmers has been suicide. In 2003, the U.S. farmer suicide rate was five times the national average. Farmers sometimes make their deaths appear accidental so that their families can collect insurance to pay off family farming debts. Other countries have also been experiencing large numbers of farmer suicides. In India there have been thousands of suicides among farmers.

Kyung-Hae Lee, a farmer who was president of the Korean Advanced Farmers Federation, killed himself with a knife as a form of protest at the World Trade Organization's convention held in Cancun, Mexico on September 10, 2003. He had written about the plight of the family farm and how "undesirable globalization" of multinational corporations is ruining the environment and killing farmers.

Farming in the U.S. changed rapidly starting in the Depression and Dustbowl periods. The government drew up a plan to help farmers by paying subsidies to those involved in growing corn, cotton, wheat, soybeans, and other crops under the farm subsidy program. Part of this involved paying farmers not to grow crops, or to destroy crops rather than to flood the market.

While the farm subsidy program may have been designed to keep family farmers in business, it quickly switched gears to benefit large industrialized agricultural businesses. These corporations began creating large, single-crop farms consisting of thousands of acres. This robbed the soil of nutrients, creating weaker plants susceptible to infestation. To improve crop harvests farms began using tremendous amounts of synthetic pesticides, fertilizers, and other chemicals made out of toxic substances developed during the World Wars.

The farm subsidy program turned into what is referred to as "corporate welfare" for the large agribusinesses. Today about 75 percent of the subsidies go to large corporate agribusinesses. These corporations rely on tens of billions of dollars in government subsidies every year to support their damaging business practices. The huge amounts of food they produce flood the world market, putting the food on the market for less than it took to grow it, and less than what farmers in other countries can get for their own crops.

The glut in American-produced grains and cottons has a negative impact on farmers and farm communities throughout the world that would be doing much better if this farm subsidy program were not so abused by corporate agriculture. Because of these subsidies, the corporations flourish, but the family farmers suffer, as does the environment.

In another way industrial agriculture subsidies also affect people of the inner cities of the U.S. When ways of cutting the budget of the U.S. Department of Agriculture are considered, often it isn't the farm subsidies that are the focus, but another part of the USDA, the school lunch programs.

Cities around the world are affected by the industrialization of agriculture. When farmers lose their farms, they often move to larger communities, such as large cities. Often they travel to other countries to find a better way of life than what they are presented with in their local towns, where many often end up working in factories producing products sold to wealthier countries. In the cities the immigrants become members of the working poor. In the country they often end up working as laborers for the industrial farms, for the factory animal farms, and for slaughterhouses. Some join the military.

The corporate agribusinesses have a big influence on what the government does because these businesses often give donations to politicians and to political parties favoring the corporations. These corporations feed off and perpetuate the lie that writer George Pyle talks about in his book, *Raising Less Corn, More Hell: The Case for the Independent Farm and Against Industrial Food*. It is the lie that the industrial agribusiness corporations are going to save the world from a food shortage. In truth, it is those corporations involved in industrial farming and the genetic engineering of food plants that are playing a major role in the world food problems, and especially in the problems being faced by family farmers and the environment surrounding them.

Rather than flooding the Third World countries with an over-abundance of crops from America, it would be better for the farmers to grow their own crops. If you give a person a piece of food, that person can eat for a day. If he is able to grow it, he can eat for a lifetime. The USDA doesn't seem to support this idea and keeps on promoting the idea that we need to bring more money into big business agriculture by exporting more and more crops.

On multiple levels the U.S. government has been no friend to family farmers.

Historically, African-American farmers have had a rougher time of it than their lighter-skinned neighbors. The promise of land and a mule that was made when the slaves were freed never materialized. Throughout the years African-American farmers have been much less likely to benefit from government programs set up to help farmers. In 1999 a lawsuit was settled between the USDA and a group of African-American farmers in which a history of discrimination was acknowledged. But few have received any part of that settlement.

There was a time when Japanese-Americans couldn't even own farmland. If they wanted to farm they had to rent land. Compounding the deprivation, many of them had lost the rented farmland they were operating when they were forced into internment camps during World War II.

Not to be overlooked are the Native peoples, not only in what is now the U.S., but indigenous peoples on every continent, and on many islands. Indigenous peoples the world over have been forced from their lands, which was then given to or sold to others, or kept by the new government. Some who have been allowed to keep their land have been taxed at stiff rates and/or subject to laws and regulations that create unreasonable hardship. Others who have had their prime farmland taken away have been moved to land that is difficult or impossible to farm.

More recently, many U.S. farmers went into debt to the federal government because the Farm Home Administration counseled farmers to take out loans in the 1970s when the value of the farms was inflating faster than the interest rates. Then the government raised interest rates on the farmers and foreclosed on family farms at record levels.

Under the massive takeover of farms by multinational corporations, family farmers are struggling to maintain and update equipment to pay for water, to keep up with packing fees, to pay for labor and transportation, and to compete with pricing. This is a driving force in the formation of rural groups who have found good reason to mistrust the government.

In addition to losing their farms to the corporate farming industry takeover, farmers have been selling out to housing developers who offer more money for the farmland than the farm can make in several years of operating at a tight budget. So the housing tracts get built on the farmland and the streets are given pleasant country names like Wildflower Lane, Cherry Orchard Court, and Apple Blossom Road.

Some U.S. farmers have moved to other countries, including Brazil where they have started *fazendas* (Portuguese for farms). They arrive with the belief that the land there will be the next leader in world produce. What they are finding is land that costs a fraction of the farming land in the U.S. There, among the tens of millions of acres in Brazil's interior, with a long and favorable season, farmers can grow a wide assortment of crops, including bananas and tropical fruits as well as coffee and sugar. While corn is being used to make ethanol in the U.S., sugar cane in Brazil is a common crop used in producing the fuel. Brazil is the world's second-largest producer of soybeans, much of which goes to feed livestock in Brazil, and is exported to feed livestock in other countries. Animal farming is huge business in Brazil, which has about 70 million cattle and an even larger population of chickens. The country exports about three billion dollars worth of beef per year to countries around the world, much of it raised on illegally-cleared rainforest land. It is a country that has an enormous export industry supplying the world food market. Unfortunately, the farmers relocating from the U.S. also are finding the same multinational farming companies working their way into the Brazilian farming industry, promoting their toxic farming chemicals, and making big plans for expansion with mechanized mono-crop farming that employs very few people. Much of this farming is being done on land that was bulldozed, chainsawed, burned, or otherwise cleared of pristine rainforest – displacing indigenous peoples, fragmenting the land, drying out surrounding forests, inducing droughts, and decimating wildlife. Cultural and language differences can require some adjustment and learning for farmers moving to new lands. Other problems include people illegally harvesting crops; labor contracting problems; squatters; hired guns; illegal logging operations; an unreliable infrastructure; a different tax structure; dishonesty in suppliers, processors, and land sales and leasing; and government bureaucracy.

Those considering a move to distant lands to start a farm may want to stay put and move toward a different way of doing business.

Some U.S. farmers have found that cooperative selling and food processing organizations are a way to do business and increase income security. Under NGCs (New Generation Cooperatives), farmers join in and own food processing and marketing associations. Under CSA (Community-Supported Agriculture), member consumers, often from nearby towns and cities, buy into the upcoming season of vegetables and fruits grown on particular farms. It is "subscription farming," and it is helping small farmers, localizing what people eat, improving nutrition, reducing pollution, and creating sustainable agriculture. More and more farmers are finding the growing demand for organically grown produce to be a way to create a brighter future for their small farms.

When you purchase organic foods, purchase non-GMO foods, purchase locally grown produce, and shop at farmers' markets, you are more likely to be supporting small farms, and less likely to be supporting the companies that have taken over family farms.

Becoming a member of a CSA is one sure way to support family farmers as well as to get food that is both locally and organically grown.

I recently spoke with some residents of Eugene, Oregon, who were planning to organize themselves into an organic CSA by turning the yards of at least a dozen homes into food gardens growing a variety of produce. They plan on selling their produce to local residents and restaurants as well as at farmers' markets. That is a wonderful idea, and a great way to both eliminate wasteful lawns and become independent from corporate farms. They will improve their environment, their health, and their community.

Plant-Based Foods and Health: Nature Provides Our Food

Inadequate nutrition and the consumption of junk food contribute to everything from skin problems to heart disease, and from depression to birth defects. Eating whole foods, such as unprocessed fruits and vegetables and whole grains, provides the body with important nutrients such as vitamins, minerals, and enzymes; and phytochemicals, such as isoflavonoids and lignans.

Studies are constantly revealing how certain fruits and vegetables (broccoli, peppers, onions, garlic, carrots, cranberries, beans, spinach, cauliflower, chard, kale, dandelion, berries, etc.) not only provide needed nutrients that are beneficial to health, but also that they contain and provide properties that prevent certain serious ailments, such as cancer and heart disease; limit intestinal exposure to carcinogens; and help the body to eliminate toxins.

> "A number of studies have shown that cancer risk is lower and immune competence is higher in individuals who consume a vegetarian diet. Epidemiological studies almost unanimously report a strong correlation between a diet high in fruits and vegetables and low cancer risk."
> — John Boik, in his book *Cancer & Natural Medicine: A Textbook of Basic Research and Clinical Research*

Eat a vegetarian diet and you will be doing what many world-class athletes are doing. For instance, Dave Scott, who has won the Hawaiian Ironman contest four times and is considered to be among the best athletes who ever lived, is a complete vegetarian.

Ultra-marathon champion Scott Jurek has won the Western States race seven straight times. In 2005 Jurek also won the grueling 135-mile Badwater race, which begins at the lowest elevation in the Western Hemisphere, in Death Valley, California, and ends 8,300 feet up a mountain, and he did it faster than anyone in the history of the race. Then he won it again in 2006. Jurek is a vegan.

> "I've found that a person does not need protein from meat to be a successful athlete. In fact, my best year of track competition was the first year I ate a vegan diet."
> — Carl Lewis, nine-time Olympic gold medal winner

Although there have always been people who have followed a diet consisting of only plant substances, the modern vegan diet is often attributed to the teachings of Donald Watson, who died at age 95 in Cumbria on November 16, 2005. He became a vegetarian after seeing his Uncle George involved in the slaughter of a pig. Hearing the pig's screams haunted him. "I decided that farms – and uncles – had to be reassessed: the idyllic scene was nothing more than death row, where every creature's days were numbered."

Eventually Watson eliminated dairy from his diet. When his elder brother and a sister also became vegetarians, his mother, who was not a vegetarian, made the comment that she felt like a hen who had hatched a clutch of duck eggs.

As an adult Watson became a woodworking instructor. In 1939 he registered as a conscientious objector and refused to go to war. At the end of the war he formed a group of "nondairy vegetarians." The group advocated the health benefits of such a diet, and taught that animal agriculture was likely to spread diseases, such as the tuberculosis that was identified in Britain's dairy cows. He concocted the term "vegan" by taking the beginning and end of the word "vegetarian." Terms that he and his group considered included "beaumangeur," "benevor," "dairyban," "sanivore," and "vitan." The first edition of The Vegan Society's *Vegan News* was published in 1944 and consisted of 12 typed pages bound using staples.

"We may be sure that should anything so much as a pimple ever appear to mar the beauty of our physical form, it will be entirely due in the eyes of the world to our own silly fault for not eating 'proper food.' Against such a pimple the great plagues of diseases now ravaging nearly all members of civilized society (who eat 'proper food') will pass unnoticed."
 – Donald Watson, founder of "veganism," acknowledging the critical microscope vegans were put under by those who consume the so-called "proper foods" of milk, eggs, and meat

When you consume a diet that consists of what Nature provides, and the closer it is to its natural state, the nearer your body will be to its natural state.

"My doctor told me to stop having intimate dinners for four. Unless there are three other people present."
 – Orson Welles

The natural state of the body is to be healthy and free from toxins and disease. The keys to health are a healthful thought pattern, a healthful exercise regimen, a healthful diet, and a healthful atmosphere. You can't eat a more healthful diet than one that consists purely of a variety of quality organically grown vegetables, fruits, herbs, nuts, seeds, and water vegetables.

To experience the abundance that Nature can provide for you, abundantly take advantage of what Nature provides. What Nature provides is a pathway to pristine health paved with nutritious foods consisting of plant substances. These are the substances that our bodies are genetically designed to eat. Anything else, such as processed foods, and those that contain artificial coloring, flavoring, textures, scents, preservatives, and so forth are not natural and should not be put into the body.

Don't try to get too complicated in regard to your food choices. Refuse to buy into the false information about various food companies trying to sell products that are filled with chemicals and chemically grown foods. Simply choose what is presented to us in Nature. Plants are in tune with Nature, and this is especially true if they are organically grown, nonhybridized, and not genetically altered.

Eating what is in tune with Nature tunes us into Nature and our natural state of being.

That is the truth about food.

It is simple. If you eat a healthful diet, you will experience better health than if you eat a diet of junk. This concept isn't part of the pop commercial diets promoted in books and through fad diet plans, which are based on ignorance and laziness. That is because people can't make money by simply telling you to eat fruits and vegetables – other than produce farmers, who deserve to be paid for their work. The most expensive diet plans out there consist of manufactured foods that have been deadened through cooking and processing. They lead to diseases of affluence, such as obesity.

> "When I buy cookies I eat just four and throw the rest away. But first I spray them with Raid so I won't dig them out of the garbage later. Be careful, though, because Raid really doesn't taste that bad."
> — Janette Barber, writer and stand-up comic

Most diet books out there are also selling something. Many have manufactured and processed food products that go with the "diet plan" that is being advocated in the books. But this book is not selling you any food products. I am simply telling you to eat organically grown plant substances. I'm also suggesting that you should grow as much of your own food as reasonable.

While acknowledging that people may not care to limit themselves to just a few types of fruits for their nourishment, it is still interesting to consider that just a few healthy fruit trees can supply a person with a lot more food than he or she could possibly eat in a lifetime. I have friends whose homes are surrounded by fruit trees. Their trees produce so much fruit that they can't give away the fruit fast enough. They get as much as they need and abundantly more. And they aren't considered to be farmers.

If you want to have a lively, vibrant body, then you should be eating living, vibrant foods. The most lively and vibrant foods you can give to your body are those found in Nature: vibrantly alive plant substances that have not been degraded by heating, chemicals, excessive hybridization, or genetic engineering.

If you are confused by all the diet and health information you have heard and read about in pop culture, there is a reason you are confused, because Nature is not confusing. Only the information put out by man is confusing. Forget about all you have heard about nutrition and eating from advertising and fad diet plans. Just stick to Nature. What Nature provides for you will not do you wrong.

Learn to eat naturally, close to Nature, and rely on foods that are as close to their natural state as possible. When you do so, your body will begin to conform to its natural state.

Stop allowing yourself to be caught up in all of the complex diets promoted by the various pop culture diet gurus and multinational food companies that want you to buy and eat their products so that they can make more money. Ignore food advertising. Skip over all of the boxed and processed foods you face at the supermarket. Go straight to the produce section. Request that your local market sell more organic and seeded produce. Shop at farmers' markets. Join or start a CSA or an organic food co-op. Grow some of your own food. Forage wild edible foods. Teach children about growing food.

Myths and Truths About Vegetarianism

"If anyone can show me, and prove to me, that I am wrong in thought or deed, I will gladly change. I seek the truth, which never yet hurt anybody. It is only persistence in self-delusion and ignorance

which does harm."
— **Marcus Aurelius**

By the term "meat," I mean all kinds of meat — cow, hog, goat, lamb, deer, turkey, chicken, duck, ostrich, fish, shellfish, and any other animals that people eat.

Those who call themselves vegetarians are not truly vegetarian if they eat fish or birds. They may not be vegetarian if they consume cheese because some cheese contains rennet, which is the stomach lining of cows.

Lacto-ovo vegetarians do not eat meat, but do consume milk and egg products.

Pure vegetarians do not eat any kind of animal product including oils or bouillon derived from animals.

The purest type of vegetarian is a vegan (VEE-gan, rhymes with begin). True vegans do not eat meat, eggs, milk products, or any kind of substance derived from animals, such as gelatin; do not consume honey or honey bee products, such as royal bee jelly, propolis, and bee pollen, as they believe it enslaves the bees; do not wear leather, real fur, or silk clothing; and avoid products that contain animal derivatives, such as some brands of soaps and cosmetics, and some types of medicine.

The Sunfood diet is a vegan diet in every way, except some Sunfoodists might consume honey, propolis, bee pollen, and royal bee jelly. Not all Sunfoodists do consume honey products. (See: Honey, Bee Pollen, Royal Jelly, and Propolis)

> "When I met my first vegetarian, he told me he had not eaten meat for fourteen years. I looked at him as if he had managed to hold his breath that entire time. Today I know there is nothing rigorous or strange about eating a diet that excludes meat."
> — **Erik Marcus,** author of the books *Vegan: The New Ethics of Eating, and Meat Market: Animals, Ethics, and Money*

Myth: Vegetarians do not get enough protein.

Truth: Vegetarians, even strict vegetarians who do not eat dairy products, get enough protein.

Protein is made up of chains of amino acids.

It is not necessary to eat animal protein to get the essential amino acids of the protein molecule. The amino acids needed to make protein in the human body can be obtained through a balanced vegetarian diet.

It is **not** necessary to combine rice with beans to get protein in a vegetarian diet.

The protein found in meat, dairy, and eggs is much more concentrated than the protein found in plants. A diet that contains a lot of concentrated protein is a burden on the body, especially on the bones, liver, blood system, digestive tract, brain, liver, and kidneys.

In John McDougall's book *The McDougall Plan*, he tells of how the studies done to determine the protein requirements of humans were actually done on baby rats. Human protein requirements are much lower than the protein requirements of baby rats. McDougall explains how there are plentiful amounts of protein in plant substances to satisfy human protein requirements.

It is pretty much impossible to be deficient in protein while following a Sunfood diet. This is because it includes such a variety of plant substances that are rich in amino acids.

> "The meat industry has raised some alarm by suggesting that protein from plant sources may not be as 'complete' as that from animal sources. Fortunately, any essential amino acids that may be missing in grains are available in legumes or vegetables and vice versa. Our liver stores and redistributes the essential amino acids where they are needed. This is precisely how the animals raised for food get their 'complete' proteins."
> — **Citizens for Healthy Options in Children's Education, CHOICE.USA**

Myth: Vegetarians often become anemic because they do not get enough iron from their diet.

Truth: Vegetables have a sufficient amount of iron. Many vegetables, such as bell peppers, broccoli, cauliflower, cucumbers, peas, spinach, and tomatoes have more iron per calorie than beef. Other sources of iron include bok choy, cashews, chard, chickpeas/garbanzo beans, dried apricots, lentils, leafy greens, quinoa, raisins, and sesame seeds (including raw tahini/sesame seed butter). Many types of fruits are also excellent sources of iron.

> "You would have to eat more than 1,700 calories of sirloin steak to get the same amount of iron as found in 100 calories of spinach."
> — **Iron in the Vegan Diet, by Reed Mangels, Ph.D., R.D.; Vegetarian Resource Group, April 2006; VRG.Org/Nutrition/Iron.htm**

The body needs vitamin C (ascorbic acid) to absorb and use iron. A lack of vitamin C can also result in anemia. Unlike some other creatures, the human body does not synthesize vitamin C, so it must be obtained through food. Cooked meat, eggs, and dairy products do not contain vitamin C; raw vegetables and fruits do. This fact supplies more evidence that we are more healthful on a raw vegan diet.

A partial list of Sunfood sources of vitamin C include the following raw foods: cabbage, cantaloupe, cauliflower, bell peppers, black currents, broccoli, Brussels sprouts, dandelion, grapefruit, guava, kiwi, red berries, rose hips, oranges, parsley, spinach, and tangerines.

Milk is *not* a good source of iron.

Meat is also *not* a good source for iron.

The iron in meat is heme iron (blood iron). A study conducted by researchers at the Harvard University School of Public Health found that high levels of heme iron raised the risk of heart disease. The iron found in vegetables is non-heme iron and is utilized by the body differently from the iron found in meat. (*Circulation*, 1994; 89:969-74)

It is pretty much impossible to be deficient in iron on the Sunfood diet. This is because it includes such a variety of plant substances that are both rich in iron and in vitamin C.

Myth: Vegetarians do not get enough B-12 from their food.

Truth: There is some truth in this, but only when you consider those who are limiting their diet to certain foods.

The statement does not take into consideration the fact that the bacteria naturally living in the mouth, throat, and intestines supplies some B-12. Many foods found in natural foods stores where vegetarians often do their shopping are fortified with vitamin B-12. But eating processed or cooked foods is not necessary to obtain B-12.

Vegetarians who do not eat a balanced diet have the potential of experiencing nutritional deficiencies much in the same way as people who are not vegetarians. The key is to eat a variety of healthful foods, and not ingest empty calories, sugary, salty, refined, processed, fried, or cooked junk.

Some people believe that vitamin B-12 supplements are not needed when a person is following a healthy vegan diet.

Sources for B-12 in a healthy vegan diet include the following foods: raw (not pasteurized) fermented foods (raw kimchi, raw sauerkraut, etc.); raw nama shoyu, a raw fermented soy sauce-like product; nutritional yeast (not brewer's yeast); organically grown raw fruits and vegetables; rejuvelac, which is also a raw fermented food; spirulina and other raw water vegetables; and grass juices using grasses grown in organic soil.

In 1996 the U.S. Department of Agriculture and the Department of Health and Human Services came out with a revised form of its Dietary Guidelines for America. The guidelines are revised every five years and are used to create federal nutrition programs, nutritional labeling, and the *Food Guide Pyramid* (which is largely influenced by the meat, dairy, and egg industries). For the first time the guidelines endorsed a vegetarian diet. But it included a message that vegetarians may need to supplement their diet with vitamin B-12.

Vegetarians often take vitamin B-12 supplements. These supplements are inexpensive and do not have to be derived from animal products. There are vegan vitamin supplements available in most natural foods stores. A person desiring to avoid animal products should make sure the label of the B-12 supplement indicates that the vitamin is derived from vegetable bacteria and not from beef liver, cod liver oil, or other part of a killed creature.

Those concerned about not getting enough vitamin B-12 can easily do away with their concerns by taking vegan vitamin B-12 supplements. There is no reason to lose sleep worrying about this issue. (See: B-12 Vitamin Sources section in this book.)

Myth: Vegetarians are short.
Truth: A 1991 study that appeared in the *European Journal of Clinical Nutrition* that involved 1,765 children found that those children who were mostly vegetarian (ate meat less than once per week) were taller than those who ate meat.

Myth: Vegetarians do not get enough cholesterol.
Truth: Cholesterol is made by human body cells, it helps the brains of babies to develop, and it is part of the cellular structure of the body. There is no need for adults to obtain cholesterol through food. Babies benefit from the cholesterol in mother's milk.

Strict vegetarians have healthier cardiovascular systems than people who regularly eat animals, milk products, and eggs – which all contain saturated fat and cholesterol.

The main reason meat eaters have heart attacks and strokes is that their cardiovascular system has been damaged by eating animals and animals products, as well as trans fats. The majority of the people waiting for heart transplants are doing so because their hearts have been damaged from years of eating meat, dairy, egg products, trans fats, and junk food, and weakened by stress and a lack of exercise.

Switching to a vegan diet can reverse much of the damage an animal-based diet has done to the cardiovascular system.

For more information on reversing heart disease through following a vegan diet and exercise regimen, see books written by Dr. Dean Ornish or Dr. John McDougall. (See the Heart section in this book.)

Myth: Vegetarian diets are not healthful.

Truth: Meats, milk products, and eggs contain saturated fat, cholesterol, and concentrated protein, have no fiber, contain no vitamin C, and are not a source of complex carbohydrates. Saturated fat, cholesterol, and animal protein play a major role in many health problems, such as obesity, gallstones, kidney stones, arthritis, osteoporosis, high blood pressure, heart disease, strokes, certain eye diseases, and hormone-dependent cancers.

Diabetics are more likely to suffer the ravages of diabetes if they consume meat and dairy products. According to the American Academy of Pediatrics, "the avoidance of cow's milk protein for the first several months of life may reduce the later development of IDDM (insulin-dependent diabetes) or delay its onset in susceptible individuals."

Vegans have lower rates of cancers of the breast, lungs, colon, prostate, and the reproductive organs. Women who eat an abundance of vegetables have a 48 percent lower risk of breast cancer (*Journal of the National Cancer Institute*, January 18, 1995). The more meat a woman eats, the more likely she is of getting breast cancer. A study led by doctors at Harvard Medical School which was published in the November 13, 2006, issue of the *Archives of Internal Medicine* concluded that women who eat more than 1 ? servings of meat per day were nearly twice as likely to develop hormone-related breast cancer than those who ate fewer than three portions per week. The study used information being gathered by the ongoing "Nurse's Health Study" that began tracking the health and lifestyles of more than 90,000 women nearly two decades ago. Even after factoring the cigarette habits and obesity issues among the women in the study, it still concluded that those women who ate more meat experienced more breast cancer than those who ate less red meat. The study also mentioned that eating red meat greatly increases the risk of colorectal cancer.

Heavy people experience more health problems than those who are reasonably thin. Vegans are less likely to be overweight than the general population (Another Reason for Vegetarianism – Reduced Health Care Costs, *Vegetarian Journal*, July-August 1996).

> "Meat and dairy products contribute to many forms of cancer, including cancer of the colon, breast, and prostate. Colon cancer has been directly linked to meat consumption. High-fat diets also encourage the body's production of estrogens, in particular, estradiol. Increased levels of this sex hormone have been linked to breast cancer. One recent study linked dairy products to an increased risk of ovarian cancer. The process of breaking down the lactose (milk sugar) into galactose evidently damages the ovaries.
> Vegetarians avoid the animal fat linked to cancer and get abundant fiber and vitamins that help to prevent cancer. In addition, blood analysis of vegetarians reveals a higher level of natural killer cells, specialized white blood cells that attack cancer cells."
> — VegInfo.Org/Health

It is true that a person can call herself or himself a vegan and eat mostly junk food, but vegans are more likely to be nutritionally aware and to eat a more healthful diet than people who eat meat, eggs, dairy products, and junk food.

Myth: All vegetarians are healthier than people who eat meat.
Truth: Some vegetarians and vegans eat a lot of junk foods containing trans fats, fried foods, processed starches, corn syrup, and artificial sweeteners. Some nonvegetarians follow a diet that is more balanced, containing fresh vegetables and fruits, while avoiding junk food. In this case, the nonvegetarians following a more healthful diet win.

Myth: You need to eat from the *Basic Four Food Groups* to be healthy.
Truth: The *Basic Four Food Groups* promoted by the animal farming industry interests were designed by the United States Department of Agriculture in 1956. They came up with the *Basic Four Food Groups* idea to increase the profits of the animal farming industry. The colorful posters, teaching materials, and coloring books that teach children to eat daily from the *Basic Four Food Groups*

are supplied free to schoolteachers in America by the groups working to promote the products of the animal farming industry. These
promotional materials should not be allowed in schools. They promote a diet that leads to a variety of diseases.

> "A vegetable-based diet for children is generally more healthful than a
> diet containing the cholesterol, animal fat, and excessive protein found
> in meat and dairy products... Children and adolescents will get plenty of
> protein as long as they eat a variety of whole-grains, legumes, vegeta-
> bles, fruits and nuts."
> — Dr. Benjamin Spock, *Dr. Spock's Baby and Child Care*

Eating the meat, egg, and dairy products promoted by the animal
farming industry increases the risks of osteoporosis, heart disease,
cancers, diabetes, arthritis, strokes, high blood pressure, etc.

> "Vegetarian diets decrease the risk of cancer."
> — The World Cancer Research Fund and the American Institute of Cancer
> Research, 1997

Sunfoodists have their own basic five food groups that are a recipe
for health: Fruits, vegetables, legumes, grains, and sea vegetables.
These should be combined with an active life that includes exercise,
the creating of a healthy atmosphere, and the utilization of talents
and intellect to build a healthy life.

Myth: Humans are carnivores; therefore they need to eat meat.
Truth: The teeth and mouths of humans are very different from
the teeth and mouths of carnivores, such as animals in the cat and
dog families. Carnivores have sharp teeth and wide mouths that can
bite, lock, and tear at meat. Some people say the omnivore shape of
human teeth suggests that humans are meant for a diet of both plant
and meat content. Other people say that because human teeth are
short and smooth, the human jaw swivels in a grinding motion, the
mouths are small and relatively weak, they therefore are more struc-
tured for eating plants. (Animals that eat plants are known as herbivores.)

> "The average adult human has 32 teeth: 4 canine (the dullest of any
> primate), 8 incisors, 20 molars: 12.5 percent dull canines, 25 percent

incisor teeth, 62.5 percent grinding teeth. This indicates that the majority of what we should eat is food which must be chewed (ground up), such as fibrous plant matter.

... The structure and function of the human's dull canines and grinding teeth, the pouch shape of the lips and cheeks, the elongated digestive canal, the sensitive nature of the sensory organs, the method of nourishment for the young, the pattern of children's development, mental set, emotional feelings, as well as the cause and cure of disease and unhappiness, all demonstrate that humans are biologically plant eaters (eaters of sweet, nonsweet, and fatty fruits along with green-leafed vegetables)."

— **David Wolfe**

Carnivores eat meat when it is raw. Humans are not natural meat eaters. When humans do eat meat they do so only after it has been tenderized or ground, then softened even more by cooking with high temperatures and then, at last, sliced with a knife.

Even after preparing, cooking, and cutting meat, humans often have a hard time chewing and swallowing the stuff – sometimes losing teeth and gagging to death during the process (the animals' revenge?).

The human mouth structures are just part of the picture. Those who say humans are meant to eat a plant-based diet may have their beliefs verified by taking the human digestive tract into consideration.

Human bowels are very different from the smooth and relatively straight bowels of meat-eating animals. The puckered, long, and curved structures of the human digestive tract indicate that humans are more attuned to eating a fiber-rich plant-based diet. The stomach acids of the human are also much weaker than those of carnivores, and are more in balance with the stomach acid levels of herbivores.

Humans need fiber to help digest food. Meat, milk, and egg products do not contain fiber. Humans who do not eat enough fiber have higher rates of serious diseases, including heart disease and colon cancer.

A healthful vegan diet contains lots of fiber.

Unlike carnivore animals, humans do not have claws that can tear into another animal to kill it and rip it open.

Humans are not carnivores. They can barely be described as omnivores.

Myth: Raw vegans are fruitarians.

Truth: Some people who consume only raw foods limit themselves to fruit. But all raw foodists, or Sunfoodists, are not fruitarians.

Some say that eating only fruit is karmically better than eating plants that have had their roots destroyed in the harvesting process because a fruit diet does not kill the plant. Examples of plants that are killed when they are harvested include onions, beets, carrots, ginger, and whole-picked green-leafed vegetables.

There are those who call themselves fruitarians who eat a more rounded diet than others. While some may seek to limit themselves to sweet fruit, which can lead to nutrient imbalances and deficiencies, other fruitarians also consume cucumbers, olives, tomatoes, peppers, squash, beans, melon, avocadoes, berries, grapes, figs, dates, carob, chocolate, goji, nuts, and even coconuts. They also include substances derived from these, such as olive oil, coconut oil, and grapeseed oil. When considering that a fruitarian diet can contain a variety of plant substances, it doesn't have to be limited to sweet fruit.

I wouldn't support a diet that consists wholly of fruits and nothing but fruit. I think it is better to include a variety of plant substances in the diet, including and especially green-leafed vegetables, grass juices, sprouts, herbs, sea vegetables, and other edible plants, such as ginger and root vegetables.

The Sunfood triangle that Wolfe uses as an example to demonstrate how someone can balance the diet includes sweet fruits, fatty fruits (and nuts), and green-leafed vegetables (including herbs, sea vegetables, and sprouts).

The roots of plants seek out nutrients. They bring the nutrients up into the highest and outermost areas of the plants – the leaves, flowers, and fruits. As the Sun and air evaporates water from the leaves of the plants, the roots are constantly bringing up more water from the ground, and within that water are more nutrients. Through this process the leaves, flowers, and fruits become amazing biospheres of nutrients. Within those leaves, flowers, and fruits are the elements that the human body needs to build healthy tissues. Considering that each plant mines a different spectrum of substances from the soil and creates its own formulation of nutrients, it is easy to understand that consuming an assortment of plant matter is the way to get a variety of nutrients.

Myth: Breatharianism (also known as Inedia) is the ultimate goal of vegans, vegetarians, and raw foodists.

Truth: That is nonsense.

There are those who promote breatharianism who say the body needs very little food. The truth of that statement depends on what they mean by "very little food." If they are saying that the body needs a lot less food than what the average American eats, the statement is quite true. Many people eat way too many calories, and don't engage in the physical activity needed to use up even a healthful amount of calories. Evidence of this is displayed in the obesity problem that is rampant in America, and an increasing detriment to the health of people in many parts of the world. As mentioned earlier in the book, there are more overweight people than starving people.

Then there are those who fraudulently claim that the body needs no food at all.

The concept that the body needs no food at all is seriously flawed. People who promote this baloney often say that if a person were spiritually enlightened he or she would not need any food. They say that a person can survive on the *prana*, which is a Hindu word that they misuse and that means "vital life force." They say this prana is available in the air and through the energy available in the light of Sun. Or they describe the ultimate nourishment as "pranic light" that is the light of God within us and that we can survive on without any additional nourishment. They claim that it is possible to survive on the nutrients in the air that include carbon dioxide, hydrogen, nitrogen, oxygen, and even pollen from plants, as well as other airborne substances.

It is true that there are nutrients in air, and that the lungs can be described as digestive organs in that they take in nutrients. But it should be blatantly clear that it is impossible to depend on air and light to provide all the nutrients the body needs to experience the best of health.

Even wild animals, beings that couldn't be living a more natural and spiritual existence, regularly eat food and drink water.

The body needs the nutrients in unheated plant substances to build and maintain healthy tissues. At the very least, these nutrients include the basics of amino acids, essential fatty acids, enzymes, vitamins, minerals, trace elements, carbohydrates, and water. When it is taken into consideration that scientists continue to discover substances in plants that benefit health, it is obvious that there are many undiscovered elements within plants that the human body utilizes and needs to maintain health.

There are those who argue that breatharianism is legitimate because it is practiced by Tibetan monks. The monks do what could be better described as fasting, and they do it for a limited amount of time. They may also follow a frugal diet.

It is said that as a young ascetic monk, Buddha survived on one hemp seed per day for several years before his enlightenment. Hemp seeds are very nutritious because they contain enzymes, amino acids, essential fatty acids, minerals, vitamins, fiber, and other nutrients. Perhaps he ate one handful of hemp seeds per day.

The sadhus (men) and sadvis (women) of the Hindu religion also practice long fasts. They spend their time in devotion to deities and are said to renunciate their attachment to the world, including material possessions and sexual relations. Some give up wearing clothes and many include the smoking or consumption of some form of cannabis to get closer to Shiva. They generally live off the donations (alms). There are a wide variety of sadhus and sadvis. They are often given as examples of breatharians. But this is hardly accurate. Those who I have seen appear to be quite well fed. A small number of them are said to eat human flesh as well as their own excrement.

Responsible fasting and following a frugal diet of quality food can help the body to cleanse and to heal. But neglecting to provide the body with adequate nutrients for a lengthy period is unwise and dangerous.

People who promote the concept of breatharianism as a theory that the body can survive on only air, light, and/or the spirit within us are either lying, being irresponsible, delusional, severely misinformed, and/or displaying a lack of understanding for the basics of life. They are promoting what can lead to, and has led to starvation, dehydration, kidney failure, infections, and death.

There are people who promote breatharianism through Web sites, publications, and seminars. Perhaps what they are best at is exposing themselves for what they are.

Some may argue in favor of breatharianism by stating that it has been the conclusion of many health studies that those who eat fewer calories tend to live longer and experience fewer health problems than overweight people. But the studies do not say that a person should eat nothing at all. The studies do not support the breatharianism concept. Those who use such studies to promote breatharianism are stretching the conclusions of the studies beyond reason.

There are an amazing number of plants that form into or produce fruits, vegetables, nuts, seeds, sea vegetables, and flowers containing nutrients our bodies need if we are to experience vibrant health.

Food is a gift from Nature, helps ground us, provides the elements for our health to blossom, and should be enjoyed.

Myth: Adolf Hitler was a vegetarian.
Truth: Hitler's favorite foods included Bavarian sausage as well as stuffed squab (pigeon or rock dove). He outlawed vegetarian groups. He also ordered that the meat supply not be reduced, even though its production used up a tremendous amount of resources during those terrible years.

Myth: George W. Bush is a vegetarian.
Truth: He's not.

"A vegetarian diet has been advocated by everyone from philosophers such as Plato and Nietzsche, to political leaders such as Benjamin Franklin and Gandhi, to modern pop icons such as Paul McCartney and Bob Marley. Science is also on the side of vegetarianism. A multitude of studies have proven the health benefits of a vegetarian diet to be remarkable."
— VegInfo.Org/Health

Back to Nature

A great and unfortunate experiment has been taking place in modern society. It's like a race and it involves hundreds of millions of people, trillions of prescription pills, billions of dollars to study where diseases come from, and trillions of dollars in medical costs to "treat" environmentally and diet-induced diseases. To support this activity there are nearly 100,000 drug sales people sent forth from the pharmaceutical companies to get American doctors to prescribe pills. Other pharmaceutical representatives focus on medical schools to make sure the students are familiar with the various drugs available to prescribe to their future patients. Doctors are also employed by the drug companies to work as "consultants" to convince other doctors to prescribe drugs. Hundreds of millions of dollars are spent to advertise pills to the public while other millions are spent to advertise the drugs in medical journals that are read by doctors. There have also been thousands of drug stores built throughout cities and towns to dispense the drugs – some of these are located in markets, on college campuses, and in shopping malls. Thousands more structures have been built to carry out medical experiments, often involving caged animals. In other structures we call "hospitals" and "medical centers," ailing people who have been eating lots of junk food are turning to doctors who prescribe drugs and perform surgery to "treat" these ills people get from eating horrible diets, not getting enough exercise, and living in unhealthful ways that are distanced from Nature.

The experiment is a big failure and nobody is winning. People keep getting more obese and sickly, cholesterol drugs made $27 billion worldwide in 2004, and the environment continues to suffer from the junk diet and the disposable and wasteful lifestyle choices of humanity. But instead of changing their eating and exercise habits, they often turn to drugs and surgery to try to improve their health. Meanwhile, the cause of their problems, as well as the answers to them, may be sitting right in front of their eyes.

People need to reconsider what they consider to be food.

"Discovery consists of looking at the same thing as everyone else and thinking something different."
– Albert Szent-Gyorgyi

While allopathic doctors release their various reports and announce "recent discoveries" showing "scientific evidence" that proves diets low in salt, sugar, oil, and animal products, and high in unrefined plant content lead to better health and lower cancer risks, the "healthfood fanatics" have always taught that edible plants contain properties that fight and heal diseases and that a diet free of junk food prevents diseases.

"There is overwhelming evidence that the consumption of a plant-based diet, which is high in fruits, vegetables, grains, and legumes, including soy, and possibly flaxseed, may reduce the risk of breast and other types of cancers."
– Clare M. Hasler, Ph.D., director, Functional Foods for Health Program, University of Illinois. Y-Me Hotline newsletter; March 1996

As the "scientific" studies supporting the role diet plays in the healing process appear more and more in allopathic medical journals, the U.S. allopathic establishment is taking the results more seriously. Dietary changes are being incorporated into the way allopathic doctors treat such conditions as arthritis, cancer, and heart disease. Nutrition is being used as a way to boost the immune system in cancer patients. Strict vegan diets are being prescribed in combination with exercise and stress reduction to reverse heart disease and to help patients avoid invasive surgery and expensive and risky chemical drugs (*Journal of the American Medical Association*, September 30, 1995).

When one considers that it costs several thousand dollars to send a patient suffering from heart disease to a health retreat, and several times that to perform bypass surgery, it is not too difficult to understand why the health insurance companies are embracing the lower-cost therapies that consist of a vegan diet, daily exercise, yoga, and intellectual stimulation through art, music, and literature.

The "healthfood fanatics" may not have had the so-called "scientific proof" of what a nutritional plant-based diet can do for the human body, but they knew all along of the health and ecological benefits of eating pure unadulterated plant-based foods that are free of animal oils and flesh. The body that is supplied with the proper fuel is healthier, feels better, and performs better than a body that has been clogged with the residues of empty-calorie, overprocessed junk foods, and heavy, disease-causing animal-based foods.

People shouldn't think about following a healthful diet as a restriction. If anything, an unhealthful diet is restrictive. An unhealthful diet restricts you from experiencing the amazing health you can experience by following a healthful diet. In fact, the more healthful your diet, the better and less restrictive your life can be. The healthful diet opens doors, and eliminates restrictions.

It is truly amazing what the body can do if it is provided with the best diet. It can rid itself of extra fat. It can eliminate toxic substances from the tissues. It can change its complexion from that of the pallid color of a person who follows an unhealthful diet to the vibrancy of a person who follows a healthful diet. The hair and nails even grow differently, taking on a more healthful appearance and texture. And these things are reflective of what is going on inside the body when a person switches from a diet that was unhealthful to a diet that is healthful. The organs themselves become cleaner and function better when a person starts eating healthfully.

Changing your diet from horrible, or even from mundane, to that which consists of exceptionally healthful foods can help your body not only to greatly improve in form and function, but can also heal ailments that may have been a problem your entire life.

The human body has an amazing power to heal. If provided the proper nutrients, exercise, and healthy environment and positive thoughts, the human body can transform from sickly to healthy in a matter of weeks or months. The longer someone goes about eating a healthful diet; carrying on a daily exercise program to strengthen, stretch, and tone the muscles, tendons, and bones; and works the mind by creating positive thoughts that drives the person to succeed in his or her goals, the more healthful and successful that person will become.

A major part of a successful life is what is put into the mouth. Without a healthful diet, people cannot succeed at experiencing their full potential in life. Anyone who has experienced the sluggishness that is a result of unhealthful food choices, and who has switched to a strictly healthful diet knows of the advantages a healthful diet provides.

> **"We must give our bodies the rich nourishment from vegetables, greens, and fruits; and sprouted seeds, beans and grains. When these foods are combined with proper rest and activity, and a healthy positive attitude, the body and will are strengthened and even the most serious health problems may be overcome."**
> **— Ann Wigmore, AnnWigmore.Org**

When you look around in Nature and see what is naturally desirable, which tastes good, which feels right to eat, and is easy to eat, you will most likely be looking at plant structures that we call fruits and vegetables. These are what Nature has provided for our sustenance, and are most often naturally created in meal-sized portions. An apple, a tomato, a bunch of lettuce, a head of broccoli, a squash, an orange, a banana, a bunch of grapes, a coconut, a carrot, a stick of celery, an avocado, and many other fruits and vegetables are produced by plants in the perfect size for humans to eat. There are berries that ripen by the handful, and nuts and fruits, such as olives, that are available for harvesting in the amount that is consistent with what is needed to create a satisfying meal. Consider that this is the way Nature intended it to be, for plants to provide humans with food.

> "And God said: Behold, I have given you every herb-bearing seed
> which is upon the face of the earth, and every tree, in which is the fruit
> of a tree-yielding seed, to be your food."
> — **Genesis 1:29**

It is certainly amazing that plants provide us with the exact nutrients that we need to survive. This is no coincidence. If we simply eat a variety of what Nature provides for us, our body gets what it needs to grow and carry on in a healthy way. It is only after humans begin to manipulate plant substances by processing them with chemicals and heat that the nutrients in the plants are damaged, and the vibrant energy within the plants is killed.

Some argue that humans have evolved to the point that they can consume things that their ancestors did not. But just because you can chew something and swallow it without vomiting doesn't mean it is good for you. The same mechanical structure that humans had thousands of years ago exists today. It is made up of the same design — the human body. Only the food has changed. The degenerative diseases caused by the unhealthful foods being consumed by today's humans has resulted in a great diversity of diseases unseen in humans who eat more natural diets.

If you were simply created fully grown and were put in a tropical area, alone, with nobody to tell you what to do, what to eat, and you simply walked around a tropical forest, most likely you would examine what was within your reach. This would include the fruits and berries hanging from the trees and vines. Most likely you would smell and taste them, and you would find that they are good. This would be your natural diet. You would be rained on from the sky, taste the rain, and know that the water is pleasant. This would be your natural source for the fluid you would desire and need.

If, while in this state of innocence, you saw animals, you would likely not taste them. If you did you wouldn't find them to be of a flavor that is desirable. They would also be difficult to eat, especially with the bones, cartilage, tendons, and skin and so forth that would be tough on your teeth. You would stick to eating the products of the vegetation — fruits, vegetables, herbs, berries, seeds, nuts, and flowers.

Even if, still in your state of innocence, you saw a dead animal, bird, or fish, and tasted the dead flesh, you would still not like the taste of that. Eating living or dead flesh simply would not taste good to you. Flesh would not be in your natural diet. This is because it is not natural for you to eat.

If, even still in your state of innocence, by some freak occurrence you came across a dead animal that somehow became burned, such as by a fire caused by a lightning strike, this cooked meat still would be tough on your teeth and jaw, and would likely not taste good to you. It would not be in your natural diet.

Those at the forefront of the raw vegan movement understand that all living things are connected and that Nature will provide us with all we need if we would work with Nature.

> "What we eat deeply and radically affects the way we think, feel, and behave. We are what we eat, and we eat what we are. Food affects every aspect of our being. Food is the physical foundation of our body. If the foundation is unstable, all that is built upon it will be unstable. Everything you physically are was once the air you breathed, the water you drank, and the food you ate. The colloidal mineral structure of your body is built out of the foods you have eaten. If there is an alteration in the food, then it is reflected in the look and function of the body. Improve your food choices and you dramatically improve the foundation upon which your body is built."
> — David Wolfe

A Sunfood lifestyle promotes a simplification of living and works toward a balance with Nature by adopting activities that contribute to a sound, clean, and natural environment. This can be done by promoting sustainable agriculture, eating only organically grown foods, using only what we need, using only what can be recycled, restoring what we have destroyed, protecting the ecosystems and plant biodiversity of the planet by not using toxic chemicals, and by not genetically altering plants. If we damage the planet we damage ourselves.

> "A vegetarian diet could support a population many times the world's present size."
> — *Take a Step Toward Compassionate Living*, by the People for the Ethical Treatment of Animals, 2004; PETA.Org

Veganism is a diet most aligned with the natural state of the planet. But it has always carried an unfair image problem. Some who hear the word "vegan" turn up their noses. They think vegan means only rice and carrots. They have not been to a gourmet vegan restaurant or to one of these large supermarket-type natural foods stores and viewed and sampled the variety of foods.

The demand for vegan food is quickly increasing. Large food companies are aware of this trend, and have begun selling products for vegans. Restaurants are eliminating the use of animal fats in their foods. Raw vegan restaurants are opening all over the world, and the chefs who work at them are publishing recipe books, teaching food prep classes, and appearing as guests on TV magazine and radio shows.

> "Veganism has given me a higher level of awareness and spirituality."
> — **Dexter Scott King**, *Vegetarian Times*, **October 1995**

Whether people seek to become healthier by improving the nutritional profile of their diet through eating more plant-based foods, or are ethically driven to eliminate all animal products from their life by becoming vegan, there are many books and Web sites on these topics listed in this book.

Some recipes for raw vegan dishes can be found in books I have listed. I suggest Renée Loux's *Living Cuisine: The Art and Spirit of Raw Foods* (EuphoricOrganics.Com); and *Angel Foods: Healthy Recipes for Heavenly Bodies*, by Cherie Soria, founder and director of Living Light Culinary Arts Institute in Fort Bragg, California (RawFoodChef .Com).

You might find some helpful recipes in a now out-of-print book written as the original companion to David Wolfe's book, *Sunfood Diet Success System*. That book is *Sunfood Cuisine*. David Wolfe and I collaborated on the book, which was compiled by Frederick Patenaude. It features artwork by Sara Honeycutt.

I had known Sara for a while and I knew she was an amazing artist. I knew that David Wolfe would really like her artwork, so I suggested her as the artist for the cover design. I had a conversation with Sara before she did the cover design. We spoke about patterns.

There are patterns in everything. There are patterns in light, in air, and in water. There are patterns in the seasons and in the day and night. There are patterns in the structures of everything that is living – patterns in the structures of the tissues and other patterns to be seen in the microscopic structures of the cells, the walls of the cells, the intercellular structures, and in the nucleus, chromatin, DNA, and in the subatomic electrons and protons. The patterns are created by energy, which is the power of Nature, which is of God, which is in us, throughout us, and surrounds us. Every thing is an expression of a pattern of this energy.

> "Every human being has etched in his personality the indelible stamp of the Creator."
> — Martin Luther King, Jr.

If you look at the Sun face on the cover of *Sunfood Cuisine* you will notice that Sara designed the face out of fruits and vegetables to show the patterns of the plants. When you eat a diet consisting of raw vegan food you are placing the patterns of Nature into your body. The patterns of Nature are healing, uplifting, vibrant, and resonate with a strong energy. These are all things that you should strive for. They are the composers of health.

When you eat only raw plant substances you are eating what is grown in Nature and what will complement the patterns of the microscopic structures and energy fields of your body tissues.

Vibrant health cannot exist without the influence of Sun. We need to be exposed to the electromagnetic wavelengths of Sun through exposure to Sun, or by eating foods grown in Sun's light. Without regular intake of solar photons to recharge our electrons, our health suffers. Cooked foods not only lack the electrons needed for health, they also clog the system, slow electrical currents, and rob the body of health. Raw plants keep our inner fuses charged.

As you sustain a diet consisting of raw plants you will be infusing your system with the wavelengths of life that permeate all life forms. If you follow a diet consisting wholly of raw plant substances that have been undiminished by heating, processing, genetic engineering, or artificial chemicals, you will be providing your body with the vital link necessary for your body to experience true health.

"Raw plant foods fall into fourteen major categories:
1. Fruits: Fruits are raw plant foods containing the seed within themselves for the reproduction of their kind. Fruits may be sweet (grapes, oranges, pears, apples, cherries), nonsweet (cucumbers, pumpkins), or fat-dominant (olives, avocados).
2. Leaves: Leaves contain life-giving chlorophyll pigments, and are the best source of minerals. Most herbs are green leaves.
3. Nuts: Nuts are the reproductive agents of certain trees. They are fat-dominant foods.

4. Seeds: Seeds are the reproductive agents of plants. Depending on the type, they may be protein-dominant or fat-dominant. Grains are seeds.
5. Legumes: Legumes include all peas, beans, and peanuts, and (in a raw vegan diet) are often sprouted before consumption. They are protein-dominant. [They are also seeds.]
6. Flowers: Flowers are the sex organs of plants.
7. Green sprouts: Green sprouts appear when sprouted seeds, or legumes, reach a certain point of growth and shoot forth green leaves.
8. Roots: Roots are the below-ground portions of plants. (Ginger, beets, radishes, and carrots are roots.)
9. Shoots: Shoots are young plants spread by underground runners from their parent plants.
10. Bark: Bark is the outer layer of trees.
11. Sap: the life-fluid of a tree.
12. Stems: Stems are the fibrous, structural pieces of plants.
13. Water vegetation: Sea vegetables (arame, dulse, kombu [kelp], hijiki, nori, and sea palm) are sea plant leaves containing bountiful minerals drawn in from the ocean, and up from the ocean floor. Spirulina and algae of all types are included in this category.
14. Mushrooms: A non-chlorophyll fungus that grows primarily in darkness, and is not directly nourished by the vibrant Sun energy, yet plays a critical role in recycling biological materials in old trees and the soil. Mushroom extracts can be an outstanding source of medicine (e.g. reishi, cordyceps, maitake, etc.)."
   — David Wolfe, *The Sunfood Diet Success System.*

Sunfood Diet

"Man is the only creature that cooks his food, and he is more subject to disease than any wild creature that dines on unrefined food."
— Dugald Semple, *The Sunfood Way to Health*

"It can be said that the greatest single cause of degeneration in man is the use of fire in the preparation of foods."
— Arnold De Vries, *The Fountain of Youth*

"Kill neither men, nor beasts, nor yet the food which goes into your mouth. For if you eat living food, the same will quicken you, but if you kill your food, the dead food will kill you also. For life comes only from life, and from death comes always death. For everything which kills your foods, kills your bodies also. And everything which kills your bodies kills

your souls also. And your bodies become what your foods are, even as your spirits, likewise, become what your thoughts are."
— The Essene Gospel of Peace, Book 1, translated by Edmond Bordeaux Szekely

When people describe themselves as Sunfoodists, or raw vegans, they mean to say that they are complete vegetarians who do not eat animal protein of any sort, including from dairy, eggs, meat, or derivatives of these. They eat only uncooked (not heated, fried, boiled, grilled, toasted, blanched, broiled, barbecued, or microwaved) food consisting of the wide variety of edible plants.

We use the term Sunfood because it indicates food grown under the vibrancy of that life-giving star, Sun.

Some people who refer to themselves as "raw foodists" include raw, uncooked meat in their diet. They are different from raw vegans and Sunfoodists, who consume no animal protein, and avoid the energy emanating from the animal farming and slaughter industries. I strongly discourage the consumption of any meat, be it fish, bird, reptile, or mammal.

Depending on whom you speak with, many who use the term "vegan" consider honey to be an animal product, and therefore not something that could be included in a vegan diet. Some Sunfoodists may consume honey, royal bee jelly, propolis, and bee pollen.

The concept behind the Sunfood diet is to provide the body only with that which is of the highest quality so that the body can function at its highest potential.

Anything less than a natural diet is diminishing your energy, essence, power, strength, and health.

"Different foods fuel different types of thoughts, potentials for success, destinies in life, and levels of health. The manifestation of our genetic and spiritual blueprint is a result of whatever we eat, assimilate, and eliminate in and out of our body and mind. What you are eating and thinking is leading you to a certain destination.
Where are you headed with your current level of nutrition and your mental diet?"
— David Wolfe

As a human being, your biology is naturally attuned to wanting to be in sync with that which is most healthful. It is the design of your cells to be in sync with Nature. The natural forces within each cell work toward cleaning out that which does not belong, and building that which is meant to be. The intricate activities that are taking place inside you at every moment constantly strive to create what is best with what is provided. It is up to you to provide the quality materials your life requires to live in the best way.

Eating a diet that consists purely of raw vegetation rebuilds your tissues at the molecular level. It does this by providing your ever-changing cellular structure with the nutrients it needs to form your body structure using the elements your body should have been pro-vided with all along. As the weeks, months and years go by, those following a Sunfood diet will find their body has been transformed into one that is healthier than the one they had when they ate low-quality foods.

It is amazing how much sedation is going on among people in Western society. Many millions of people are taking prescription sedatives that their doctors say will help them. They feel eager or anxious, unable to suppress their urge for something that they can't define. Their body is trying to tell them something, trying to get a message across. But instead of working through and discovering what the message is, they suppress it by using some sort of drug from which pharmaceutical companies are making millions and billions by selling them through toxic stores we call "the drug store," or "the pharmacy." What people really need to do is to stop putting artifi-cial food substances into their bodies and to eat a more natural diet so their bodies can function better. When your body functions bet-ter your life functions better.

"Every living organism is vibrating at a certain metabolic level. If the internal energy of the organism drops below a certain level, then the immune system is compromised. Illness is an energy crisis in the body – the body no longer has enough energy to hold together its integrity. Purifying the body through a balanced Sunfood diet raises the energy vibration, thus increasing the immune system."
– David Wolfe

A healthful diet based on high-quality raw plant foods tunes your body into the powerful energy that exists in Nature. Plants vibrate with a living energy. Following a Sunfood diet transfers this energy into your system. The energy will work within your body to get each and every cell to work better. The high-quality nutrients obtained by eating a wide variety of living plant foods transfer into your body and they are then used by your body to allow your cells to function bet-ter with a stronger resonance in tune with a higher power. Damaging residues left over from low-quality foods begin to get pushed out of your system. As your cells become cleaner, the energy that was previously spent by each cell to deal with the junk you were eating finally becomes an energy you can use to work your life better.

By following a Sunfood diet you will be stimulating your life with the positive, alive, and vibrant energy of Nature. The tissues of your brain, including the pineal gland, begin to function better because your brain will be cleaner and the cells within it will function better. Your thinking will become clearer, your intuition will awaken throughout all of the cells of your body, and your perceptions will change to tune into your instinct. You will have a stronger desire to work with your talents and to succeed. You can work with the energy you will experience to propel you into a better life situation. Your very essence will be permeated with the energy and nutrients provided by Nature and created by the energy of Divinity.

A diet relying purely on plants benefits the planet in many different ways. It eliminates the reliance on the wasteful meat and dairy industries; it requires that more fruiting trees be planted. Because of this the soil becomes richer with minerals that the roots of the trees mine from the ground. When the leaves, stems, bark, and branches eventually make their way back to the ground they compost into a rich soil base. All of the trees help to keep the air clean, provide oxygen, generate water, become homes to wildlife, and create a more healthful environment for all forms of life.

As every cell in the body works like a little factory to maintain health, including by eliminating waste products formed within the cell, eating a clean diet gives the cells a rest. With less junk going into the body in the form of cooked and processed foods, and the chemicals in junk food, the cells do not have to work so hard to maintain health.

> "The form, function, and food choices of every plant and animal are not determined by evolution or adaptation over time. But each organism has a form, function, and food supply ordained by design. When humans follow their dietary design, the result is extraordinary."
> — **David Wolfe**

As you take care to eat higher-quality foods to get yourself in better physical health, and to attain your goals by using your intentional thoughts and given talents to live up to your potential, your life will work like a symphony with all your instruments being fine-tuned. On a Sunfood diet you will be better able to perform and function at a healthful level.

Clearing damaging, artificial, and overly processed foods from your life degunks your system and opens up your being to your potential. The benefit of healthful eating is that it unlocks dormant powers.

On a Sunfood diet the power contained in your body will awaken from its dormant state that was induced by unhealthful eating and lack of use. You can begin to radiate health, reflect your happiness out into the world and people around you, and become in tune with who you are.

Living healthfully through eating right, taking care of your physical body, and working to succeed at your life awakens your instincts.

Once you get a "taste" of how good your life can become, you will instinctively want to increase the good. Your perceptions of what you are capable of accomplishing and your abilities to do so awaken and become clear to you.

By working with the natural resources within you that instill the desire to succeed, you can experience happiness, your life can improve in ways you may have thought were not possible, or that you thought were beyond your reach.

This radiant health of Nature is what people have become detached from, and need to attach to. It is the energy, wisdom, reasoning, and consciousness that is in all, through all, and of all. It is within and without the animals, the plants, the ground, the water, the air, the universe, and us.

> "The whole field of Darwinism/evolution is based on the critical assumption that life is shaped by the outer environment. This generated the sociology of 'the environment' as determining the character of living beings. And yet, in a pure sense, what is life? Life is the unfolding of the inner potential. Potential is fulfilled by action, just as a seed, with its inward certainty of bursting life and future fruit generation, is fulfilled by action through water, soil, and Sun. The environment does not determine the inner potential – it can only help or hinder its expression. The physical world of Nature is in reality the materialization of the inner spiritual potential of all living things. The inner world creates the outer world."
> **– David Wolfe**

Realize that life is full of possibilities for those who believe in their divinity, who cherish the strengths of their spirit, who honor their body by providing it with the best nutrition and quality activities, and who seek and believe and work toward making things happen in alignment with their talents and intellect.

Just as a plant grows from the ground into a thing of beauty, humans can grow from a diet of plants, taking the elements of the plants to form themselves into beautiful, healthy beings. It is from within that the exterior is formed.

The Sunfood diet beautifies the body, the mind, and the spirit. It brings you to experience the vitality that you should be experiencing. Sunfood is fuel from Nature, and is grown under the Sun, which nourishes all life on Earth. By infusing the body with the healthiest nutrients from the foods that Nature creates, the body can overcome health challenges. When a person's health improves, every other area of that life improves.

All that is beautiful, nourishing, kind, loving, and vital to building a healthful life is advocated in this lifestyle.

On a Sunfood diet your life and love become alive.

Earth, Air, Water, Bacteria, Fungi, Sun, and Vitamin D

Just as the plants need Sun, so do you. All life on the planet relies on Sun. Even the forms of life that are not directly exposed to Sun are still dependent on Sun. The plants that give us oxygen to breath could not do so without Sun. The photosynthesis that happens within the plants is powered by Sun energy.

It can be said that we are partially made up of Sun. We are also made up of Earth, of plants, of water, of air, of fungus, and of bacteria. If any one of these were missing, all life as we know it would die. We are actually all of these elements transformed. Fungus and bacteria help aid in the existence of healthy soil and in transforming elements that can be absorbed into plants and into our bodies that become the fabric of our tissues. As plants are the transformed elements of fungus, bacteria, water, soil, Sun, and air (which all consist of many elements), we and animal life are these elements transformed into our structures.

Sun also triggers the formation of hormones in your brain and body tissues that lift the spirit and spread throughout all of the tissues. Those who live in regions of the world where Sun light is limited often experience depression, and all that goes along with that malady.

Exposure to Sun light and the consumption of raw fruits and vegetables go hand-in-hand. Beta-carotene and other carotenoids, substances in the fruits and vegetables we eat, protect us from damaging ultraviolet rays. They protect both the cells of the plants, and within our bodies they protect the cells of our tissues.

> "A diet high in cooked fat (free radicals), chemicals, and low in green leaves has been positively linked to skin cancer. This is because free radicals and toxins in the unprotected skin are baked and mutated by the Sun's rays.
> Researchers at Baylor College of Medicine found that people on a low cooked-fat diet had a greatly reduced risk of developing pre-malignant growth and nonmelanoma skin cancers."
> — David Wolfe

Just as Sun light helps to bring nutrients into the leaves of plants through evaporation of water from the leaves, which pulls more water with nutrients into the plant through the root and stem systems, Sun light creates nutrients in our bodies. Sun light also triggers us to drink water, thus bringing that nutrient into our bodies. Sun light also helps our body to metabolize sugar, which is interesting in that sweet fruits are more common in the sunny months when we also tend to get the most amount of Sun exposure.

Sun light also draws toxins out of the skin as the water evaporates from our skin during Sun exposure. This is why you may feel like rinsing off after you Sun bathe – your skin becomes coated with the toxins being brought to the surface.

Reasonable Sun exposure can help to heal the skin of bruises, rashes, and other skin injuries. Sun exposure stimulates the flow of blood through the capillaries within the skin, and this works to eliminate discoloration within the skin caused by fungus, bruises, rashes, and other skin issues. Sun light can also kill bacteria that exist in skin infections, such as ingrown nails, acne, and sties.

As mentioned elsewhere in this book, those with candida strongly benefit from reasonable amounts of Sun exposure because it helps to both metabolize sugar and kill mold. Those with candida and/or yeast infections benefit from Sun bathing while following a low-sugar and highly alkalizing diet.

If we don't get exposure to Sun, our health suffers. Exposure to the ultraviolet rays of Sun stimulates the creation of Vitamin D 3 (cholecalciferols) in our skin, and Vitamin D 2 (ergocalciferols) in plants. D vitamins are steroid compounds that absorb and transfer calcium, phosphorus, and magnesium through the intestines, and work to deposit these minerals in the bones. A lack of Vitamin D, which is rare, results in rickets, a condition of undermineralized bones and teeth. Vitamin D also plays a part in maintaining healthy levels of calcium in the blood, and is vital for healthy kidney, parathyroid, and immune cell function.

Too much vitamin D can result in increased levels of calcium in the blood, which can result in kidney stones. It also can cause calcification (hardening) of the arteries, as well as general physical weakness, fatigue, bone pain, nausea, vomiting, and heart rhythm irregularities.

Through reasonable amounts of Sun exposure, the body has an amazing ability to create and maintain healthy levels of vitamin D. It is when people take vitamin D supplements, and eat lots of foods with added vitamin D, that problems of an overdose may occur. Those countries where drinking lots of dairy products, and especially of foods that contain added vitamin D, are also the countries with the highest levels of arteriosclerosis (thickening and hardening, and loss of elasticity, of the arteries). So it is important to get your vitamin D in a natural manner, through Sun exposure, and not to rely on food additives and vitamin D supplements.

Exposure to Sun light is important. As part of your health maintenance regime, be sure to get reasonable exposure to Sun. Just remember, overexposure is not a good thing. Just as too much water and food, as well as too much sleep, or even being awake too long, are not good for you, too much Sun also works against you. Be reasonable about the amount of Sun exposure you allow onto yourself. Even wild animals seek shade and are wise enough to limit their exposure to Sunshine. Let them be your guide.

Eating citrus fruits, berries, and other vitamin C-rich foods works in conjunction with Sun exposure because vitamin C enhances vitamin D activity.

In the winter, a good source for vitamin C is rose hips, which can be gathered throughout the year from organically grown and wild rose bushes. It is important to avoid eating rose hips from bushes that have been treated with chemical fertilizers, insecticides, fungicides, and/or herbicides.

One way to use rose hips is to split them open, put them in a bottle of water along with mint leaves and shavings of ginger root. Let the bottle remain in the winter Sun for three or more hours when temperatures are above freezing, then drink this winter Sun tea. (Be sure not to let the water freeze in the bottle as it can cause the glass to break.)

Colors in Plants Infuse Health

"Beauty and vitality are gifts from Nature, for those who live by her laws."
— **Leonardo da Vinci**

I like to visit and support animal sanctuaries where animals that were once sickly from being caged or mistreated are able to live in natural surroundings and reclaim their health by eating a natural diet. Many of the animals that I have visited on these sanctuaries were once on the brink of death and have truly been transformed into healthy beings with a zest for life.

Just as the animals that have been rescued from the horrible living and diet conditions of factory farms can become healthier through improved nutrition and more healthful surroundings, the human body that has been mistreated and/or neglected can also regain much of its luster and vigor. This is obvious in those who have gone from obesity to a healthy weight simply by changing their food choices, increasing their physical activity, improving their atmosphere and restructuring their thought processes to become more positive and successful.

"That which we persist in doing becomes easier for us to do; not that the nature of the thing itself is changed, but that our power to do is increased."
— **Ralph Waldo Emerson**

The body works to generate health. The microscopic activities deep in the cells work toward health in the best way possible using whatever nutrients that are provided.

Health is something that comes from within. To assist this activity, the person should supply the body with the best form of nutrients available. Doing less than that is limiting the ability of the body to produce vibrant health.

Raw plant substances are what the body needs if a person desires to experience the best health.

Picture the colors on fruits and vegetables. Would you consider the unadulterated, undamaged, vibrant botanical colors to be nutrients? There is more than meets the eyes to the colors within plants that we eat.

The spectrum of botanical pigments existing inside plant cells contain molecules that absorb specific wavelengths of Sun light and energy. In turn the cells of the plant store and carry different levels of vibrational energy fields. These frequencies contained in the unheated substances of plants have a function when a person consumes them.

Your body wants and desires to be around certain colors of Nature. You automatically are attracted to the piece of fruit that has reached its peak level of ripeness, be it the radiant peach, the passionately red strawberry, the gleaming plumpness of melon, the practically glowing yellow of a ripe banana, or the rich green of fresh vegetables. Once fruits and vegetables have passed their prime and their colors have begun to fade, they don't elicit the same response from us.

The pigments synthesized within plants often work as defense mechanisms for the plants much in the same way the immune system of the human body works to protect health. The plant chemicals have been described as "plant antibiotics." They work to protect plants from the elements, such as fungi, bacteria, tissue damage, extreme temperatures, and ultraviolet light. It is understood that there is some interaction between the plant and a pathogen that will trigger the manufacture of certain chemicals within the plant to defend it against the pathogen. Plants will also manufacture certain chemicals when the plant is exposed to certain stresses, such as wind, temperatures, moisture, and dryness.

Plants that are not provided with sufficient nutrients and conditions through soil, light, water, and temperature become weak and do not produce the chemicals they need to protect themselves from pathogens and environmental stresses.

Amazingly, when humans consume plants, the very same chemicals that protect the plants have been found to protect human health. They lower cholesterol, prevent heart disease, regulate blood sugar, and function as antioxidants.

Similar to plants, a human body that is not provided with the right combination of nutrients and atmosphere will also fail to defend itself from pathogens and stresses.

There are thousands of plant chemicals that benefit human health.

Probably the most commonly known beneficial plant color is the beta-carotene that is found in apricots, cantaloupe, carrots, peaches, pumpkin, and spinach. There is also alpha-carotene that is found in carrots, red and yellow peppers, and in pumpkins. Lutein, a carotenoid that is found in avocado, corn, kale, and spinach, has been found to prevent cataracts. Zeaxanthin is a carotenoid that helps give color to corn and saffron, and has been found to protect age-related macular degeneration (age-related blindness). Then there is lycopene in pink grapefruit, guava, tomatoes, and watermelon, and many other plant colors. They are only a few of over 600 identified plant chemicals that give plants their colors. Many more are being discovered. With each new discovery comes research that looks into the health benefits of the phytochemical, how the chemical works with others, and how the enzymatic systems of the human organs metabolize them.

One plant chemical that is currently getting a lot of attention as an antioxidant is one given the tongue-twisting name pterostilbene (pronounced tero-still-bean). This chemical is present in colorful fruits like blueberries. It is sensitive to light and air, which means it is more present in fruits that have not been processed or heated.

Another plant chemical that is rightly touted as a health-enhancer is resveratrol. This chemical is present in the skin of grapes, cranberries, and in some berries. It has been shown to improve liver and neuron tissue health, and may contribute to a longer life among those who consume an abundance of plants that contain it.

Resveratrol survives the wine-making process, and is present in red wines, which is a raw food. (If you purchase wine, make sure it is organic and that the company does not use any animal by-products in their processing. Some wines will indicate on the label that they are "vegan.")

Each edible plant consists of a different variety of healthful, natural chemicals that work as nutrients when consumed by humans. To gain the benefits of these chemicals, eat a variety of unheated, raw, organically grown vegetables, fruits, nuts, seeds, sea vegetables, and an occasional edible flower. Select from a variety of plants, allowing your diet to consist of a kaleidoscope of colors. The biological functions the colors play within the plants will also play a part in maintaining your health.

Remember that many nutrients are transported into the system by way of dietary fats. Carotenoids are fat-soluble. Including a little bit of quality oil in some part of a meal can aid in the assimilation of the nutrients. In this way, an oil, such as unheated, organically grown olive oil, hemp oil, or grapeseed oil, flax oil, or coconut oil, added to a salad is a perfect match. The oils in olives, avocado, and nuts in a salad also work to help the body absorb the nutrients of the foods accompanying those plant substances. Raw seeds, such as sesame or hemp, have a bit of quality oil and these work well in fruit salads (they can be ground first to increase the availability of the nutrients). This is also why we put a few drops of oil into the juices and smoothies that we make.

We know that humans respond both emotionally and physically to colors. Being around certain colors can trigger emotional responses, such as alarm or calm that illicit changes among the molecules within body tissues. When you consider that the molecules within living plants carry specific color ratios and that these are resonations of energy, you can understand that there is an interaction going on between the frequencies of the molecules within the plants and the molecules within your body.

The energy frequency of the foods you eat is reflected in your body tissues, from your skin to your bones. It becomes quite obvious who is eating a deadening diet consisting of cooked starches and heated oils with little to no fresh plant matter as much as it is obvious who is eating an abundantly nutritious diet that is rich in fresh, raw plant substances.

When you cook plants, the colors throughout the plant tissues change, the order of the molecules changes, and the energy fields die. When you are putting deadened plants inside a body that relies on living plants to bring in nutrients, you are not getting the benefit of the plants.

In other words, plants collect elements from the soil, air, atmosphere, and light and turn these into their structures, which nourish us when we eat them — if we eat them when they are unheated and fresh. The raw plant matter carries a resonating energy that is in tune with the quality of nourishment they received as they grew.

To experience vibrant health, partake of foods that contain their full spectrum of colors and living frequencies of energy. Eat vibrant, radiant, raw, living plant matter that has been organically grown in healthy soil.

Shed the False Self and Transform on Sunfoods

When a person does not supply the body with what it needs, the body draws from its tissues to try to produce the best health that it can from what it can access. If a person follows an unhealthful diet for a long period, the body cannot generate health, and degeneration occurs as the tissues weaken and become clogged with residues of an unhealthful diet.

When the body starts to degenerate because the person is not supplying the body with quality nutritional food, and because the foods that are eaten contain artificial and harmful substances (chemical dyes, flavorings, sweeteners, highly processed ingredients, heated oils, cooked starches, saturated fat, farm chemical residues, and so forth), the body's ability to rid itself of waste products is hampered. Then the system starts to become clogged on a cellular level. In this state the person gains weight, toxins collect in the cells, the blood system of arteries and veins become coated with cholesterol, the lymph system slows, the organs don't function as they should, the joints become rigid and arthritic, and the organs begin to break down and become misshapen, the body shape becomes distorted, and the person becomes essentially crippled by his or her diet.

The accumulation of toxins and excess fat in the body can cause people to carry what amounts to the weight of a dead person inside them. They have their living body that is working to generate health, but it is bogged down by this saturation of accumulated garbage that interferes with and gets in the way of every effort the body is trying to make to generate health. This accumulation of toxins, residues, and excess fat can weigh even more than the person's natural body. In this day of junk food and sedentary people who spend their days sitting on their fannies, it is not unusual to hear of people who weigh more than twice their ideal weight.

If people with these degenerative diseases go to a standard American (allopathic) doctor, they are labeled "patients." Then they will likely be told that they need to take various chemical drugs to treat their condition, and perhaps will need to undergo surgery to "correct" their health situation. They will most likely not be told that they need to make radical changes to their diet and exercise regimen (if an exercise regimen is even part of their daily activities). A major reason for the cluelessness of allopathic doctors is that allopathic medical schools focus their teaching on working with high-tech medical equipment, on surgery, on chemistry, and on prescription drugs, and not on diet, exercise, stress relief, detoxification, the mind/body connection, or on health.

One clue to how much allopathic hospitals know about the importance of real nutrition in health can be found in nearly every hospital cafeteria. It is there that you will find junk food, meat, candy, soda, and all the foods you need to eat to fall into the pattern of illness, disease, chemical drugs, and surgery.

Allopathic doctors give each health condition a label, and for each label there is a drug or a surgical procedure. Evidence of this can be seen in the amount of people being labeled "morbidly obese," and who then undergo expensive and risky surgery on their stomach and intestines to reduce their ability to eat large amounts of food.

Those who find themselves obese would do much better by following a balanced Sunfood lifestyle than they would by undergoing surgery and/or trying to control their weight with toxic drugs.

The amazing thing about the body is that it can generate health. The body can reverse diseases. The body can become healthier and shed the accumulation of fat deposits and plaques formed during years of unhealthful eating and lack of exercise. But it can only do so if it is supplied with what it needs to do so, if the damaging substances are no longer put into the body, if the person begins to take in lively vibrant foods, if the body gets the movement it needs, and if the person begins to think in a way that generates the flow of good things in his or her life and creates the atmosphere of health.

Putting meat and dairy out of your life clears your spirit, and detoxifies your body from the bad energy associated with the entrapment and suffering of farm animals, from the horrors of the slaughterhouse. It releases you from the bad energy of misusing Earth's resources the way it is done by the farming, killing, packaging, marketing, and consumption of meat.

When you work your life in tune with the energy of Nature, you are tuned into your natural instinct. You will be able to think more clearly. You will be healthier and have more energy. You will experience a synchronicity with your thoughts, actions, feelings, goals, and talents. A healthier you will manifest from inside as you shed the physical and spiritual residues you carried from living and eating an unhealthful life.

When you eat only raw plant substances you are eating what is grown in Nature and what will symphonize with the patterns of the microscopic structures of your body tissues. As you sustain a diet consisting of raw plants you will be infusing your system with the wavelengths of life that infuse all life forms.

The longer you maintain a diet of healthful foods, the sooner you will be able to detect the changes in your body when you don't eat the best quality of foods. When you are eating a very healthful diet your body can better communicate what is good and what is not. As you become attuned to how your body feels after certain foods, you will naturally want to stick with the foods that make you feel good. Your body will acclimate to eating and desiring that which is healthy.

Following a Sunfood diet increases your vibrancy. By eliminating the deadness of cooked food from your diet, you will be subsisting on the unadulterated nutrients of plant matter radiant with the vibrational patterns of Sun and Nature. You will experience a new health destination and your life will align in accordance with it.

On a Sunfood diet your life and love become alive.

Once you get a taste of how good your life can become you will instinctively want to increase the good. Your perceptions of what you are capable of accomplishing and your abilities to do so awaken and become clear to you.

By working with the natural resources within you that give you the desire to succeed and experience happiness, your life can improve in ways you previously may have thought were not possible.

Realize that life is full of possibilities for those who believe in their divinity, and who seek and believe and work toward making things happen.

> **"Let food be thy medicine and medicine be thy food."**
> **– Hippocrates**

Transform your life.

Be daring, brave, and wise. Bring yourself out of the box you have kept yourself in. Break down the walls of dullness. Decide now to enliven your energy. Stop eating dead foods. Allow yourself to experience the benefits of the Sunfood diet. It will ignite your life and propel you into experiencing amazing things.

Be strongly involved in the Sunfood revolution.

Heal, enliven, and elevate your health, consciousness, and spirit through the Sunfood diet.

Visualize a healthier world, and work toward it.

Take care of your body and work to create a healthful atmosphere by nurturing success and happiness.

Accept and manifest your divinity by expressing your talents and intellect.

Be a persistent advocate for good things to happen in your life.

Let your healing be the healing of the planet by helping to replenish Nature in your region of the world. Respect and protect wildlife and wild land. Plant native trees, bushes, and wildflowers. Grow a food garden and share it with your neighbors.

Run for office.

Work to rid your communities of billboard blight.

Legalize hemp farming.

As Earth revolves around Sun, let your life revolve around Sunfoods.

Please, don't eat animals. They are you.

Evolve through love.

John McCabe
Turtle Island, 2007

Direction

"I find that the great thing in this world is not so much where we stand, as in what direction we are moving."
— **Oliver Wendell Holmes**

Sunfood Living Directory

N one of the companies, individuals, or organizations listed here paid to be mentioned in this book.

Those that have been listed appear in all sincerity to be working to provide services, products, or information that can help a person to live a healthier life closer to Nature, to heal Earth, and to provide ways to make good things happen.

The author does not necessarily agree with or endorse all of the practices, philosophies, or views of all those who are listed.

The scope of the topics covered makes it difficult to check the accuracy of all of the information shared, or the claims of the various persons, organizations, and companies listed.

When using this guide, work to determine the ethics of the listed on a case-by-case basis.

If you believe there is a company, organization, or person who should be included in future editions of this guide, please send the information to John, c/o Caremania, POB 1272, Santa Monica, CA 90406-1272, or email to Info@SunfoodLiving.Com.

Activist Directories

"You must be the change you wish to see in the world."
— **Mahatma Gandhi**

"Activism is getting off your ass and working to try to better some-thing that really bothers you. Something that you know is undoubtedly unfair, corrupt, unjustifiable, or simply wrong. It's being a strong voice for a cause and taking action into your own hands – not assuming that others will do it for you. It's being a missionary – spreading your mes-sage no matter how others might judge you or how uncomfortable and alienated you may feel doing it. It's being righteous."
— **Jenny Brown, co-founder of Woodstock Farm Animal Sanctuary, WoodstockSantuary.Org; WoodstockFAS.Org; as quoted in** *Herbavore* **magazine, Fall 2006**

"The penalty good people pay for not being interested in politics is to be governed by people worse than themselves."
— **Plato**

"I am only one, but I am still one. I cannot do everything, but I can do something."
— **Helen Keller**

"We must use time creatively, and forever realize that the time is always ripe to do right."
— **Martin Luther King, Jr.**

"Politics is democracy's way of handling public business. We won't get the type of country in the kind of world we want unless people take part in the public's business."
— **David Brower, first executive director of the Sierra Club; founder of Friends of the Earth; founder of Earth Island Institute; father of the modern environmen-tal movement**

"It is one of the most beautiful compensations of this life that no one can sincerely try to help another without helping himself."
— **Ralph Waldo Emerson**

"This country, with its institutions, belongs to the people who inhabit it. Whenever they shall grow weary of the existing government, they can exercise their constitutional right of amending it, or their revolution-ary right to dismember or overthrow it."
— **Abraham Lincoln, First Inaugural Address**

Adbusters, 1243 W. 7th Ave., Vancouver, BC, V6H 1B7, Canada; 800-663-1243; AdBusters.Org

Albion Monitor, AlbionMonitor.Com
Alternative newspaper on the Internet.

Animal Rights Action Network, Kildare, Ireland; ARAN.Ie

Animal Rights Canada, AnimalRightsCanada.Com

Animals Australia, North Melbourne, Victoria, Australia; AnimalsAustralia.Org

Center for the New American Dream, NewDream.Org

CivicMediaCenter.Org

Compact, SFCompact.BlogSpot.Com; Groups.Yahoo.Com/Group/TheCompact
Perhaps best described as an anti-shopping group, Compact is a growing group of people involved in not shopping, and helping each other find stuff or give away stuff that they need or no longer have use for. The group was started by a group of people in the San Francisco area who agreed that consumer culture is destroying the world. They vowed to not purchase anything new other than health and safety items and underwear. Getting used items from swap meets, garage sales, and second-hand stores or Web sites, such as the free stuff section on CraigsList.Org, and FreeCycle.Com doesn't count. They also vowed to support local farms rather than to purchase food grown thousands of miles away, and to simplify their lives.

DawnWatch.Com
Karen Dawn became involved in the animal rights movement after reading Peter Singer's book *Animal Liberation*. Her site covers animal issues that appear in the international media. You can sign up for her news alerts to be emailed to you. She includes a list of suggested books. There is also information about fur, leather, wool, down (feathers ripped off animals), and on animal-safe clothing.

Deep Ecology Index, Home.C2I.Net/DEI
DEI is an index of deep ecology resources.

DroppingKnowledge.Org

Earth First! Journal, Daily Planet Publishing, 831 East 47th St., Tucson, AZ 85713; EarthFirstJournal.Org
The *Earth First! Journal* publishes a directory of environmental activist organizations, organizers, and associations. Earth First! has many branches in various regions working to defend Earth.

Eco-Action, Eco-Action.Org; Eco-Action.Net

The Environment Directory, WebDirectory.Com

Fairness and Accuracy in Reporting, FAIR.Org

Global Action Network, Montreal, Canada; GAN.CA

TheGreenPages.CA
The Green Pages is a Canadian network of eco-minded individuals whose mission is to empower and support students, educators, and communities by connecting them to environmental information for the purpose of making meaningful contributions towards environmental sustainability.

Greenpeace International, Ottho Heldringstraat 5, 1066 AZ, Amsterdam, The Netherlands; +31 20 7182000; Greenpeace.Org/International/

GreenVolunteers.Org

HerbivoreMagazine.Com
A vegetarian activist quarterly.

The Independent Media Center, IndyMedia.Org/EN/Index.shtml
Indymedia is a collective of independent media organizations and hundreds of journalists offering grassroots, noncorporate coverage.

Mindfully.Org

The National Environmental Directory, EnvironmentalDirectory.Net
Lists more than 13,000 organizations in the United States concerned with environmental issues and environmental education.

NeighborhoodsOnline.Net

Northwest Earth Institute, 317 SW Alder, Ste. 1050, Portland, OR 97204; 503-227-2917; NWEI.Org

OldDogDocumentaries.Com

Oxygen Collective, POB, 533, Ashland, OR 97520; O2Collective.Org

Pacifica Radio, Pacifica.Org

Portland Independent Media Center, Portland.IndyMedia.Org

Protest.Net

Radio 4 All, Radio4All.Org
Working to reclaim the airwaves from corporate occupation.

Radio-Locator.Com

Resist, Inc., ResistInc.Org

Robin Wood, RobinWood.DE
European environmental concerns.

Rocky Mountain Peace and Justice Center, POB 1156, Boulder, CO 80306;
303-444-6981; RMPJC.Org

TreeHugger.Com

Vermont Law School's Environmental Law Center, POB 96, Chelsea St., South
Royalton, VT 05068; 800-227-1395; VermontLaw.Edu

Activist Film Festival

The Artivist Collective, POB 910, Hollywood, CA 90028; Artivists.Org
International activist film festival held every year in Los Angeles. Addresses human
rights, children's advocacy, animal rights, and environmental preservation while raising awareness for global causes.

Animal Protection

Also see:
- Circus Animals
- Foie Gras
- Fur
- Rodeos
- Veal
- Vivisection
- Waterlife Protection

Book:
- *Wildlife Wars: My Fight to Save Africa's Natural Treasures*, by Richard Leakey with
  Virginia Morell

> **"I will cease to live as a self and will take as my self my fellow crea-
> tures."**
> **— Shantideva**

"Isn't man an amazing animal? He kills wildlife – birds, kangaroos, deer, and all kinds of cats, coyotes, beavers, groundhogs, mice, foxes, and dingoes – by the million in order to protect his farm animals and their feed. Then he kills farm animals by the billion and eats them. This in turn kills man by the million, because eating all those animals leads to degenerative – and fatal – health conditions such as heart disease, kidney disease, and cancer. So then man tortures and kills millions more animals to look for cures for these diseases. Elsewhere, millions of other human beings are being killed by hunger and malnutrition because food they could eat is being used to fatten domestic animals. Meanwhile, some people are dying of sad laughter at the absurdity of man, who kills so easily and so violently, and once a year sends out cards praying for 'Peace on Earth.' "
   – **C. David Coats, in the preface of his book** *Old MacDonald's Factory Farm: The Myth of the Traditional Farm and the Shocking Truth About Animal Suffering in Today's Agribusiness*

"The time will come when men such as I will look upon the murder of animals as they now look upon the murder of men."
   – **Leonardo da Vinci**

"Non-violence leads to the highest ethics, which is the goal of all evolution. Until we stop harming all other living beings, we are still savages."
   – **Thomas Edison**

"Until man extends the circle of his compassion to all living beings, he himself will not find peace."
   – **Albert Schweitzer**

Humans moving into and building on untouched land has shrunk the habitats of many animals. When humans move into an area they build roads, clear land for homes and structures, erect fences, and often proceed to kill animal species that have lived on the land for many thousands of years. Not only do the large animals lose land, they are often harmed or killed by vehicles on the highways, by barbed wire fences, and by disruption of their natural behavior. Many hundreds of thousands of others lose their lives every year through hunting, poisons, and traps. The rivers, streams, ponds, and lakes where the animals found food and water are often drained, rerouted, dammed, and/or polluted.

During the building booms of the 1900s many acres of virgin land in many parts of the U.S. were developed into tract housing as well as industrial and commercial centers. Most recently there have been incidents where mountain lions have attacked residents of newer rural homes in the Southwest. Time and again the people react as if the mountain lions are some sort of monsters invading human territory.

Some people speak of the nature preserves that already exist as if these are enough and we do not need to set aside more land for nature preserves. The land that has been set aside is a very tiny amount of land compared to what is needed to preserve the wildlife that is rapidly becoming endangered all over the world. Setting aside small bits of land here and there is not enough. When a whole species of animal is forced to live on one bit of land we risk losing the species to fires, storms, or disease. The preserves are often not enough land for the animals to carry out their natural migration patterns. Corridors are shut off by human sprawl and the animals are unable to forage for food or nest in anyplace but a small area. They are also only able to breed with a small number of others in their species who live in the small area of land set aside for them, which greatly limits their gene pool. It is amazing that many more animals are not already extinct.

ActionAgainstPoisoning.Com

Action for Animals, AFA-Online.Org

AdoptATurkey.Org

Advocates for Animals, Edinburgh, Scotland; AdvocatesForAnimals.Org

African Wildlife Foundation, AWF.Org

Alley Cat Allies, 1801 Belmont Rd. NW, Ste. 201, Washington, DC 20009; 202-667-3630; AlleyCat.Org
Promotes nonlethal control for feral and stray cats with trap-neuter-return (TNR) programs that reduce their population by sterilization - not euthanasia.
Did you know that one of the main reasons that songbird populations of North America are declining is because of cats killing them? There is an overpopulation of cats in North America. A major way to help this situation is to sterilize cats through the trap-neuter-return program of Alley Cat Allies. You can also help prevent the damage to songbird populations by having your cat wear a collar that has a bell on it so that it can't sneak up on birds. Other reasons for songbird decline include the destruction of forests throughout North, Central, and South America, the blight of broadcast and cell phone towers, skyscraper buildings, and lights on at night, all of which play a part in the death of hundreds of millions of birds every year.

Allied Efforts to Save Other Primates, AESOP-Project.Org

American Anti-Vivisection Society, AAVS.Org

American Museum of Natural History, AMNG.Org
Abundant information about specific animals that are endangered.

American Tortoise Rescue, Malibu, CA; 800-938-3553; Tortoise.Com

Animal Alliance of Canada, Toronto, Ontario; AnimalAlliance.CA

Animal Concerns Community, AnimalConcerns.Org

AnimalCruelty.Com

Animal Defense League, POB 1587, Huntington, NY 11743;
AnimalDefense.Info

Animal Defense League, Los Angeles; ADLLA@AnimalDefense.Com
On Thursday, September 8, 2005, the *Los Angeles Times* published an article critical of those protesting the Los Angeles Animal Services Department's way of killing
tens of thousands of dogs every year.

"Regarding the article written by Andrew Blankstein and Steve
Hymon which was on the front page of the California section in yester-
day's L.A. Times, we have this to say...
If underground animal rights activists use illegal tactics and vandalize
property, then so did the conductors of the Underground Railroad, the
colonists who participated in the Boston Tea Party, and the Allies who
liberated the inmates and destroyed the gas chambers of the Nazi concentration camps.
Once and for all, let's recognize that those who are responsible for
and who neglect, abuse and kill animals at their jobs are the REAL
criminals and terrorists.
Animal Defense League of Los Angeles (ADLLA) is an above-ground
animal rights group whose protests are, admittedly, noisy and con-
frontational – but always legal. The group does not engage in, have
foreknowledge of, or incite others to commit – illegal activities.
It does, however, understand that some activists are driven to 'take it
a step further.' Years of 'please' and 'thank you' have done little for the
animals – and the consequent frustration impels some to adopt those
'tougher tactics.' ADL-LA philosophically supports the anonymous brave
warriors who risk their freedom to employ 'more convincing measures'
to fight against the animal killers – or to directly liberate animals from –
the interminable abuse.
History has shown that the animal rights movement is the ONLY
social justice endeavor that has NOT resorted to violence against its

opponents. It has, in fact, been remarkably and admirably restrained in this regard. Some underground activists damage property because they perceive that it is the only medium of 'communication' – the only form of 'dialogue' – to which abusers pay attention.

Put in a nutshell, the only thing that seems to mean anything to the torturers and murderers of animals is their money, ego, and power. It is they, therefore, who determine that economic sabotage is the only language in which some animal rights freedom fighters feel they can meaningfully – and successfully – converse.

The government enacts laws that protect the corporations who torment animals and rape the Earth. The police and courts are their henchmen who enforce those laws. The public flippantly bandies about the 'terrorist' buzzword when activists obey the 'higher law' that decries the suffering of sentient beings.

For most people, the world stretches no farther than the lengths of their own selfish noses. They are oblivious to suffering – with the duly noted exception of their own, of course!

Thus, an hour's clamor in their neighborhoods once or twice a month sends them into a tizzy – but the execution of over 44,000 puppies, kittens, dogs, cats, rabbits, and wildlife every year in the six city shelters leaves them unmoved.

Indeed – those who are silent toward the pain of others cry the loudest at their own."
— **Animal Defense League-LA**

Animal Legal Defense Fund, POB 96041, Washington, DC 20090-6041; 127 Fourth St., Petaluma, CA 94952; 707-769-7771; ALDF.Org

Animal Legal and Historical Center, Michigan State University College of Law; AnimalLaw.Info

AnimalNews.Com

Animal Outreach of Kansas, Lawrence, KS; AnimalOutreach-KS.Org

Animal Place, 3448 Laguna Creek Trail, Vacaville, CA 95688; 707-449-4814; AnimalPlace.Org

Animal Protection Institute, Sacramento, CA; API4Animal.Org

AnimalRescueSite.Com

AnimalRightsHawaii.Com

Animals Asia Foundation, AnimalsAsia.Org

AnimalsVoice.Com

Anonymous for Animal Rights, Israel, Anonymous.Org.IL

Ape Alliance, Action for Apes, 4Apes.Com

Ape Foundation, AAP Sanctuary for Exotic Animals,
AAP.NL/Int_English/Index.php

The Association of Sanctuaries, TAOSanctuaries.Org

Association of Veterinarians for Animal Rights, POB 208, Davis, CA 95617-0208; 530-759-8106; AVAR.Org

The Bat Conservation Trust, Bats.Org.UK

Bite Back, 222 Lakeview Ave., Ste. 160-231, W. Palm Beach, FL 33401;
DirectAction.Info

Bleating Hearts Sanctuary, Boulder, CO; Info@LeadingVeg.Com

Bonobo Species Survival Plan, Zoological Society of Milwaukee,
ZooSociety.Org/Conservation/Bonobo/SSP.php

Borneo Orangutan Survival Foundation, SaveTheOrangutan.Org.UK

BornFree.Org.UK

BornFreeUSA.Org

BuffaloFieldCampaign.Org, Buffalo@WildRockies.Org
  Working to protect the last wild herd of buffalo in the U.S.

Bush Meat Crisis Task Force, BushMeat.Org

CaliforniaWildlifeCenter.Org

Cambodia Wildlife Sanctuary, POB 7033, Los Angeles, CA 91357-7033;
CambodiaWildlifeSanctuary.Com

Canadian Endangered Species Coalition; 800-267-4088; ExtinctionSucks.Org;
Zoology.UBC.CA/~Otto/Biodiversity/CESC.html

Canadian Great Ape Alliance, Great-Apes.Com

CarnivoreConference.Org

Cayman Turtle Farm, POB 645 GT, Grand Cayman, British West Indies; 345-949-3894; Turtle.KY

Center for Great Apes, Prime-Apes.Org

Center for the Expansion of Fundamental Rights, CEFR.Org

Centro de Rescate y Rehabilitación de Primates, MACACOS.CL

The Chimpanzee Collaboratory, ChimpCollaboratory.Org

The Chimpanzee and Human Communication Institute, Central Washington University, CWU.Edu/~CWUCHCI/

The Chimpanzee Collaboratory, Washington, DC; ChimpColLaboratory.Org

Chimpanzee Cultures, Chimp.ST-And.AC.UK/Cultures

Chimps-Inc.Org

China Bear Rescue, AnimalsAsia.Org/Index.PHP?Module=2&1g=EN

Citizens for Animal Rights of Eastern Iowa, CARE-IA.Org

Coalette's Connection for Action, CCForAction.Com

Coalition of Animal Rights Education, Purdue University, IN; StudentVeg.Com

Compassionate Action for Animals, POB 13149, Minneapolis, MN 55414; CA4A.Org

Compassion in World Farming, CIWF.Org.UK
   Anna and Peter Roberts, farmers who became vegetarians, started this organization. Appalled by the way farm animals were being treated, they successfully worked to outlaw veal and sow gestation grates in England.

CornwallWildlifeTrust.Org.UK

Doris Day Animal League, DDAL.Org

Desert Tortoise Council, POB 1738, Palm Desert, CA 92261; DesertTortoise.Org

Endangered Primate Rescue Center, PrimateCenter.Org

The Endangered Species Coalition, 1101 14th St., NW, Ste. 1400, Washington,

D.C. 20005; 202-682-9400; StopExtinction.Org

Elephant Nature Park, Thailand, ElephantNaturePark.Org
   In 1900 there were an estimated 10,000,000 elephants on the planet. As of 1995 there were an estimated 400,000. In the past three decades there has been a decrease of about 1/3 of the world's population of elephants. Despite a 1989 global ban on killing elephants for the ivory tusks, the killing continues.

FactoryFarming.Com

FactoryFarming.Org.UK

Farm Animal Reform Movement (FARM), POB 30654, Bethesda, MD 20824; 888-FARM-USA; FarmUSA.Org

Farmed Animal Watch; AnimalPlace.Org; FarmedAnimal.Net

Farm Animal Welfare Network, Iowa City, IA; IowaFawn@Yahoo.Com

Farm Sanctuary, POB 150, Watkins Glen, NY 14891; 607-583-2225; POB 1065, Orland, CA 95963; 530-865-4617; FarmSanctuary.Org; FactoryFarming.Com; NoVeal.Org

FaunaFoundation.Org

FirePaw.Org

Florida Voices for Animals, POB 17523, Tampa, FL; FloridaVoicesForAnimals.Org

Food Animal Concerns Trust (FACT), POB 14599, Chicago, IL 60614; 773-525-4952; FACT.Com

Dian Fossey Fund, The Gorilla Organization, DianFossey.Org/Home/

Friends of Animals, 777 Past Rd., Darien, CT 06820; 230-656-1522; FriendsOfAnimals.Org

FriendsOfWashoe.Org

The Fund for Animals, 200 W. 57th St., Ste. 705, New York, NY 10019; 888-405-FUND; FundForAnimals.Org

Fund for Wild Nature, POB 42523, Portland, OR 97242; FundForWildNature.Org

Georgia Animal Rights and Protection; GARPAtlanta.Org

The Jane Goodall Institute, 8700 Georgia Ave., Ste. 500, Silver Spring, MD 20910; 240-645-4000; JaneGoodall.Org

> "Chimpanzees suffer in captivity... imprisoned, in the name of science, in tiny barren cages. I am haunted by dull, blank eyes staring out onto a world that offers them no hope. The least I can do is speak out for them. They cannot speak for themselves."
> — Jane Goodall

The Gorilla Foundation, Gorilla.Org

Gorilla-Haven.Org

Gorilla Help Site, Kilimanjaro.Com/Gorilla/

Grassroots Animal Rights Conference, GrassrootsAR.Org

GreatApeProject.Org

The Great Ape Project – Brazil, ProjectoGAP.Com.BR

Great Apes Survival Project of the United Nations Environment Programme, UNEP.Org/Grasp

The Great Ape World Heritage Species Project, 4GreatApes.Com

Green People, GreenPeople.Org
Listings of animal protecting organizations.

GreenPets.Com

Greyhound Protection League, Greyhounds.Org

> "Far from the cheers of the crowd, thousands of greyhounds who don't finish 'in the money' are often sold or donated to schools and laboratories for experimentation, dissection, and surgical training.
> In the U.S. each year, an estimated 20,000 to 30,000 greyhounds are killed, including thousands of puppies."
> — New England Anti-Vivisection Society, NEAVS.Org

Humane Farming Association, POB 3577, San Rafael, CA 94912; 415-485-1495; HFA.Org

The Humane Society Legislative Fund, Fund.Org/Index.html

The Humane Society of the United States, HSUS.Org

Hunt Saboteurs Association, HuntSabs.Org.UK

In Defense of Animals, 131 Camino Alto, Mill Valley, CA 94941; IDAUSA.Org

In Defense of Animals – Africa, IDA-Africa.Org

The International Fund for Animal Welfare, IFAW.Org/IFAW/General

International Primate Protection League, IPPL.Org

The International Union for Conservation and Natural Resources, World Conservation Union, IUCN.Org

Ironwood Pig Sanctuary, Marana, AZ, IronPigSanctuary.Org

Journal of International Wildlife Law and Policy, JIWLP.Com

Jumping Frog Research Institution, POB 1416, Angels Camp, CA 95222; JumpingFrog.Org

Last Chance for Animals, LCAnimal.Org

Leicestershire Primate Concern, LeicPrimateConcern.FSNET.CO.UK

Liberation Magazine, Liberation-Mag.Org.UK

Lubee Bat Conservancy, Lubee.Org

Lucky Parrot Refuge & Sanctuary, POB 110334, Naples, FL 34018-0106; LuckyParrot.Org

Mercy for Animals, MercyForAnimals.Org

Mindy's Memory Primate Sanctuary, MindysMem.Org

Mona Foundation, FundAcionMona.Org/Final/English/

Monkey World Ape Rescue Center, MonkeyWorld.CO.UK/Main.pnp

National Audubon Society, 700 Broadway, New York, NY 10003; 212-979-3000; Audubon.Org

The National Sanctuary for Retired Research Primates, PrimateSanctuaryNSRRP.Org/

National Wildlife Federation, NWF.Org/NWF

New England Anti-Vivisection Society, 333 W. Washington St., Ste. 850, Boston, MA 02108-5100; NEAVES.Org; ReleaseChimps.Org

No Compromise, 740 A 14th St., San Francisco, CA 94114; 831-425-3007; NoCompromise.Org

NoPuppyMills.Com

OpposeCruelty.Org

Orange County People for Animals, OCPAUSA.Org

Orangutan Conservancy, Orangutan.Com

Orangutan Foundation International, Orangutan.Org

OranUtanRepublik.Org

PawProject.Org
Do not declaw a cat! Declawing cats is a disgusting and torturous procedure that mutilates the highly sensitive toes of the cat. A cat that has been declawed will not be able to defend itself, is more likely to bite and attack, and will experience bone misalignment and other health problems. Work to make cat declawing illegal. The Paw Project has produced a documentary titled *Cat Fight: Exposing the Brutal Secrets of Veterinary Medicine.*

Peaceful Prairie Sanctuary, Dear Trail, CO; PeacefulPrairie.Org

People Against Chimpanzee Experimentation, PACE.Care4Free.Net

People for the Ethical Treatment of Animals, 501 Front St., Norfolk, VA 23510; 757-622-PETA; PETA-Online.Org

PetCoSucks.Com

Pigs Peace Sanctuary, POB 155, Arlington, WA 98223; 360-435-5435; PigsPeace.Org

Poplar Spring Animal Sanctuary, POB 507, Poolesville, MD 20837; 301-428-8128; AnimalSanctuary.Org

Primate Rescue Center, PrimateRescue.Org

Project R&R: Release and Restitution for Chimpanzees in U.S. Laboratories, ReleaseChimps.Org

RedPandaProject.Org

RhinoRescue.Org

Rhino-Trust.Org.NA

Rocky Mountain Animal Defense, Boulder, CO; RMAD.Org

RomaniaAnimalRescue.Com

San Diego Animal Rights Advocates, AnimalAdvocates.Org

Save Animals from Exploitation, SAFE.Org.NZ

SaveTheChimps.Org

SaveTheRhino.Org

SaveTheSheep.Com

"Most people have no idea that sheep raised for wool are often mutilated and castrated without painkillers, then disposed of by being shipped thousands of miles on open-deck, multitiered ships through all weather extremes, and eventually slaughtered while fully conscious... There are plenty of durable, stylish, and warm fabrics available that aren't made from animal skins. Please join the millions of people who know that compassion is the fashion. Save a sheep – don't buy wool."

Save Vietnam Primates, Coombs.ANU.Edu.AU/~Vern/Hnu/Primates.html

SaveWildElephants.Com

SaveZooElephants.Com

Shac7.Com, NJARA, PO Box 174, Englishtown, NJ 07726
Learn about how the government is working against the free speech of those working to shut down animal testing (torture) labs, and how there have been laws passed to protect corporations at any cost to the point of imprisoning those who speak out against horrible business practices and grotesque animal abuse.

"Militant activism took a blow when six activists from the Stop Huntingdon Animal Cruelty (SHAC) campaign received the first ever conviction under the 1992 Animal Enterprise Protection Act and were sentenced to years in prison. Their campaign aimed to shut down the notorious Huntingdon Life Sciences laboratory. It was initially inspired

by undercover video that showed a Huntingdon scientist punching a beagle puppy in the face, and a monkey on a Huntingdon operating table with her chest cut wide open, conscious and lifting her head. Acts against Huntingdon and associated companies included pipe bombings and notes sent to employees threatening their children. The SHAC prisoners were not charged with or convicted of those acts but with running a Web site that was alleged to have encouraged or inspired them."
  — **DawnWatch.Com; December 2006**

"The term Green Scare refers to the Red Scares of the early twentieth century, made famous by the McCarthy hearings and the House Un-American Activities Committee. The Green Scare demonstrates a similar systematic criminalization of dissent as the U.S. government is using all its tactics (e.g., grand juries, specialized legislation, paid agents provacateurs) to target the radical environmental and animal rights movements, those who publicly support them, and others who struggle for a healthy, diverse eco-system and the rights of animals."
  — **Shac7.Com**

Showing Animals Respect and Kindness, Geneva, IL; SHARKOnline.Org

Sinapu, 1911 11th St., Ste. 103, Boulder, CO 80302; 303-447-8655; Sinapu.Org
  Named after the Ute word for wolves. Dedicated to the restoration and protection of native carnivores and their wild habitat in the Southern Rockies, and connected high plains and deserts.

Society and Animals Forum, Psychologists for the Ethical Treatment of Animals, PSYETA.Org

STOP Hunting and Trapping on National Wildlife Refuges; Refuges.Org
  Unbeknownst to most Americans, recreational hunting and trapping are allowed — even encouraged — on more than half of the nation's 540 national wildlife refuges.

Stop Primate Experiments at Cambridge, POB 6712, Northampton, NN2 6XR, England; PrimatePrison.Org

Stray Cat Alliance, FeralCatAlliance.Org

Student Animal Rights Alliance, DefendAnimals.Org

Sumatran Orangutan Society, Orangutans-SOS.Org

TakingActionForAnimals.Org

Tribe of Heart, POB 149, Ithaca, NY 14851; 607-275-0806; TribeOfHeart.Org

The Turtle Foundation, Turtle-Foundation.Org

Turtle Trax, Turtles.Org

Tusk Trust, Tusk.Org

United Poultry Concerns, POB 150, Machipongo, VA 23405-0150; 757-678-7875; UPC-Online.Org

US McLibel Support Campaign, POB 62, Craftsbury, VT 05826-0062; 802-586-9628; E-mail and listserve DBriars@World.STD.Com; McSpotlight.Org

Viva USA, POB 4398, Davis, CA 95617; VivaUSA.Org
Works on behalf of animals killed for food.

WegmansCruelty.Com
About egg farm conditions.

Wildlife Conservation Society – Congo, WCS-Congo.Org/About/About.htm

Wildlife Rescue and Rehabilitation, Inc., Kendalia, TX 78027, Wildlife-Rescue.Org

Woodstock Farm Animal Sanctuary, WoodstockFAS.Org

World Animal Net Constitution Project, WorldAnimal.Net/Constiution.htm

The World of Chimpanzees, Jinrui.Zool.Kyoto-U.AC.JP/ChimpHome/ChimpanzeeE.html

World Society for the Protection of Animals, London, WSPA.Org.UK

The Xerces Society, 4828 SE Hawthorne Blvd., Portland, OR 97215-3252; Xerces.Org

Zoopharmacognosy, Jinrui.Zool.Kyoto-u.ac.jp/CHIMPP/ CHIMPP.html
Article about the medicinal use of plants by chimpanzees in the world.

B-12 Vitamin Sources

B-12 comes from microorganisms. It is good to include several sources of B-12 in the diet so that there is no possibility of B-12 deficiency. Nutritional yeast is often given as a good source of B-12.

Where do vegans get B-12?

- Algae: Spirulina, wild blue green algae, etc.
- Fermented seed cheeses containing nutritional yeast.
- Intestinal flora: The good bacteria in your digestive tract.
- Kimchi: A fermented vegetable salad. Best if made using raw, unheated, organically grown ingredients. See Sauerkraut, below.
- Nama shoyu: A raw, fermented, soy sauce-like product made with wheat, soy beans, salt, and a bacterial starter. (Only buy if it says it is raw, and has not been heated. Although the product is made using cooked wheat and soy, the sauce is the product of months of fermentation, which results in a vat of enzymes, amino acids, good bacteria, and other nutrients, including B-12.)
- Nutritional yeast: Grown on mineral-enriched molasses. It is also rich in other B-complex vitamins as well as in amino acids. Nutritional yeast is NOT baker's yeast, which is different.
- Rejuvelac: See the Rejuvelac section in this book.
- Organically grown raw fruits and vegetables: Soil organisms are on the leaves and skins of these.
- Sauerkraut: A fermented cabbage salad that may also contain other vegetables. It should be made using raw, unheated, organically grown ingredients. Sauerkraut sold in your market is likely to have been pasteurized, which kills the enzymes and bacteria. Sauerkraut is relatively easy to make. Some natural foods stores now sell raw sauerkraut. If you happen to live near a raw restaurant, they may have it on their menu, or may make it for you if you request it several days in advance.
- Sea vegetables: Dulse, nori, kelp, wakame, etc.
- Wheat, barley, and other grass juices made from grass grown in soil.
- Vegan B-12 supplements: For those who have any concern at all that they are not getting enough B-12 through their food choices. Companies that make vegan B-12 supplements include Freeda, Nature's Bounty, Solgar, and Veg Life.

The lack of B-12 could lead to hyperhomocystemia, which is a condition defined by an elevated level of homocystine in the blood, which can lead to heart disease and stroke. Vitamin B-12 deficiency can also cause fatigue, depression, upper respiratory infection, nerve damage, and anemia. Most people get enough B-12 to avoid these health issues.

Dr. Michael Greger, DrGreger.Org

Dr. Michael Klapper, VegSource.Com/Klaper/

VeganHealthStudy.Com

VeganSociety.Com/html/Food/Nutrition/B12/

Baby Care Books:

- *Mother's Pearls: The Revival of Parenthood*, by Chava Dagan
- *Primal Mothering in a Modern World*, by Hygeia Halfmoon, Ph.D.
- *Transitioning to Health: A Step-by-Step Guide for You and Your Family*, by Beth Montgomery

Since they came on the market in the 1960s, disposable diapers have grown into a major ecological concern with some municipalities reporting that disposable diapers take up as much as 2 percent of their landfill space. By the year 2000 it was estimated that diaper manufacturing was using an estimated 250,000 trees (for wood pulp fiber), and up to 100,000 tons of plastic.

Some brands of disposable diapers contain toxic chemicals that may cause cancers, glandular disorders, breathing difficulties, and learning disabilities, as well as damage to the environment and wildlife. These chemicals, including what are called volatile organic compounds (VOCs), include dopentene, ethylbenzene, toluene, and xylene, are not only absorbed into the tissues of the baby, but also end up in the environment as the disposable diapers break down. The absorbent filler used in many disposable diapers, sodium polyacrylate, may cause breathing problems. These chemicals are in addition to the heavy metals and solvents that are released into the environment during the manufacturing of disposable diapers as well as in the harvesting, drilling, and production of the raw materials used in the diapers. The pollution caused by the packaging, shipping, and marketing of billions of disposable diapers should not be overlooked when considering the total amount of pollution that disposable diapers cause.

Dioxin is a long-lasting carcinogenic and hormone-disrupting chemical that causes endometriosis. It is a byproduct of chlorine bleaching. It is a concern with both cloth and disposable diapers as it may be present within the diapers, and may react with other chemicals in the diapers. Disposable diaper companies use chlorine bleach in the manufacturing process, and most cloth diapers are made out of bleached fabric. A solution is to use non-chlorine bleached diapers made of organic cotton and/or hemp.

If you use disposable diapers, at least use the brands that are highly biodegradable. Biodegradable diapers are often made from a cornstarch base, and this breaks down faster than other disposable diapers. It is also safer for the environment. But some so-called biodegradable disposable diapers still may contain plastic and other substances that are not truly biodegradable.

Even though cloth diapers are better for the baby, can be used more than 100 times, which is beneficial, and they are more environmentally friendly than disposables, cloth diapers are not free of environmental concerns. They take water to clean, which must be heated and mixed with some sort of cleaning agent. Some people have concluded that cloth diapers cause more pollution than disposable biodegradable diapers because cloth diapers use more water per change, and the cleaning solution and drying methods create more pollution. But these concerns can also be partially addressed by using non-chlorine bleached diapers made of organically grown fabrics; by using cleaning solutions that are both plant based and biodegradable; and by hanging the diapers to dry instead of using a dryer.

Additionally, on the topic of baby care pollution, some of the most commonly used lotions and oils that people put on babies contain derivatives from crude (petroleum) oil. Would you rub petroleum gasoline or diesel fuel on your skin? Then why would you put petroleum-based oils on your baby? Look for baby lotions that contain only plant derivatives, or use organically grown olive, hemp seed, grapeseed, or coconut oil.

> "A baby is born with a need to be loved and never outgrows it."
> — **Frank A. Clark**

Eating a healthful diet is particularly important for expectant mothers, as well as women who believe that they may soon become pregnant. As the fetus depends on nutrients from the mother, if the mother's system has a lack of certain nutrients, the fetus is affected.

Because all of the tissues that become the whole baby are formed in the womb, the mother's diet has a huge influence on every area of that formation, from the heart and brain to the bones and what will become the teeth. This is why it is important for soon-to-be pregnant, and pregnant mothers to truly eat the foods of the highest nutritional quality.

> "Yoga improvements in pregnancy outcomes include increased blood flow to the placenta, decreased transfer of maternal stress hormones, and decreased premature release of hormones that trigger the onset of labor."
> — *Journal of Alternative and Complimentary Medicine;* May 2005

Love, be kind to, protect, and nurture your baby with gentle hugs, good words, encouragement, nice music, pleasant stories, and excellent nutrition.

BabyWorks.Com

ChooseyDiapers.Com

EarthBaby.Com

EcoBaby.Com

GreenPeople.Org/Search2nd.cfm?type=Baby_Care
Site lists a slew of companies and information having to do with natural baby care around the world, including organic baby clothing, bedding, diapers, skin care, and toys.

InOtherWords.Org
Women's books and resources.

Mothering.Com

MotherSNature.Com
Mothers sharing information about baby care.

National Association of Diaper Services, DiaperNet.Org

NaturalBaby-Catalog.com

Nature Boy & Girl, Gamlavärmdövägen 10, 13137 Nacka, Sweden; +46-8-6449696; Naty.SE/
Sells diapers that are fully biodegradable because even the plastic is made from corn, and not from petroleum.

SeventhGen.Com

Tushies.Com
Uses hydrogen peroxide instead of chlorine bleach in their wood pulp processing.

Bags: Use Cloth, Not Paper or Plastic

- In New York City alone one less grocery bag per person per year would reduce waste by five million pounds and save $250,000 in disposal costs.
- Plastic bags carry 80 percent of the nation's groceries, up from 5 percent in 1982.
- When one ton of paper bags is reused or recycled, three cubic meters of landfill space is saved and 13 to 17 trees are spared. In 1997, there were 955,000 tons of paper bags used in the United States.
- When one ton of plastic bags is reused or recycled, the energy equivalent of 11 barrels of oil are saved.
  - SierraClub.Org/Bags/Index.asp

Did you know that there are billions of plastic shopping bags used in California every year alone? According to *National Geographic*, somewhere between 500 billion and a trillion plastic shopping bags are used worldwide every year. Many of these bags end up as litter, clogging water systems, flapping in bushes, trees and landscapes, and playing a part in the death of wildlife. Many of the plastic bags can take more than 1,000 years to decompose.

In January 2002, Bangladesh put a complete ban on store plastic bag use. Many shoppers have gone back to using fabric bags made out of the fiber of the jute plant. And that is where the cloth shopping bags got their nickname, even though most are made of other fabrics.

In 2002, Ireland markets started charging 15¢ for each shopping bag a customer uses. Since this law went into effect, many stores in Ireland have reported that their bag use has decreased by over 95 percent. (Mindfully.Org/Plastic/Laws/Plastic-Bag-Levy-Ireland4Mar02.htm)

Imagine how many bags could be eliminated if people would simply used cloth shopping bags! Even better if those shopping bags were made out of pure plant fabrics, such as from jute, hemp, sisal, ramie, or flax.

If you can't make a cloth shopping bag, or purchase one at your local store, you can order one through one of the following companies (order several, and give them away to friends):

Carbon Canyon Hemp Company, Seattle, WA; CarbonCanyonHemp.Com/catalog/item/1423414/913189.htm
Sells at least one type of hemp shopping bag.

ChicoBag.Com

Earthwise Reusable Bags, EarthWiseBags.com

Ecobags.Com, 800-720-2247; Ecobags.Com
Ecobags sells a variety of bags in various shapes, sizes, and fabrics made of organic cotton and/or hemp (including mesh fabric).

Environ Gentle, 543 S. Coast Hwy. 101, Encinitas, CA 92024; EnviroGentle.Com

GreenBag.Info
Sells a variety of shopping bags, including one that folds and zips into a small pocket.

GreenFeet, 1360 E. 1st Ave., Chico, CA, 95926; 888-562-887 [U.S. only]; 530-894-5255; GreenFeet.Com/Hemp-Shopping-Bag.html

HempBags.Com

Hemp Basics, 888-831-3747; HempSupply.Com/bags/2101.asp
Sells a hand-crocheted hemp shopping bag.

Hemp Utopia, 22256 100th Ave., Langley, British Columbia, Canada, V1M 3V5; Canada-Shops.Com/Stores/HempUtopia

ReusableBags.Com; 888-707-3873
Sells a variety of cloth shopping bags, including those made from organic cotton and hemp.

Shopping.Com, Shopping.Com/xGS-Hemp_Shopping_Bag~NS-1~Linkin_id-3068575
Sells a variety of cloth shopping bags that are more stylized than most others.

Sunfood Nutrition, 11653 Riverside Dr., Lakeside, CA 92040; 800-205-2350; 888-RAW-FOOD; International: +001-619-596-7979; 888-raw-food; Sunfood.Com
Sells a sturdy hemp/cotton blend shopping bag.

VeganEssentials.Com, VeganEssentials.Com/Catalog/Hemp-Shopping-Bag.htm
Sells hemp shopping bags, backpacks, and totes in various styles, including some partially made of recycled materials.

Bamboo: The Environmentally Safe Wood Alternative

Also see:
• Building Materials and Supplies

Books:
• *Bamboo Construction Manual*, O. H. Lopez
• *Designing and Building with Bamboo*, Jules A. Janssen
• *Grow Your Own House: Simon Velez and Bamboo Architecture*, Simon Velez

Bamboo is a fast-growing, renewable, environmentally safe alternative to wood. It can be used for paper, furniture, flooring, fences, countertops, and cutting boards. It is stronger than concrete, and has a similar tensile strength-to-weight ratio as steel. It is a food and medicine, and bamboo fiber can be made into fabric. The growing plants can be used to prevent soil erosion, to create a wind block for farms and gardens, and to provide oxygen while absorbing air pollution. It can be used to make beautiful musical instruments, including flutes, organs, and the bases of drums, as well as the sticks to play the drums. Some types of bamboo grow more than 50 feet in a season. In comparison, it takes a tree decades to grow the same amount of marketable material that a bamboo plant can provide in less than a year.

American Bamboo Society, AmericanBamboo.Org

"Bamboo is just grass, but it varies in height from dwarf, one foot (30 cm) plants to giant timber bamboos that can grow to over 100 feet (40 m). It grows in a lot of different climates, from jungles to high on mountainsides... Bamboo is both decorative and useful. In many parts of the world it is food, fodder, the primary construction material and is used for making a great variety of useful objects from kitchen tools to paper to dinnerware."

ASOSISMica.Org

Bamboo Buzz, 503-351-7143; Canby.Com/BambooBuzz

BambooDirect.Com

BambooOfTheAmericas.Org

Bamboo.Org

Bamboo Web, Kauai.Net/BambooWeb/Bamboo.html

Bamboo2000.Com
Bamboo flooring.

BambuHome.Com

BuildingGreen.Com

Deboer Architecture, DeboerArchitects.Com/BambooThoughts.html

Environmental Bamboo Foundation, POB 196, Ubud 80571, Bali, Indonesia; 62-361-974-027; BambooMan.Com.AU/BambooTreatment/EBF.php

International Bamboo Foundation, BambooCentral.Org

International Network of Bamboo and Rattan, POB 100102-86, Beijing, 100102, PR China; INBAR.Int

PandaBamboo.Com

Smith & Fong, 866-835-9859; PlyBoo.Com
Bamboo plywood.

WFIBamboo.Com

Battery Recycling

Also see:
• Electronics Recycling

Batteries contain heavy metals and other toxic substances. If you use batteries, please do not throw them into the trash. Instead, take them to a battery recycling center.

Want to help prevent pollution caused by disposable batteries? Start a used battery collection box in your community.

BatteryRecycling.Com

Earth911.Org

RBRC.Org

Beds and Bedding

Also see:
• Paints and finishes

Consider for a moment how many beds there are on this planet. Now consider how long those beds last, how often they are thrown away, and how much pollution this causes. Those beds that contain springs and other metal parts as well as plastics and synthetic fabrics made from petroleum create an enormous amount of pollution.

Many beds are also made with bed frames made out of tree wood treated with and/or coated with toxic preservatives and finishes that are not a good choice for those interested in sustainable materials and protecting the environment. A better choice would be bed frames made out of bamboo wood or compressed hemp fiberboard, which are both sustainable and biodegradable.

Now consider how long you spend sleeping every day. Would you rather be surrounded by nontoxic materials during this important time when your body is at rest?

Safe choices in bedding include futons, pillows, and fabrics that contain no metals, plastics, or petroleum-derived fabrics or chemicals. Safe fabrics include those made from organically grown cotton, sisal, flax, jute, ramie, bamboo, and hemp.

For information on safe bedding, see the sections in this book headed Bamboo, Cotton, and Hemp.

AbundantEarth.Com

Coyuchi.Com

EcoChoices.Com

Gaiam.Com

GreenSleep.Com

HeartOfVermont.Com

LifeKind.Com

NaturalHighLifestyle.Com

NaturesBedroom.Com

NonToxic.Com

TribalFiber.Com

WhiteLotus.Net

Biking

Books:

- *Asphalt Nation: How the Automobile Took Over America, and How We Can Take It Back*, by Jane Holtz Kay
- *Divorce Your Car! Ending the Love Affair with the Automobile*, by Katie Alvord

It is estimated that
- Americans make about 125 MILLION CAR TRIPS EACH DAY that are within two miles of their homes.
- 33 percent of all trips in Amsterdam are made by bike.
- Less than .5 percent of all trips in Los Angeles are made by bike.
- 27 tons of trash is created to manufacture one car.

According to a report by *Environmental Defense* published in June 2006, Americans own 30 percent of the 700 million cars in use on the planet, and emit nearly half of the carbon dioxide (greenhouse gasses) caused by the world's automobiles. Americans cars and light trucks traveled about 2.6 trillion miles in 2004, which equals 470 trips back and forth to and from Pluto. About one third of the global warming toxins spewed by American cars, light trucks, and SUVs came from those made by General Motors, the biggest seller of vehicles in the U.S. Because there are more small vehicles than there are SUVs, it is the smaller vehicles that create the most amounts of environmentally damaging gasses, and part of the reason for this is that there are many older small vehicles that get low gas mileage.

Meanwhile, the car industry keeps fighting every step of the way to prevent laws being put into effect that would place limits on the amount of toxins vehicles can emit.

"Getting kids to ride their bikes just half an hour each day helps them to burn hundreds of calories a week and reduces their risk of developing Type 2 diabetes by up to 50 percent."
  — **These Roads Were Made for Biking**, by Linda Baker; *OnEarth* **magazine, Summer 2006**

By riding a bike instead of driving a car:
- You don't pollute the air.
- You slow global warming.
- You don't have to pay for parking.
- You aren't using or paying for gas.
- You aren't paying for car insurance.
- You aren't making car payments.
- You aren't paying for car repairs or maintenance.
- You can whiz past traffic jams.
- You have a better connection to your community.
- You can quickly stop by places.
- You are getting exercise.

Did you know that one gallon of used motor oil can pollute one million gallons of water?

Did you know that 43,000 Americans were killed in automobile accidents in 2005?

Adventure Cycling Association, 150 E. Pine St., Missoula, MT 59807; 800-721-8719; AdventureCycling.Org

American Cycling Association, 7781 E. Jarvis Pl., Denver, CO 80237; 303-458-5538; AmericanCycling.Org

Ashland Community Bike Program, Ashland, Oregon; AshlandFreeSkool@Hotmail.Com

Better World Club, 20 NW 5th Ave., #100, Portland, OR 97210; BetterWorldClub.Com

Provides everything from an "auto club" membership for roadside assistance for bikes and cars; auto insurance for the environmentally minded traveler; maps and travel services aimed at eco-travel; car rental discounts; and discounts for owners of hybrid vehicles.

Bicycle Civil Liberties Union, BCLU.Org

BicycleKitchen.Com

Bicycle Paper, 68 S. Washington St., Seattle, WA 98104; BicyclePaper.Com

Bicycle Transportation Alliance, BTA4Bikes.Org

Bicycling magazine, Magazine-Director.Com/Bicycling.htm

BikeLeague.Org

BikeNow.Org

BikeRides.Com

BikesBelong.Org

BikeSummer.Org

Boston bike maps, CityOfBoston.Gov/Transportation/Bike.asp

CarFree.Com

Chicago bike map, CityOfChicago.Org/Transportation/BikeMap

Citizens of the Road, EasyToShare.Com

Critical Mass, Critical-Mass.Org
    Biking, bikers' rights, biker documentaries, city biking events, biking activist posters and fliers, information about reversing car culture: the trend to purchase cars, rely on them, and build roads for them. There are Critical Mass groups in many cities around the world.

Culture Change, Fossil Fuels Policy Action, POB 4347, Arcata, CA 95518; 707-826-7775; CultureChange.Org
    Formerly the *Auto-Free Times*, this publication covers issues relating to energy consumption, the paving over of land with roads, parking lots, and buildings, and other issues relating to the damage caused by a society that relies on engines and on the fossil fuels to run them. It focuses on alternatives to sprawl and petroleum dependence while fighting new road construction and designing creative alternatives to auto addiction.

> "At the turn of this century there was little or no asphalt paving. Now there are millions of square miles of it. In many metropolitan areas the square footage of asphalt is many times greater than the square footage of what is left there of the natural Earth.
>   Next summer go stand in the grass with no shoes on. Then walk out onto the pavement on a hot day and you will see what I am getting at."

CycleSantaMonica.Org

Cyclists Inciting Change through Live Exchange, Cicle.Org

LAPostCarbon.Org

League of American Cyclists, BikeLeague.Org/Coqs/Resources/FindIt/Index.php

Los Angeles bike map, LABikePaths.Com

Los Angeles County Bike Coalition; 634 S. Spring, Suite 821, Los Angeles, CA 90014; LABikeCoalition.Org

Midnight Ridazz, Sports.Groups.Yahoo.Com/Group/Ridazz/
A growing number of Los Angeles-area bicyclists meeting once a month for an all-night bike rides. Similar groups are forming in other cities.

New York area bike maps, TransAlt.Org/Map

Ohio Bicycle Federation, OhioBike.Org
Site contains a lot of links to other bike organizations.

Portland City Repair Project, CityRepair.Org

Raging Bike; RagingBike.CO.UK
An England-based Web site where people post their rants about their biking experiences. Also contains environmental news.

San Francisco bike map, SFBike.Org

Seattle bike map, CI.Seattle.WA.US/Transportation/BikeMaps.htm

Velo Vision, The Environmental Community Center, St. Nicholas Fields, York; YO13-3EN UK; Calhoun Cycle, 3342 Hennepin Ave., S., Minneapolis, MN 55408; 612-827-8000; CalhounCycle.Com; VeloVision.CO.UK

World Car-Free Network, WorldCarFree.Net

WorldNakedBikeRide.Org

XtraCycle SUB, 888-537-1401; XtraCycle.Com
The world's first sport utility bicycle meant for carrying large loads, such as groceries and work gear.

Biodegradable

Biodegradable products are becoming more common on store shelves. They are those that degrade into soil, and leave no harmful residues in the environment.

The Biodegradable Products Institute, BPIWorld.Org/BPI-Public

Recyclaholics.Com

Biofuels

Also see:
- Hemp
- Peak Oil

Books:
- *Biodiesel America: How to Achieve Energy Security, Free America from Middle-east Oil Dependence and Make Money Growing Fuel*, by Josh Tickell
- *From the Fryer to the Fuel Tank: The Complete Guide to Using Vegetable Oil as an Alternative Fuel*, by Joshua Tickell
- *Powerdown: Options for a Post-Carbon World*, by Richard Heinberg

Documentary:
- *Who Killed the Electric Car?* In 1996 electric cars started appearing on the roads – especially in California where the state had set a goal to create a market for zero emissions vehicles. Ten years later, the electric vehicles were almost entirely gone as they were taken back and crushed by the cars' makers who would only lease the vehicles. Watch this documentary to get an idea of the corruption carried out by the oil companies and the G. W. Bush administration.

One day I was on a very long jog on a road in the coastal rainforest area of the Big Island of Hawaii when I heard the distant sound of a diesel engine. I dreaded that the diesel engine was going to ruin the air for my jog. But when the car finally drove past, all I could smell were French fries. It was a diesel engine running on fryer oil.

Biofuel is a fuel that is not fossilized, or that is made up of a mix of fossil- and plant-based fuels, including corn, soy, sugar cane, hemp, palm, flax, rapseed, switchgrass, or canola, and even lawn clippings. Used restaurant fryer oil can also be utilized as a biofuel in diesel vehicles. Running engines on 100 percent plant-based fuel is carbon-neutral, which results in cleaner air.

Petroleum (gasoline and diesel) and coal are fossil fuels.

Biodiesel is a mix of diesel fuel with plant oil. It releases about 40 percent fewer emissions than regular diesel fuel, and is safer for the environment in all areas. Producing biofuel locally makes us less dependent on foreign oil (and all the problems that can lead to), creates jobs where it is produced, and reduces the trade deficit.

Landscape clippings are the most widely produced plant substance in America, but nearly all of them get thrown in the garbage, which ends up in landfills.

Biofuels can be used to reduce pollution, and can run all sorts of engines, from trucks and buses to boats and generators.

Rudolph Diesel, inventor of the diesel engine, designed his engine to run on plant oils, not on petroleum fuel, which he considered to be a filthy fuel. When he demonstrated his engine, he used peanut oil. He considered hemp seed oil to be the ideal fuel for the engine he invented.

Henry Ford also meant for his cars to run on plant fuels in the form of ethanol, and not on petroleum gasoline. Ford also wanted the bodies of his cars to be made out of fiberglass made from plants, including hemp, and not out of metal. He viewed the mining of metal to be environmentally destructive and wanted the metal parts in his cars to be limited.

Imagine what the world would be like if we didn't use petroleum fuels for cars or trucks and instead used low-polluting ethanol and plant oils!

A study conducted by Cornell University determined that refining corn-based ethanol burns 29 percent more fossil-fuel energy than the amount of energy that is produced by the fuel. Ethanol replacement of regular gasoline reduces greenhouse gas emissions by about 12 percent.

A study released in July 2006 concluded that soybean biodiesel yields a 93 percent return on the energy used to produce it, and that ethanol's return is 25 percent. The study also concluded that if all of the corn and soybeans grown for human consumption in the U.S. were used for fuel instead, the crops would produce only 11 percent of gasoline and less than 9 percent of diesel.

Corn-based ethanol also is not the most environmentally sound fuel. Nor is soybean oil. The way most corn and soybean crops are grown uses a tremendous amount of fossil fuel fertilizers and other toxic farm chemicals that are not good for the environment, and help cause dead zones in the ocean, extreme storms, and global warming. Corn is the most tax-subsidized crop, and the corn industry is currently experiencing tremendous growth as the demand for ethanol increases. While soy releases lower rates of nitrogen, and phosphorus and fewer pesticides are used on it than corn, soy is still not the best crop to grow for fuel.

We need to do better than that. We need to legalize hemp for fuel. Hemp grows faster than corn, provides more biomass per acre than corn, uses fewer resources to cultivate, leaves the soil in better shape than corn, absorbs more heat than corn, absorbs more air pollution per acre than corn, puts out more oxygen per acre than corn, and provides more dietary nutrients than corn.

It is currently illegal to grow hemp in the U.S. and many other countries. The laws need to be changed so that we can grow hemp for fuel oil (to replace petroleum diesel) and for ethanol (to replace petroleum gasoline). It can also be used to replace coal, can be used for food, fabric, fiber, building materials, paint, fiberglass, and furniture. Hemp can help family farmers and their communities become more independent. It can help us to become less dependent on foreign oil. At this stage it is outrageous that we can't grow hemp for industrial uses. Work to change the laws banning industrial hemp farming.

Berkeley Biodiesel Collective, BerkeleyBiodiesel.Org

Better World Club, 20 NW 5th Ave., #100, Portland, OR 97210; BetterWorldClub.Com
  Provides everything from an "auto club" membership for roadside assistance for bikes and cars; auto insurance for the environmentally minded traveler; maps and travel services aimed at eco-travel; car rental discounts; and discounts for owners of hybrid vehicles.

BioBling.Com

BioDieselAmerica.Org

BioDieselCommunity.Org

BioDiesel-CoOp.org

BiodieselNow.Com
  Site contains a link to locations where biofuel is available.

BioDiesel.Org

BioDieselSolutions.Com

BioFuelOasis.Com

BioFuels.Ca

BoulderBioDiesel.Org

ClimateCrisis.Net

CoalitionForCleanAir.Org

EndOfSuburbia.Com

GoldenFuelSystems.Com

GreaseCar.Com

HempCar.Org

HempOilCanada.Com

JourneyToForever.Org

LABioFuel.Com

LiveGreenGoYellow.Com

LoveCraftBioFuels.Com

MakeBioDiesel.Com

Mayors for Climate Change, 436 14th St., Ste. 1520, Oakland, CA 94612; CoolMayors.Org

Piedmont Biofuels, Pittsboro, NC; BiofuelsCoOp
This site provides a good variety of information on how to create biofuels.

PathToFreedom.Com

StopGlobalWarming.Org

SustainableOptions.Com

SustainableTransportClub.Com

TerraPass.Com
Company funds clean energy projects through donations and buyback programs. You can purchase a pollution buyback that is equivalent to the amount of pollution your vehicle creates every year.

VieggieAvenger.Com

Yokayo Biofuels, YBiofuels.Org

Blood Sugar Issues

The human body runs on sugar and oxygen. But the wrong kind of sugar sources can damage the body. Choose to get high-quality sugars into your system through raw plants.

Low-quality sugars can be addictive, and work like a drug by rapidly changing the body chemistry. This happens when a purified sugar, such as corn syrup or white sugar, is consumed and rapidly enters the bloodstream, giving the person a "sugar high." Candy, soda, cake, beer, and similar products that contain large amounts of processed sugar can cause this. In addition, cooked grains as well as cooked hybrid vegetables (beets, carrots, corn, and potatoes) can also lead to a sugar rush.

A person experiencing a sugar rush can then experience the subsequent "hangover" that happens after the hyperinsulization of the blood. Feelings of this hangover include drowsiness, fatigue, and a lack of dietary satisfaction – which leads to more eating, too many calories, and eventually to obesity – with all of its degenerative complications.

The endocrine system becomes overstimulated and can be damaged by a diet that is consistently high in sugar. The bones also suffer on a high-sugar diet as the body relies on the calcium and other alkaline minerals stored in the bones and tissues to alkalize the system.

A sugar rush may also occur when someone drinks beet, carrot, apple, orange, and other types of sweet juices. Many of these fruits and vegetables have been hybridized to increase their sweet taste. Seedless fruits (seedless grapes, seedless oranges, seedless watermelon, etc.) are particularly sweet, not natural, lacking in adequate levels of trace minerals, and carry a less vibrant energy. For this reason people should avoid getting into the habit of drinking lots of sweet juices.

It is better to make the base of a juice drink largely out of something like cucumber and green-leafed vegetables, with a relatively lesser amount of sweet juice added only to adjust the taste. Adding a raw green nutrient powder can help alkalize the juice. Adding the powder of freshly ground raw flax seeds, pumpkin seeds, or hemp seeds to your juice adds high-quality essential fatty acids, amino acids, enzymes, and trace nutrients. Using seeded (as opposed to "seedless") grapes to sweeten a vegetable juice provides some essential fatty acids because these substances are in grapeseeds.

Most everyone presented with a sugarcoated doughnut and a ripe pear would be able to point out what is better for the body. The sugars of processed foods – such as cane sugar and corn syrup – are pure forms of sugar. The sugars available to the body in a piece of fruit are better because they are accompanied by beneficial substances – such as vitamins, trace minerals, and enzymes – and therefore are more healthful for the body.

One way of determining if a fruit is not in its natural state is that the fruit will be seedless – such as seedless watermelon, seedless oranges, seedless grapes, seedless lemons, etc. Look for fruits that contain their seeds. If your natural foods store does not carry them, you may find it helpful to ask the produce manager if they can order some seeded fruit (especially seeded watermelon). Farmers' markets often have farmers who specialize in organically-grown, seeded fruits so you may try your local farmers' markets to find the produce you are seeking (better yet, grow your own!).

If you are someone who followed a high-sugar diet, work to keep your system balanced by consuming plentiful amounts of quality green-leafed vegetables. If you are experiencing health issues such as diabetes and hypoglycemia, and even alcoholism, it is best to avoid all refined sugars, cooked grains, and both cooked and raw overly hybridized fruits and vegetables. Stick to natural (seeded) fruits, and balance the diet with high-quality greens and raw plant fats (olive oil, flax oil, hemp oil, grapeseed oil, pumpkin seed oil, coconut oil, etc.).

> "Refined and hybrid sugars in the form of sucrose actually take water away from the body. In order to break down sucrose into two molecules of glucose, a molecule of water is required. Thus, drinks or smoothies containing refined or hybrid sugar can actually make you thirstier. This is why I believe it is best to rehydrate the body with fresh green-leafed vegetable juice rather than with fruit juice. A juice made from celery and cucumber juices blended with kale is particularly useful in rehydrating the body."
> — **David Wolfe**

Those who are experiencing such conditions as hypoglycemia, diabetes, or candida can find relief in a raw vegan diet. These health conditions are both aggravated and triggered by the consumption of meat, dairy, cooked starches, and processed sugars. Meat and dairy are not good for those with sugar issues because animal flesh and milk contain the body hormonal chemistry of animals, and this clashes with human chemistry. Cooked starchy foods are not good for those with sugar issues because the starch turns into sugar in the system. Processed sugars simply aggravate the system and wreak havoc on the pancreas. All four categories of these foods — meat, dairy, cooked starches, and processed sugars — are not part of the raw vegan diet.

Overly sweet fruits can be a problem for someone whose system has been damaged by the consumption of the five damaging food categories of meat, dairy, cooked starches, heated oils, and processed sugars. Those with blood sugar conditions can greatly improve their health by sticking to a diet consisting of a healthy ratio of raw plant fats, green foods, and the right amount of quality fruits.

Along with diet, physical activity is an important part in bringing health to a person who is experiencing blood sugar issues.

A good example of how a healthful diet can transform health is evident in the Boutenko family.

Sergei Boutenko was diagnosed with diabetes when he was nine years old. This was after he had collapsed when he binged on Halloween candy. Doctors told him that he would be dependent on insulin for the rest of his life. His sister, Valya, had been diagnosed with asthma, couldn't sleep, was having a horrible time in school because she couldn't concentrate, had a bad memory, and could barely read or write. Their father, Igor, suffered from arthritis, and had surgery scheduled for hyperthyroidism. Their mother, Victoria, had a heart condition called arrhythmia, which is an irregular heartbeat. They were overweight, depressed, unhealthy, and things were not good.

Weeks after Sergei's collapse, Victoria was standing in line at a natural foods store when she randomly struck up a conversation with a woman in line, telling her about Sergei's health. The woman told Victoria about the raw vegan diet, and suggested that Victoria read raw vegan books, such as those by natural foods advocate Ann Wigmore.

After Victoria began eliminating meat from Sergei's diet, his health began to improve.

The entire family began to follow a raw vegan diet and their health improved to the point of going off medications, and they no longer depended on doctors.

When they were eating unhealthful foods they had no energy, were overweight, and struggled with boredom and depression. After they began eating only raw vegan cuisine, they had so much energy that they began jogging, their weight dropped, and their moods stabilized.

Valya, who formerly had little interest in school and reading, began to read books cover-to-cover, and her grades greatly improved. She has excelled in many areas, including art, which she now sells (RawFamily.Com/Valya.htm). Along with her brother, she wrote their wonderful recipe book, *Eating Without Heating: Favorite Recipes from Teens Who Love Raw Food*.

> "I didn't know that I was sick until I became healthy. I didn't know that I was sad until I became happy. Who would have thought that something as small as diet could change my life so much! I realize that if we do not change our diets, we will all get sick. It is inevitable. How many completely healthy people do you know? Let us not wait until we have no other choice. Sometimes we try to take the easy way out. There is no easy way. There is only the hard way, and the harder way. We only get one chance to live each moment. Let us never miss a chance to change or do something better right now, because this is the only now we have."
> **— Valya Boutenko, RawFamily.Com**

The Boutenko family has traveled to several continents to teach people about the benefits of raw veganism. They have also become excellent raw vegan chefs. I have visited with them in their home and have been blessed to enjoy food prepared by their hands. They all have a natural gift for preparing amazing foods. Their story is told in the book *Raw Family: A True Story of Awakening*.

Victoria wrote the popular raw vegan book *12 Steps to Raw Foods*. Her latest book, *Green for Life*, does a great job of explaining the importance of green vegetables in the diet to maintain a healthful pH balance. The book details a study conducted by the Boutenko family that involved 27 people who drank one quart of freshly made green smoothie every day for one month. "This project started on April 29, 2005. My whole family took turns blending many gallons of the green drink. Igor drove the valuable load 240 miles round trip, every other day. It was quite a commitment, not only for my family, but also for all the participating people and even their families."

More information about the Boutenko family and the books they have written is available through their Web site, RawFamily.Com; or write Raw Family, POB 172, Ashland, OR 97520. Their books are also available in many natural foods stores.

Sergei conducts Nature hikes; access his Web site at HarmonyHikes .Com.

Brain

When it is taken into consideration that the mind alone can bring disorder to the body (psychosomatic illness), it should also be considered that bad diet (lack of quality nutrients, including a lack of enzymes and of Sun photons from not eating uncooked plant matter) can play a huge role in bringing the brain and body away from health.

A bad diet results in low energy, and this is felt not only through the body, but also within the brain.

A diet that is in alignment with that advocated in this book will help the brain to function better.

A chief culprit working against health is cooked food. Cooked foods lack electrons and clog the system, slowing electrical currents. Cooked fats end up in the cell membranes, where they interfere with the electronic charge essential to cell health throughout all of the tissues.

If you want your brain to function better, then you should eat healthfully and exercise your mind through intellectual stimulation, practice your talents, engage in daily physical activity, and increase your will to improve by setting goals and working to achieve them.

The living enzymes and unheated plant oils of a Sunfood diet are especially beneficial to the function of the brain.

Nearly 4,000 older adult residents of Chicago were studied for six years. It was found that those who consumed two or more servings of vegetables every day had increased mental capacity by about 40 percent. The study was conducted by the Rush University Medical Center's Rush Center for Healthy Aging and was published in the October 24, 2006 issue of *Neurology*, the scientific journal of the American Academy of Neurology. The study concluded that those who did not eat a significant amount of vegetables improved their brain function by increasing their daily intake of vegetables. Another study, the Nurses Health Study, which involved 120,000 nurses, found similar results.

Vitamin E, which is more common in vegetables than in fruits, is beneficial to brain health, as are raw oils, which prevent damage from free-radicals, help transport nutrients, and are needed to maintain healthy cell membranes. Vitamin E, raw oils, and other antioxidants found in raw fruits and vegetables play a part in neuron health.

Victoria Boutenko of RawFamily.Com points out in her book, *Green for Life*, that the essential amino acids found in raw green vegetables are used by the body to produce neurotransmitters "like tyrosine, trypto-phan, glutamine, histamine, and others. Neurotransmitters are the natural chemicals that facilitate communications between brain cells. These substances govern our emotions, memory, moods, behavior, learning abilities, and sleep patterns."

You can choose to eat healthful foods that nourish your brain. With a healthier brain you can think better.

When you eat unhealthful foods, not only are you clogging your system with residues of low-quality foods, you are also limiting your ability to tune into the source that can guide you into a better life.

A bad diet has a particularly negative effect on the hypothalamus, thalamus, and pineal glands in the brain. They are the receivers and managers of information. They are in the center of the brain and nothing in the body goes on without their input.

When a person eats an unhealthful diet, all organs and tissues of the body are negatively affected, including the power center of the brain. Like all parts of the body, the brain gets tarnished by an unhealthful diet, and this lowers one's capabilities.

Your organs, including the brain, cannot function at their full potential if you are not supplying your body with the fuel it needs to function at its full potential.

Think of it this way: When you eat a diet that is not healthful, your organs wither in health, and become saturated in stress and residues that lead to illness. On a healthful diet consisting of raw plant substances, your body becomes saturated in health, and toxic residues are eliminated, allowing your body and brain to function at a higher level.

Since the brain, like all organs, responds to the quality of the diet, it is only natural for an unhealthful diet to result in an unhealthful mind that produces withering thoughts of failure, self-doubt, world-weariness, morbidity, despair, regret, and sorrow.

When a person cleanses the body through following a pure diet, regularly fasting, getting colon hydrotherapy, and working out to eliminate toxins and keep the body tissues in shape, it is greatly beneficial to the brain and all its connected parts, including the hypothalamus, thalamus, and pineal glands. People who lose weight and begin to follow a healthful diet feel lightened, have more energy, and feel they can think more clearly. The person who loses the weight notices it, and the people around them notice it.

When the subconscious mind is burdened, the mind cannot function at a healthy level. Losing excess weight, organizing your life, getting adequate amounts of daily exercise, and eating only healthful food clears the fog from the system by essentially cleaning the circuitry of the mind/body connection.

A diet that is in alignment with that advocated in this book will bring the brain to function better. The living enzymes of a raw vegan diet are especially beneficial to the function of the brain. When one considers that the mind alone can bring disorder to the body (psychosomatic illness), one should also consider that bad diet (lack of quality nutrients, including enzymes and raw essential fatty acids from uncooked plant matter) can play a huge role in bringing the brain and body into a healthy order.

Breeding and Cloning Pets

Millions of dogs and cats are killed each year because they have no homes, because their owners didn't want them, or because they were abused. Even some of the smallest U.S. cities kill more than 10,000 cats and dogs every year. Some dogs and cats that end up in pounds are sold off to science labs for a profit and some are subjected to horrible, terrifying, and torturous experiments. At the same time breeders are breeding cats and dogs to sell to pet stores, to science labs, and to individuals seeking their version of the ideal pet.

Don't support pet breeders. Work to get pet breeding businesses shut down in your area, and stop pet stores from selling dogs and cats.

If you want a pet, adopt one from the pound or an animal shelter.

Work to get spay/neuter services promoted in your community. Get your family, friends, and neighbors to spay or neuter their pets.

Work to get your local animal shelter to provide better services for the animals in their care. Many city animal shelters are horrible places. They need to be redesigned, or moved, to provide natural, open environments that don't traumatize the animals.

Alley Cat Allies, AlleyCat.Org

Best Friends Animal Society, BestFriends.Org

Companion Animal Protection Society, CAPS-Web.Org

Doris Day Animal League, DDAL.Org

Last Chance for Animals, LCAnimal.Org

NoPetCloning.Org

Pet Savers Foundation, PetSavers.Org

PetSmart Charities, PetSmart.Com

Pets911.Com

Prevent a Litter Coalition, PALC.Org

SpayUSA.Org

Building Materials and Supplies

Also see:
- Bamboo
- Beds and Bedding
- Gardening and Farming
- Paints and Finishes

Books:
- *Building With Hemp*, by Steve Allin
- *Good Green Homes*, by Jennifer Roberts
- *Green Building Products*, edited by Mark Piepkorn
- *Green Remodeling: Changing the World One Room at a Time*, by David Johnston and Kim Master
- *The New Ecological Home*, by Dan Chiras
- *Solar Living Source Book: The Complete Guide to Renewable Energy Technologies and Sustainable Living*, edited by John Schaeffer

> "What use is a house if you haven't got a tolerable planet to put it on?"
> — **Henry David Thoreau**

Of course it would be nice if people would work with the structures we already have, and the footprints of the buildings that have already been built, before considering using any more land for houses and buildings.

If you are going to build or remodel a structure, seek out materials and ways of building that do the least amount of damage to the environment.

Be careful of companies that say they are selling green-building products when they are not, but are only working to cash in on this growing market.

When building and remodeling green, consider:
- Tankless hot water systems.
- Low-flow toilet that uses less water.
- Exterior urinal or waterless urinal. Why do we use so much water to simply wash away our urine? The average American flushes away a few thousand gallons of water every year after urinating. An exterior urinal surrounded by bushes or other privacy design and that goes down into a base of pebbles or gravel can save a lot of water. Some places have laws against composting toilets, but urine is not held to the same standards. So, pee outside and save water.
- Graywater systems.
- Rainwater harvesting system.
- Low-impact structures, such as yurts or stilted "tree houses" that don't destroy land.
- Regionally-produced materials that don't have to be shipped long distances.
- Natural insulation from recycled natural fabrics, ground-up newspapers, or hemp fiber.
- Using recycled, second harvested, or fallen wood.
- Wood windows, not vinyl or other toxic materials. Prefab windows may be made from wood treated with petrochemical glues, pesticides, and other toxic substances that off-gas such substances as formaldehyde, which can cause nose and throat cancer. Using windows taken from older structures is one solution, but they must be cleaned of old paint that may contain lead. Learning carpentry or hiring a carpenter to make your windows from scratch may be the best solution.
- Using nontree wood, such as bamboo, hemp fiberboard, etc.
- Solar energy.
- Solar heating.
- Radiant heat using a solar-powered system.
- Natural wax candles (not petroleum wax) with lead-free hemp wicks. See the Candles section in this book.

- Energy-saving light bulbs.
- Reverse osmosis water system.
- Utilizing natural light.
- Nontoxic finishes, plant-based stains, and no-VOC paints
  (VOC = Volatile Organic Compounds: toxic chemicals often found in petroleum paints, thinners, fuels, dry cleaning agents, and hair spray).
- Biodegradable fabrics (hemp, organic cotton, bamboo, jute, ramie, flax, and sisal).
- Laundry hanging lines made from hemp, which naturally resists mold, mildew, and lasts longer in the Sun than other ropes.
- Shower curtain of hemp fabric. Plastic/vinyl shower curtains contain carcinogenic and hormone-disrupting chemicals. As mentioned, hemp fabric is naturally resistant to mold and mildew. Hemp shower curtains last for many years.
- Organic mattresses and/or futons. Keeping your mattress wrapped in a hemp or organic cotton barrier cloth will prolong its life and help prevent bed mites.
- Furniture that is free of foam. Foam is made from petrochemicals, often treated with chemical fire retardants, and degrades into particles that result in toxic dust.
- Nontoxic floor coverings (coconut husk carpet [coir], bamboo flooring, jute, sisal, hemp, sea grass, natural linoleum, etc.).

Bamboo is a popular environmentally sustainable wood for floors, even though it is actually a type of grass. It is twice as strong as oak and harder than maple.

Cork is another alternative flooring material that can also be used as a wall and ceiling covering (helps with sound and insulation). It is hypoallergenic, absorbs sound, resists water, repels insects, and repels fire. It is the bark of trees that is cut off the tree without killing the tree, which simply grows more bark.

Natural linoleum (Marmoleum is one brand) is made of linseed oil, pine rosin, jute, wood flour, and limestone. It repels water, resists mold, and comes in a variety of colors.

If you do want carpeting, seek out those that are free from volatile organic compounds (VOC), and also look for those that are made without polyvinyl chloride (PVC), a known carcinogen. PVC requires large amounts of fossil fuels and chlorine to produce. It leaches dioxin into the environment. PVC is not a good thing. Shaw Carpet of Dalton

Georgia is one that no longer uses PVC in their carpeting.

- Agricultural fiberboard (strawboard, wheatboard, and plyboo [bamboo plywood]) cabinetry. Most particleboard contains formaldehyde, which is classified as a carcinogen, and can lead to allergies, burning eyes, headaches, and nausea. As mentioned earlier, it can also lead to nasal and throat cancers. The U.S. allows formaldehyde-emitting wood to be imported from countries that won't even allow the wood to be sold in their stores. If you purchase plywood or compressed and fabricated wood products, look for those that are free of formaldehyde.

- Natural plasters that use organic and nontoxic substances. Traditional plaster is safe because it is made with sand, rock, gypsum, and water. When you purchase premixed plasters they may contain petrochemical preservatives and volatile organic compounds that are not good to have as part of your home.

- Permeable pavement, open block/soil center pavement, or no pavement. Open block paving "bricks" allow grass or other plants to grow through. This allows the soil to breath, the rain to seep in, and reduces heat.

- Using native plant species in landscaping, including on a sod-covered roof.

- Native wildflower area to attract native bees and helpful insects.

- Landscape mulch to conserve water.

- Providing space for a food garden with compost and gray water systems.

- Rain collection watering system.

- Percolation gravel pit where rainwater from pavement and roofing can be guided to drain into the soil rather than into sewers or storm drains.

- Vegetable-based cleansers and glues.

- Plant- and/or turf-covered roofing with native plants.

- Hempcrete brickwork and roofing, and hemplaster. This is stronger, lighter, more flexible, and more environmentally sustainable than regular concrete.

AdobeBuilder.Com

Architects, Designers & Planners for Social Responsibility, ADPSR.Org

Bamboo2000.Com
Bamboo flooring.

Bonded Logic, 480-812-9114; BondedLogic.Com
Recycled cotton carpet and insulation.

BuildingForHealth.Com, 800-292-4838

BuildingGreen.Com

BuildItGreen.Org

BuildNaturally.Com

Cape Fear Green Building Alliance, CFGBA.Org

Chanvre-Info.CH/Info/Fr/Procede-Isochanvre.html
The site for the French company that makes patented hemp cement. The site can be read in French or English.

Colorado Yurt Company, ColoradoYurt.Com

Crest.Org

DECAT.Net

DirtCheapBuilder.Com

EarthFriendlyGoods.Com

EcoBuilderNetwork.Org

EcoFriendlyFlooring.Com
Tiles made of recycled metal, stone, and glass. Also sells bamboo, linoleum, cork, and reclaimed wood.

EcoHome.Org

Eco-Living.Net

EcoProducts.Com
Wheatboard and strawboard cabinetry.

EcoSmartInc.Com

EcoTimber, 415-258-8454; EcoTimber.Com

EnergyTaxIncentives.Org

Environmental Building News, BuildingGreen.Com

Environmental Construction Outfitters, EnvironProducts.Com

EnvironmentalHomeCenter.Com

El Paso Solar Energy Association, EPSEA.Org/Straw.html

Expanko, 800-345-6202; Expanko.Com
  Recycled rubber and cork flooring.

Forbo Flooring, 800-842-7839; TheMarmoleumStore.Com
  Natural linoleum.

Furnature.Com

Globus Cork, 718-742-7264; CorkFloor.Com

Goodwin Heart Pine Company, 800-336-3118; HeartPine.Com

TheGreenBuilder.Com

GreenBuilder.Org

Green Building Council, USGBC-LA.Org

Green Building Press, NewBuilder.Co.UK

GreenFloors.Com, 703-691-1616

TheGreenGuide.Com
  Numerous listings for green home supplies as well as informative articles.

GreenHome.Com

HealthyHome.Com

Healthy House Institute, HHInst.Com

HempBuilding.Com

iFloor.Com
  Sells bamboo, cork, and tile flooring.

International Cellulose Corporation, 800-444-1252; Spray-On.Com
Insulation.

Jefferson Recycled Woodworks, 530-964-2740; EcoWood.Com

Lars' Yurt Page, RDrop.Com/~Glacier/Yurt.htm
Shows how he built the yurt that he lives in on an organic farm in Oregon.

The Last Straw, The International Journal of Straw Bale and Natural Building,
StrawHomes.Com

LivingArchitectureCentre.Com

Living Architecture Centre Dot Com, Ireland, LivingGreen.Com
Internet-based school of sustainable building design and construction.

Lowen.Com
Windows.

Marvin.Com
Windows.

Natural Carpet Company, 310-447-7965; NaturalCarpetCompany.Com

NaturalHomeMagazine.Com

Natural Lawn of America, NL-Amer.Com

NewDream.Org

NorthWest Builders Network, 888-810-8296; NWBuildNet.Com

Northwest EcoBuilding Guild, EcoBuilding.Org
Publishes the *EcoBuilding Times*.

Oikos.Com

OrganicInteriorDesign.Com

Palmer Industries, 800-545-7383; PalmerIndustriesInc.Com
Insulation.

ParamountWindows.Com, 204-233-4966

Permaculture Magazine, England; PermaCulture.Co.UK

PhoenixOrganics.Com

ReBuildingCenter.Org

Sierra Pine Co., 800-676-3339; SierraPine.Com
  Formaldehyde-free, medium-density *Medite II* fiberboard.

Smith & Fong, 866-835-9859; PlyBoo.Com
  Bamboo plywood.

StrawBuilding.Org

SustainableABC.Com

SustainableFlooring.Com

Tamalpais Natureworks, 415-454-9958; Tamalpais.Com
  Furniture kits.

TerraMai.Com
  Reclaimed wood flooring and for other uses.

Thermal Line, 800-662-1832; TLWindows.Com

Traditional Lime Company, Ireland, TraditionalLime.Com

U.S. Green Building Council; 202) 82-USGBC or 828-7422; 1015 18th Street, NW, Ste. 508, Washington, DC 20036; USGBC.Org

WeatherShield.Com, 800-477-6808
  Windows.

Yurts.Com

YurtWorks.Co.UK

Candles

If you buy candles, avoid those that are made out of petroleum wax (paraffin). Paraffin is one of the leftover byproduct residue extracts of petroleum (crude) oil. Other extracts of crude oil include gasoline, jet fuel, kerosene, diesel fuel, and asphalt.

When you burn paraffin wax candles in your home, you are essentially poisoning your air. The soot given off by a paraffin wax candle is similar to the soot given off by engines that burn fossil fuels.

Contaminates in the smoke of paraffin wax candles include benzene, methyl ethyl keyton, naphthalene, and toluene, which are also found in lacquer, paint, and varnish removers, and are known to cause cancer, birth defects, and learning disabilities.

If you purchase candles, buy those that contain lead-free wicks (non-metallic cores), and are made out of such things as hemp oil, soy, vegetable glycerin, and beeswax, palm wax, or vegetable wax. If you are a vegan you may want to avoid beeswax candles.

If the candle says it contains scented oils, find out if the oil is petroleum based, or if it is a plant oil. Some scents used in oils are also toxic and contain hormone-disrupting phthalates. Choose plant-based oils and scents.

Be aware that even some soy candles contain such toxic substances. Solvent extraction using petroleum chemicals is often part of the manufacturing process.

In addition, avoid candles that have leaded wicks. Candle companies use leaded wicks because they are easier to keep straight. Candles with leaded wicks emit lead into the atmosphere, creating a health hazard.

Canteens: Reducing Plastic Throwaway Bottle Use

A mericans use about 2.5 MILLION PLASTIC BOTTLES EVERY HOUR. This is creating an enormous amount of trash that will tarnish Earth for thousands of years.

HempBags.Com
Sells a water bottle sling with shoulder strap and zippered compartment.

Klean Kanteen, 800-767-3173; KleanKanteens.com
Sells canteens made from stainless steel and nonleaching materials.

Car Sharing

FlexCar.Com

Chef Training

Many of the raw vegan restaurants teach food prep classes. Sometimes they have authors of popular raw vegan recipe books teach the classes. Some of the health retreats listed in the book also do the same.

Living Light Culinary Arts Institute, 301-B N. Main St., Fort Bragg, CA 95437; 800-816-2319; 707-964-2420; RawFoodChef.Com
This is Cherie Soria's certified raw vegan chef school. She is the author of *Angel Foods: Healthy Recipes for Heavenly Bodies, and The Raw Food Diet: Feast, Lose Weight, Gain Energy, Feel Younger!* They also run Living Light Events, which offers event planning and catering, chef placement services, and healthy retreats.

Chicken and Eggs

Book:
• *Bird Flu: A Virus of Our Own Hatching*, by Michael Greger, M.D.

Compassion Over Killing, POB 9773, Washington, DC 20016; 301-891-2458; TryVeg.Com; COK.Net; EggScam.Com

United Poultry Concerns, POB 150, Machipongo, VA 23405-0150; 757-678-7875; UPC-Online.Org

Children & Young Adults

Books:
• *Baby Greens: A Live-Food Approach for Children of All Ages*, by Michaela Lynn and Michael Chrisemer, N.C, with a preface by Gabriel Cousens, M.D.
• *The Kid's Guide to Social Action*, by Barbara A. Lewis
• *The Power of Positive Talk*, by Douglas Block, M.A., and Jon Merritt, M.S.

Campaign for a Commercial-Free Childhood, CommercialExploitation.Com

Center for Ecoliteracy, Berkeley, CA; EcoLiteracy.Org

Children for a Clean Environment, KidsFACE.Org

Children's Eternal Rainforest, Monteverde Conservation League, POB 124 - 5655 Monte Verde Puntarenas, Costa Rica; ACMCR.Org/Rain_Forest.htm

CollageFoundation.Org

Works to show youth they have choices about their role in the world, and the power to make a difference in a variety of ways.

Citizens for Healthy Options in Children's Education, 877-6choice; ChoiceUSA.Net

Promotes vegetarian and vegan options for school lunch programs. Works to prevent the sale of fast-foods and foods of low-nutritional quality in schools.

- School children are routinely served meals with excess protein, saturated fats, cholesterol, hormones, pesticides, and pathogens, and few vegetables and fruits.
- School lunches contain 33 percent calories from fat, including 12 percent from saturated fat.
- 90 percent of our children consume amounts of fat above the recommended level.
- Only 17 percent of our children eat the minimum daily recommended servings of vegetables, and 20 percent eat no vegetables on a given day.
- Less than 15 percent of our children eat the minimum daily recommended servings of fruit, and 35 percent eat no fruit on a given day.
- 25 percent of children ages five to ten have high cholesterol, high blood pressure, or other early warning signs for heart disease.
- As many as 30,000 children have Type 2 diabetes, once limited largely to adults.

Eco-Schools.Org

Eco-Schools.Org.UK

EdibleSchoolyard.Org

FarmToSchool.Org

Graduation Pledge Alliance, GraduationPledge.Org

Aims to get new graduates to "pledge to explore and take into account the social and environmental consequences of any job" they consider and work to "try to improve these aspects of any organizations for which" they work.

***Green Teacher* magazine**, Canada: Green Teacher, 95 Robert St., Toronto, ON M5S 2K5; United States: Green Teacher, POB 452, Niagara Falls, NY 14304-0452; 416-960-1244; 888-804-1486; GreenTeacher.Com

Know a grade-school teacher? Gift them with a subscription to *Green Teacher*.

HealthySchoolLunches.Org

In Defense of Animals, The Guardian Campaign, YouthForAnimals.Org

KidActivists.Com

KidsGardening.Com

Leonardo DiCaprio's children's Web site, LeonardoDiCaprio.Org/Kids

NaturalPlay.Com

The School Garden Project of Lane County, Eugene, OR; EFN.Org/~SGP/

SFGreenSchools.Org

Student Environmental Action Coalition, POB 31909, Philadelphia, PA 19104; SEAC.Org

TreeInABox.Com

Tree Musketeers, TreeMusketeers.Org
  A kid-centered urban forestry-planting organization empowering young people to work to rescue Earth.

Urban Nutrition Initiative, Franklin Building Annex, 3451 Walnut St., Ste. P-117; Philadelphia, PA 19104; 215-898-1600

YES!, 420 Bronco Rd., Soquel, CA 95073; 831-465-1091; YesWorld.Org
  YES! is a nonprofit organization that connects, inspires and empowers young changemakers to join forces for a thriving, just, and sustainable way of life for all. YES! is directed by the husband-wife team of Michele and Ocean Robbins. *Food Revolution* author John Robbins is Ocean's father.

YoungReporters.Org

Chocolate

Book:
• *Naked Chocolate*, by David Wolfe and Shazzie

Yes, it is true, chocolate has some beneficial properties, including methylxanthines, which stimulate the transmission of nerve signals. But, if you choose to eat chocolate, stick to dark chocolate that is free from milk and milk extracts, corn syrup and other processed sugars, lecithin, artificial flavorings and colorings, and other additives. Raw chocolate is the best of all.
  Understand that it is very important that your chocolate come from an organic, slave-free farm.
  Yes, slavery still exists.
  Many companies are selling chocolate and coffee that have been grown using slave labor, including farms where children and other

workers are horribly abused, beaten, and sometimes killed if they cannot, or do not, work as hard as the farm owners want them to.

Read the article by John Robbins: *Is There Slavery in Your Chocolate*, by accessing: FoodRevolution.Org/Slavery_Chocolate.htm.
If you purchase chocolate or coffee, only purchase that which is labeled "fair trade" and organic.

Fair Trade; Store.GlobalExchange.Org/Chocolate.html

Sunfood Nutrition, 11653 Riverside Dr., Lakeside, CA 92040; 800-205-2350; 888-RAW-FOOD; International: +001-619-596-7979; Sunfood.Com
The raw chocolate they sell is grown on organic farms in Ecuador.

Cigarette Butt Litter

CigaretteLitter.Org
"It is estimated that several trillion cigarette butts are littered worldwide every year. That's billions of cigarettes flicked, one at a time, on our sidewalks, beaches, Nature trails, gardens, and other public places every single day. In fact, **cigarettes are the most littered item in America and the world**. Cigarette filters are made of cellulose acetate tow, NOT COTTON, and they can take decades to degrade. Not only does cigarette litter ruin even the most picturesque setting, but the toxic residue in cigarette filters is damaging to the environment, and littered butts cause numerous fires every year, some of them fatal."

Circus Animals

Also see:
• Animal Protection
• Vivisection

E lephants are among the most common animals used by circuses. They are caught in the wild when they are toddlers. In the wild, elephants will nurse for up to three years, and spend the first dozen years with their mothers. When they are taken from their mothers at a young age the mother has often been killed. Social skills from interacting with their family are arrested. Sold to a zoo or a circus, the elephant struggles to function in a foreign environment, learning what they can from their surroundings. As they are trained to perform in a circus they are often bound at the ankles with chains; hit with bull hooks or beaten with sticks; kept in cages; and food and water are often kept from them as a way to break their will. As they travel they may be kept in dirty train cars for days at a time. During this time they may be exposed to extreme temperatures.

"If animals in circuses are the 'most enriched animals on the face of the Earth,' as John Kirtland, Ringling Bro.'s executive director for animal stewardship contends, trainers would be armed with treats and other forms of positive reinforcement. Instead, circuses pack an arsenal of bull hooks, chains, ropes, cinch collars, chock prods, axe handles, baseball bats, metal pipes, and whips."
— KinshipCircle.Org

"The idea that it is funny to see wild animals coerced into acting like clumsy humans, or thrilling to see powerful beasts reduced to cringing cowards by a whipcracking trainer is primitive and medieval. It stems from the old idea that we are superior to other species and have the right to hold dominion over them."
— Dr. Desmond Morris, anthropologist, animal behaviorist, author

"The Cruelty Connection: What most people don't know is that there is a revolving door between the world of entertainment and the research laboratory. Many chimpanzees used in entertainment have been sent to research labs when they were no longer 'cute,' easy to handle, and profitable."
— The Fauna Foundation, FaunaFoundation.Org; New England Anti-Vivisection Society, NEAVS.Org

Circuses.Com

CircusWatch.Com
"Whips, bullhooks, chains, and electric shock prods! That's right: Behind all that glitter lies a dirty secret. To force animals to perform stressful and frightening acts, trainers use whips, electric prods, and sharp metal bullhooks that they jab into the sensitive skin out of sight behind an elephant's thighs, ears, and knees. In Nature, animals are free to walk and run, choose lifetime companions, and raise their families. The circus forces animals to perform demeaning tricks night after night for 48 to 50 weeks every year. Between acts, elephants are kept chained by two feet, unable to take two steps in any direction and bears and tigers are 'stored' in cages barely large enough for them to turn around in."

KinshipCircle.Org

Starbreezes.Com/11/CircusAbuse.html

Cleaning, Soaps, and Detergents

Also see:
• Cosmetics
• Laundry and Dry Cleaning

Did you know that the most common cleaning substances contain chemicals that can poison you? The colorings, astringents, scents, and other substances found in soaps and detergents are often made out of carcinogenic and hormonal disrupting chemicals that can cause birth defects, learning disabilities, and other health problems. Disinfectants may contain phenol and cresol, which can cause fainting, diarrhea, and dizziness and well as damage to the kidneys and liver. Additionally, wood and floor polishes may contain nitrobenzene, which is a carcinogen that can also cause birth defects. Metal polishes may contain petroleum distillates that interfere with vision and cause damage to the kidney and nerves.
Safer choices for cleaning include vinegar and baking soda. Non-chlorine bleaches and hydrogen peroxide can be used as disinfectants.

Avoid soaps and detergents made out of petrochemicals. Either make your own cleaner, or purchase those that are more environmentally safe.

Look for cleaners that are made of plant substances, and that are from companies that do not test their products on animals. Many of these may be found in your local natural foods market.

Bi-O-Kleen, 503-557-0216; NaturallySafeCleaning.Com

Bio-Pac.Com

Citra-Solv, 800-343-6855; Citra-Solv.Com

DrBronner.Com

Earth Friendly Products, Ecos.Com

Ecover, 323-720-5730; Ecover.Com
Ecover produces a full line of biodegradable household cleaners.

Earth Friendly Products, 847-446-4441; Ecos.Com

GreenEarth.Com

Mountain Green, 866-686-4733; MtnGreen.Com

SeventhGeneration, 802-658-3773; SeventhGeneration.Com

WildOats.Com/U/Health100599

Clothing: Natural and Organic Fiber

Also see:
• Cotton: Seek Organic
• Hemp Farming: Work to Legalize It
• Laundry and Dry Cleaning
• Vegetarian Groups, Web Sites, Restaurants & Stores

One of the best ways to protect the environment is to limit your clothing choices to those that are made of organically grown fiber. It has only been since the drilling of oil began on a major scale in the 1800s that fibers started to be developed from fossil substances. And those are the worst fibers of all as they are not sustainable, are not biodegradable, and are often treated with health-damaging chemicals that are absorbed into the skin of the wearer, as well as into the environment. The drilling, mining, and processing of petroleum, coal, and shale is massively destructive to the environment.

Most cotton grown on the planet is also damaging to health and the environment because cotton is most often grown using large doses of defoliants, fertilizers, herbicides, insecticides, and pesticides. Most cotton is also bleached during processing, which releases dioxin, a long-lasting toxic chemical. Altogether, the cotton industry releases hundreds of millions of pounds of toxic chemicals into the environment in the form of farming chemicals, chemical dyes, and finishing agents. When buying cotton fabrics, seek those made from cotton grown organically and that are dyed with natural coloring agents.

A safe clothing fiber is hemp. It produces more fiber per acre than cotton and does not require the use of the chemicals used in intensive cotton farming or processing. Hemp is naturally whiter than cotton, so it is easier to whiten using safer bleaching agents than those that are used on cotton. Hemp clothing is currently costly in the U.S. because the ridiculous laws that have been created using lies and political and corporate corruption prevent U.S. farmers from growing hemp. Because of this, all hemp fabric is imported from other countries. Industrial hemp farming needs to be made legal in the U.S.

Not to be overlooked in the form of natural fabrics that are environmentally safe are those made from bamboo. It is growing in popularity.

Tencil is a newer fabric that is made from managed tree farms. There are some chemicals used in the manufacture of tencil, but it is still a safer choice than petroleum fibers and chemically grown cotton.

AHappyPlanet.Com

All Vegan, San Diego, CA; AllVeganShopping.Com

AmericanApparel.Net
Carries a line of organic cotton clothing.

ArtisanGear.Com

Center for the New American Dream, NewDream.Org
Information about sweatshop-free clothing.

Conscious Clothing; 505-982-7506; GetConscious.Com
Creates hemp/tencel blend wedding dresses.

Decent Exposures, 206-364-4540; DecentExposures.Com

EarthCreations.Net

EarthRunnings.Com
Hemp furnishings and linens.

EarthSpeaks.Com

Earth-Wear.Com

The Emperor's Clothes, EmperorsHemp.Com
Hemp clothing made in Montana.

Environ Gentle, 543 S. Coast Hwy. 101, Encinitas, CA 92024; EnvironGentle.Com

Evergreen Hemp Co., EverGreenHemp.Com

FaeriesDance.Com

GlobalHempStore.Com

GreenPeople.Org/OrganicCotton.htm
This Web site lists a slew of sources for organic cotton products.

Heartland Products, 515-332-3087; TRVNet.Nets/~HrtLndp

HempBags.Com

HempBelts.Com

HempFabric.Com

HempShoes.Com

HempStores.Com

Hemp Utopia, 22256 100th Ave., Langley, British Columbia, Canada, V1M 3V5; Canada-Shops.Com/Stores/HempUtopia
   Donates a portion of all sales to famine relief, hemp re-education, and environmental causes.

HempWallets.Com

Hempys.Com

HerbivoreClothing.Com

International Hemp Fair, CannaTrade.CH

KasperOrganics.Com

Kentucky Hemp Outfitters, KentuckyHemp.Com

LoomState.Org

Maggie's Functional Organics, MaggiesOrganics.Com

MamasEarth.Com

MooShoes.Com

NaturalHighLifestyle.Com

OfTheEarth.Com

OrganicClothes.Com

OrganicCottonAlts.Com

OrganicCottonPlus.Com

OrganicThreads.Com

PlanetHemp.Net

Rawganique.Com

SaharaOrganics.Com

SweatshopWatch.Org
Information about sweatshops and issues relating to workers' rights in clothing manufacturing.

SweetGrassFibers.Com

TwoStarDog.Com

UnderTheCanopy.Com

UtopianLiving.Com

VeganStore.Com

Vegetarian-Shoes.Co.UK

Vital Hemptations, VitalHemp.Com

Vreseis.Com

WildlifeWorks.Com

Communes: Intentional Living Communities

There are a variety of intentional communities throughout the world. Some are truly "communes" where members share incomes and may work for a community business in exchange for the room, sustenance, and sometimes a stipend. In the majority of intentional communities, members are self-supporting through their personal income, investments, or savings while participating in communal upkeep and activities.

Communities – Journal of Cooperative Living, 138 Twin Oaks Rd., Louisa, VA 23093; 828-863-4425; IC.Org/Resources/CDir1995/CommunitiesJournal.html
Web site contains information about communes around the world. The online database of intentional communities can be searched by topic, such as location, and diet type (vegan, raw vegan, etc.)

CommunityMade.Com
Crafts and creations from U.S. intentional communities.

Global Eco-Village Network, Findhorn, Scotland; EcoVillage.Org

International Communities Publication, RadicalCaring.Org

Lost Valley Education Center, Dexter, Oregon, LostValley.Com

Composting

BioCycle: Journal of Composting & Organic Recycling,
JGPress.Com/BioCycle.htm

CompostingCouncil.Org

EcoCycle.Org

HowToCompost.Org

Cosmetics

Books:
- *Drop Dead Gorgeous: Protecting Yourself from the Hidden Dangers of Cosmetics*, by Kim Erickson
- *Eating for Beauty*, by David Wolfe
- *Mother Nature's Guide to Vibrant Beauty & Health*, by Myra Cameron
- *The Truth About Beauty: Transform Your Looks and Life from the Inside Out*, by Kat James and Oz Garcia

> "It is amazing how there is such a lack of regulation when it comes to cosmetics. Many ingredients in cosmetics contain toxic substances that are on the Environmental Protection Agency's lists of hazardous wastes and hazardous substances. Since there was the long-ago myth that the skin is an impermeable barrier, cosmetics laws became a low priority – much to the chagrin of the American people."
> — **Elizabeth Howard, RawRawGirls.Com, a living foods catering and cosmetics company**

Did you know that many of the skin, hair, and oral care products sold in stores today contain toxins that can cause cancer and that also poison our lakes, rivers and oceans; and can cause birth deformities, miscarriages, and learning disabilities in both humans and wildlife?

Many of these products contain petroleum-derived parabens. These are known carcinogens and are used as preservatives in the products. Parabens are known to mimic estrogen and disrupt testosterone levels. Many of the same chemicals used on insecticides are often used in body scents and other cosmetics. Other chemicals used on the most popular cosmetic products include coal tar coloring, labeled as D&C and FD&C colors; formaldehyde, a known carcinogen; lead, phthalates; and nonylphenols, chemicals that disrupt hormonal balance and that are contained in many shampoos, shaving creams, and hair dyes.

Perfumes and colognes are some of the most toxic substances people put onto their skin. They often contain chemicals that are derived from petroleum and coal and that can interfere with respiratory function, hormonal balance, and the function of the brain and neurons. Additionally, many of the chemicals in perfumes and colognes are known to cause asthma, birth deformities, and cancer. When the chemicals are put onto the skin they are absorbed into the body where they collect in fat cells and in the blood.

Perfumes and colognes contain so many toxins that municipalities advise people to avoid disposing the products by pouring them into the sink or toilet, but to take them to the nearest hazardous-waste collection center.

Many people think that the Food and Drug Administration is a gatekeeper that protects consumers from exposure to toxins by not allowing companies to use them. The truth is that the FDA does not get involved until a problem arises. And even then they may have to be dragged into it through lawsuits and consumer outrage.

The body care product companies that make the products may conduct some testing, but they are known to use some of the most toxic chemicals in their products. Some of the very same chemicals have been identified by the U.S. Environmental Protection Agency as hazardous to the health of humans and wildlife.

Why are companies permitted to use these chemicals in their personal care products, and advertise them using "super models"? Good question. I don't have the answer other than that the industry trade group for the hair, skin, nail, and oral care product companies, the Cosmetic, Toiletry and Fragrance Association, may like the way things are done.

There is no government agency testing the combination of chemicals used as ingredients in body care products. Nobody knows what happens when you mix some of the chemicals with others because testing has never been done.

Meanwhile, those who use the products are absorbing the synthetic chemicals into their tissues, and the chemicals often end up lingering in the fat cells of the body, where they can cause or contribute to an assortment of ailments.

Remember that what you put on your skin, hair, nails, and use to care for your teeth ends up in your body, and in your environment.

When you purchase skin, hair, and oral care products, choose those that contain ingredients that have not been tested on animals, do not contain toxic chemicals, and that are biodegradable. Steer clear of products containing petrochemicals (chemicals derived from petroleum), synthetic dyes and fragrances, phthalates, mineral oils, artificial preservatives, and derivatives of coal.

When purchasing cosmetic products, look for those that use natural preservatives, such as grapefruit seed extract, peptides, vitamins, essential oils, herbs, and plant alcohols.

Many natural foods stores now have skin, hair, oral, and other personal care products that are free of toxic chemicals. Even when purchasing your products from these stores, you should read the labels to see what ingredients are in the products.

Avoid cosmetics that contain any of the following:
- **Benzoic acid** – derived from vertebrates, unless the label states it is derived from plants
- **Butylated hydroxytoluene (BHT)**
- **Butyl paraben**
- **Carbomer 941**
- **Carmine, carminic acid, or cochineal** – a red color derived from crushed cochineal beetles
- **Cetyle alcohol** – unless the label states that it is derived from coconut or a vegetable source, assume that it is derived from murdered dolphins or sperm whales
- **Diazolidinyl Urea** – a preservative that causes cancer
- **Dimethicone**
- **DMDM hydantoin**
- **FD & C yellow no. 6**
- **Ethyl paraben**
- **Glycerin** – if the label doesn't say it is "vegetable glycerin," it is likely to be derived from the fat of slaughtered animals
- **Hydrolized animal protein**, also called hydrolyzed collagen –it is derived from the tendons and bones of slaughtered animals, and also from pets killed in animal shelters as well as from roadkill sold to rendering companies.

- Imidiazolidinyl urea
- Imidazolidinyland diazolidinyl urea
- **Keratin** – this is often an ingredient in shampoos. It is derived from the feather, hair, hooves, horns, and quills of killed animals
- **Lanolin** – an emollient used as an ingredient in skin care products, it is derived from sheep wool
- **Laureth sulfate or sodium lauryl** – a surfactant that is an irritant
- **Methyl paraben**
- **Mineral oil** – refined liquid hydrocarbon
- **Padimate-O** – found in sunscreens and can damage DNA
- **Parabens**
- **PEG-50 almond glycerides**
- **Phthalates** – a chemical that is known to cause birth defects
- **Propolyn glycol** – petrochemical derivative solvent that is harsh and an allergen
- **Royal jelly** – if you are opposed to using bee products, you will want to avoid this. It is a form of concentrated honey fed to queen bees.
- **Silk powder** – a secretion of the silkworm
- **Stearalkonium chloride** – used in creams and conditioners, this chemical is a known carcinogen
- **Stearic acid** – derived from the fat of slaughtered animals, from pets killed in animal shelters, and from roadkill collected by cities, towns, and counties and then sold to rendering plants
- **Synthetic colors** – often consisting of cancer-causing chemicals that are bad for people, animals, and wildlife
- **Synthetic fragrances** – often consisting of chemicals that are neurotoxins, can trigger asthma attacks, and may cause birth defects as well as other serious health problems
- **Sodium laureth sulfate (SLS)**
- **Triethanolamine (TEA)** – often contains nitrosamines, is toxic and irritates the skin
- **Urea** – derived from the urine and body fluids of animals

Avoid toothpaste that contains fluoride.

If you are vegan, you want to read labels of cosmetics to make sure they don't contain beeswax or other bee products, as well as animal products. Also, many of the most popular cosmetic products contain ingredients derived from processing the remains of animals from slaughterhouses as well as roadkill and dead animals from animal shelters sold to rendering plants. (See Howard Lyman's book *Mad Cowboy*.)

Beware that the skin of some people may also react to certain natural skin and hair care products. Find what products work for you.

Also note that some companies that sell themselves as "natural" hair and skin care product companies do use animal by-products and other ingredients that are not so good for you, for wildlife, or for the planet.

Check out the cosmetics at your local natural foods store. Look for those that state on the label that they consist of organic ingredients, do not contain animal by-products, synthetic chemicals, or ingredients that were tested on animals.

Better yet, learn to make your own cosmetics. You may invent new types of cosmetics using the substances of Nature. Some of the ingredients can be found in your kitchen, your garden, nearby wildlands, and the local farmers' market, or the produce section of your natural foods store.

The following companies are less likely to make products that contain harsh chemical agents, animal by-products, or ingredients that have been tested on animals.

Because companies change ownership, or company policy, it is good to keep informed about what their products may or may not contain before you purchase them.

AlbaBotanica.Com
See Avalon Natural Products below.

AllForAnimals.Com
Lists cosmetic companies that do not test on animals.

AngelHeart.Com

Avalon Natural Products, Petaluma, CA; AvalonNaturalProducts.Com
Skin, hair, body, and "un-petroleum" lip care, as well as Sun lotion. 100 percent vegetarian ingredients that are not tested on animals and do not contain petrochemicals.

Aveda, Minneapolis, MN; Aveda.Com

Azida.Com

Aztec Secret, Parhump, NV; Aztec-Secret.Com
Facial cleanser made of betonite clay.

Bare Essentials, Emeryville, CA, BareEscentuals.Com
Mineral cosmetics.

Beeswork, Novato, CA; BeesWork.Com
Skin and hair products using beeswax, herbal extracts, and plant oils.

Better Botanicals, Herndan, VA; BetterBotanicals.Com
Skin products.

The Campaign for Safe Cosmetics, SafeCosmetics.Org

ChooseCrueltyFree.Org.AU

The Coalition for Consumer Information on Cosmetics, Washington, DC;
LeapingBunny.Org
This organization is a partnership of animal rights groups that has established a "cruelty free" standard for cosmetics and toiletries. The leaping bunny logo found on products from companies that don't test on animals (vivisection), is from this organization.

Crystal, Burlingame, CA; TheCrystal.Com
Fragrance and deodorant products.

Derma e, Chatsworth, CA; DermaE.Net
Organic bodycare products.

Dr. Bronner's Magic Soaps, Escondido, CA; DrBronner.Com
Hemp-based soaps in recycled plastic bottles.

Earthly Delights, Cedar Creek, TX; EarthlyDelightsUSA.Com
Water-based nail polishes that don't contain toxic toluene, formaldehyde, or other hardeners and chemicals commonly found in popular nail polish.

Earth's Beauty, Dewey, AZ; EarthBeauty.Com
Non-synthetic cosmetics.

Ecco-Bella, Wayne, NJ; Eccobella.Com
Skin care and cosmetics.

Ejuva.Com

The Environmental Working Group, Washington, DC; EWG.Org
Source for information on phthalates.

EO, Corte Madera, CA; EOProducts.Com
Products include soaps, shampoos, conditioner, essential oils, bath salts, perfume, lotions, and foot balm.

FlourideAlert.Org

The Fluoride Education Project, Bruha.Com

Giovanni Organic Hair Care, Long Beach, CA; GiovanniCosmetics.Com

Grateful Body, Berkeley, CA; GratefulBody.Com
Herbal skin and body care products.

Green Products Alliance, Middlebury, VT; GreenProductsAlliance.Com
Cosmetics manufacturers working for socially responsible business practices. The members have agreed to avoid animal testing, animal by-products, petrochemicals, and other harmful chemicals. They also agree to use organic ingredients and recycled or reusable packaging.

Hemp Organics, San Francisco, CA; ColOrganics.Net
Lip colors that don't contain mineral oil, FD&C colors, parabens, or other coal tar or petroleum derivatives.

Jade & Pearl, Hawthorne, FL; JadeAndPearl.Com
DEET-free insect spray; natural tampons; bath and personal care products.

Jakare, Bozeman, MT; Jakare.Com
Skin care using wildcrafted and organic plant oils and herbs.

Jason Natural Cosmetics, Culver City, CA; Jason-Natural.Com
This company recently reformulated their products to make them safer.

Kiss My Face, Gardiner, NY; KissMyFace.Com
Company headquarters are on an organic farm with a barn once used as a hospital during the revolutionary war.

Lilly of Colorado, Henderson, CO; LilyOfColorado.Com
Botanical personal care products using ingredients from the company's organic farm.

Living Nature, Kerikeri, New Zealand; LivingNature.Com
Natural personal care products in glass bottles.

Lotus Brands, Twin Lakes, WI; Internatural.Com
Henna in various shades.

Lunapads International, Vancouver, BC, Canada; LunaPads.Com
Organic cotton menstrual pads.

Mad Gab's, Westbrook, ME; MadGabs.Com
Skin salves and lip care products.

John Masters Organics, New York, NY; JohnMasters.Com

Skin and hair care using plant extracts.

Mera Naturals, Circle Pine, MN; 800-752-7261
Haircare products.

Moom, Point Roberts, WA; IMoom.Com
Haircare and hair removal products.

Morganics, Phoenix, AZ; DrRickettsNutri.Com
Skin, hair, and bath products.

Natural Dentist, Englewood Cliffs, NJ; TheNaturalDentist.Com

Nonie of Beverly Hills, Los Angeles, CA; NonieOfBeverlyHills.Com

Omega Nutrition, Bellingham, WA; OmegaNutrition.Com
Face and body soaps.

Paul Penders, San Pablo, CA; PualPenders.Com
Hair coloring as well as skin and hair products.

PleasureHeals.Net

Sunfood.Com

RawRawGirls.Com
Elizabeth Howard sells cosmetics free of toxic chemicals. She is also a raw chef. Because she worked in the field of hazardous waste compliance she knows a lot about toxic substances, including those that are found in the most popular brands of cosmetics and toiletries. Her enewsletter is available through TheRawRawGirls@Yahoo.Com.

Real Purity, Grass Lake, MI; RealPurityTM.Com
Cosmetics and personal care products.

Recycline, Somerville, MA; RecyCline.Com
Oral care products.

SandyOrganics.Com

Sappo Hills Soapworks, Ashland, OR; 541-482-4485

TerrEssentials, Middletown, MD; TerrEssentials.Com
Skin, hair, and bodycare products.

Tisserand, Petaluma, CA; Tisserand.Com
Hair and bodycare and aromatherapeutic essential oils.

Tom's of Main, Kennebunk, ME; TomsOfMain.Com
Oral and body care products.

Trillium Herbal Company; Sturgeon Bay, WI; AromaFusion.Com

Vermont Soap Works, Middlebury, VT; VTSoap.Com

Vita-Myr, Las Vega, NV; VitaMyr.Com
Makes oral care products free of fluoride, alcohol, artificial sweeteners, and sodium lauryl sulfate.

V'tae, Las Vegas, NV; V'tae.Com
Perfumes, body, and bath products using essential oils.

Weleda, Germany; Weleda.Com
Natural skin and hair products.

Cotton: Seek Organic

Also see:
• Clothing
• Hemp

Cotton is most often grown using a variety of toxic chemical fertilizers, insecticides, and pesticides. This poisons the air, land, and water for many years to come.

Many cotton seeds end up in cattle feed, contributing to toxic farm animals. Other cotton seeds are turned into oil that is used in food processing. The cotton fiber ends up largely being made into fabric, which carries residues of the toxic chemicals used in the farming of the cotton.

When you purchase anything made of cotton, seek that which has been organically grown, and that has not been put through a manufacturing process where chlorine bleach is used. The bleaching used in fabric manufacturing is also damaging to the environment.

When you purchase anything made of any fabric, go for natural fabrics, and not those made out of synthetic fibers created from fossil fuels. Synthetic fabrics may be less expensive to purchase, but the environmental cost of these fabrics is multilayered and terrible.

Natural fabrics include those made from organic cotton, hemp, sisal, jute, ramie, flax, and bamboo.

GreenPeople.Org/OrganicCotton.htm

This Web site lists a slew of sources for organic cotton products.

OrganicExchange.Org

SustainableCotton.Org

Cultured and Fermented Foods

Books:
- *Live Kim-Chee and Cultured Veggies*, by Victoria and Valya Boutenko
- *Living Cuisine: The Art and Spirit of Raw Foods*, by Renée Loux

Cultured foods can be highly nutritious, rich in enzymes, and provide healthful probiotic bacteria (L. acidophilus, L. bifidus, etc.) that gather in the intestines as "intestinal flora." This helps us to assimilate nutrients provided by other foods, and brings the system into healthy pH balance. Fermentation also breaks down complex proteins into the simpler amino acid compounds, making them easier to digest for those with a digestive tract that has been weakened by sickness or bad diet.

To experience vibrant health you need to have a population of good bacteria taking up residence in your intestines. A good base of intestinal flora is important for our immune system; helps fight off bad bacteria that cause disease; provides and creates nutrients, such as the B-complex vitamins; and provides for healthy elimination of toxins. Fermented Sunfoods provide these.

Cultured foods include the traditional Korean food called kimchi (also spelled *kim-chee*), as well as a raw food more common to North America, sauerkraut, which is from Eastern Europe. Kombucha tea is also a cultured food. A cultured, nonheated soy sauce called nama shoyu is cultured. Miso, a salty paste made from beans, is cultured (but make sure it is made from raw beans, or make it yourself). Raw apple cider that has been fermented is also a cultured food, as is wine, which is fermented, not brewed.

Cultured foods are relatively easy to make and rely on naturally present cultures that are in the air. They can also be made using a non-dairy source of kefir culture.

Make your cultured foods with organically grown raw vegetables, not with those that have been heated, boiled, or otherwise cooked.

When you make cultured foods, do so under sanitary conditions to avoid molds and harmful bacteria that can spoil your creation.

When making fermented foods, the area where the crock or other container sits should be out of direct Sun light, in an area free from dust and disturbance, and where the container can remain for several days as the food ferments (some people ferment kimchi and sauerkraut for up to several weeks, and even longer – but start simple, and learn from there).

Be aware that many types of cultured foods sold in stores have been pasteurized (heated). If you buy cultured food, make sure the label says "unpasteurized" or "raw vegan." These will be found in the refrigerated section. Cultured foods, in their unheated state, are becoming more popular in natural foods stores.

You can also make cultured seed and/or nut cheeses by mixing soaked pine nuts, almonds, macadamia, or others blended with nutritional yeast, sea salt, and cultured rejuvelac water. This raw vegan cheese can be used soft, or dehydrated into a crisp cheese similar to Parmesan. The soft cheese can also be flavored with Italian herbs. See the Rejuvelac section in this book. See Renée's book, *Living Cuisine*.

A tool helpful in making fermented foods is a kimchi crock. They are often sold in Asian markets. It has a lip around the edge that gets filled with water so that the lid fits into this lip, preventing air from getting in, but allowing gas to escape.

Never eat food that you are unsure about. If the fermented food you are making ends up smelling rotten rather than tangy, and especially if the vegetables turn brown or even black, toss them away.

Read the book by the Raw Family, or Renée's book, to learn more.

Gold Mine Natural Food Co., 7805 Arjons Dr., San Diego, CA 92126; 800-862-2347; GoldMineNaturalFood.Com

RawFamily.Com

Renée Loux, EuphoricOrganics.Com

Dating

Concerned Singles, POB 444, Lenoxdale, MA 01214; 413-445-6309; ConcernedSingles.Com

Green Singles NATURAL Friend; Natural-Friends.Com

HappyCow.Net

Living and Raw Foods Personals; Living-Foods.Com/Personals

Organic Weddings, 617-367-1807; OrganicWeddings.Com

RawFoodChat.Com

Sunfood.Com

VegetarianMeetup.Com

Dehydrated Foods

Also see:
• Recipe Books for A Raw Vegan Kitchen

Dehydrated foods in Sunfood cuisine include common dehydrated foods like raisins, Sun dried tomatoes, dried figs, and prunes. They also include dehydrated, but not cooked or heated, dessert crusts; dehydrated flat breads; dehydrated chips; dehydrated sweet cookies; dehydrated veggie burgers; dehydrated pizza crusts; seed and vegetable crackers; and even granola mixes.

Dehydrating food is an excellent way to create foods that can be stored for lengthy periods. They also provide quality foods that can be taken on trips so that you don't have to depend on lower-quality foods.

It is good to eat dehydrated foods with those that are in their fresh state, such as by spreading guacamole, or raw vegan pates, or sauces on dehydrated seed and vegetable crackers. With Sunfood pizza, the crust is dehydrated, but the topping consists of a variety of regular but uncooked and thinly sliced toppings, as well as raw vegan pesto sauce. Dehydrated pine nut cheeses can be used in green salads. Dehydrated "sweet breads" (made out of fruit and soaked oats, for instance) can be eaten with raw vegan berry cream sauces (berries blended with soaked nuts, agave nectar, cinnamon, and a pinch of salt).

If you eat too many dehydrated foods, you may end up feeling dehydrated. Water or other fluid, such as vegetable juice, or lemon-infused rejuvelac (See Rejuvelac section in this book), are good to drink when eating dehydrated foods. Otherwise you may experience rough digestion and flatulence if you eat too much dehydrated food by itself.

Dehydrated foods in Sunfood cuisine are made using low heat to preserve the nutrients, and especially the enzymes, of the living plant substances. There are many figures thrown around as to what is the maximum temperature to use when dehydrating foods without damaging the nutrients. Various raw vegan recipe books state that the figure is 108° F, and others say it is 120° F. The temperature at which the enzymes are damaged depends on which plant substance you are dehydrating.

As an experiment I put flax seeds, sunflower seeds, and pumpkin seeds in a 125° F dehydrator for 24 hours, then I took the seeds and kept them moist. They sprouted. David Wolfe has conducted a similar experiment with rye seeds, some of which sprouted after being exposed to temperatures over 120° F.

While 125° F may not harm some seeds, including those that survive through forest fires and desert heat, that temperature is probably too high to use when dehydrating things like fruits and vegetables and their pulp. I use a lower temperature, below 110° F, for those types of foods.

Ideally, dehydrating will remove only the water from the food you are dehydrating, while preserving nutrients. What is left over is a much smaller piece of food with an intensified taste.

The first time I ate gourmet raw vegan pizza crust I was convinced that dehydrated foods were something to look into. The scrumptious "raw pizza" was made by Jeremy Safron during one of his speaking engagements. His recipe book *The Raw Truth: The Art of Preparing Living Foods* contains the recipe for his raw pizza (as well as a lot of other excellent recipes).

Those who are used to eating cooked food may need to adjust their expectations of what crackers, flat breads, and cookies will taste like when they first take a bite out of those that are made using low-heat dehydrators. Some foods may taste very familiar, while others may provide a new taste experience.

As in any other type of food, there are dehydrated foods that are quite satisfying, and others that you may not enjoy so much. The key is to explore and find the ones that work for you. I have found some I like, and some I'd rather never taste ever again.

If you are used to eating cooked foods, you may find that the density of dehydrated foods will satisfy that feeling of fullness that you are used to. But it is good not to rely so much on dehydrated foods, and to make your diet consist largely of fresh foods.

To increase the nutritional quality of the nuts and seeds you may be using in such things as dehydrated crackers, crusts, biscotti, and cookies, soak them in water for several hours, then rinse and let them sprout for a day. This will trigger the nutrient-making machinery in the nuts and seeds, providing more enzymes and other nutrients that are less present in unsprouted nuts and seeds.

You can dehydrate any food, from fruit to vegetables to herbs and edible flowers to sea vegetables and sprouts.

There are many dehydrators on the market, but the most common tool for dehydrating foods is one that has been used since the earliest of times. That tool is called Sun.

Ancient people, and some even today, prepare dehydrated foods using Sun by laying them on top of such things as rocks, adobe bricks, dried tree bark or wood, or on metal sheets or ceramic flats or plates.

Someone I know dehydrates foods using a shallow box he made out of wood, with a ceramic plate at the bottom. A suspended screen in the center acts as a shelf to put the food on. A screened lid keeps out bugs.

When dehydrating food using Sun, you need to learn to prevent the food from baking, as a base of metal or a ceramic plate can get quite hot when Sun is at the day's zenith.

You may be able to find people selling used dehydrators by checking the community board of your local natural foods store.

Because each type of fruit and vegetable, and the various types of raw recipes for dehydrated foods, contain different amounts of water, some foods take longer to dehydrate than others. The temperature plays a big part in how long it takes to dehydrate a food. But it is best to dehydrate the foods at very low temperatures so that the nutrients, such as the enzymes, are not damaged. Simply leave in a dehydrator until the desired level of dryness is reached, then store in a sealed container in a cool, dry place.

Many of the raw vegan recipe books contain recipes for dehydrated foods. Check out *Living Cuisine: The Art and Spirit of Raw Foods*, by Renée Loux.

Detox and Fasting

Books:
- *The Detox Book*, by Bruce Fife, N.D.
- *The Detox Miracle Sourcebook*, by Robert Morse, N.D.
- *Detox Your World*, by Shazzie
- *The Fasting Handbook: Dining from an Empty Bowl*, by Jeremy Safron
- *Fasting Can Save Your Life*, by Herbert Shelton
- *Fasting and Eating for Health*, by Joel Fuhrman, M.D.

- *Fasting for Renewal of Life*, by Herbert Shelton
- *Golden Path to Rejuvenation*, by Morris Krok
- *Master Cleanser*, by Stanley Burroughs
- *The Miracle of Fasting*, by Paul Bragg, N.D. and Patricia Bragg
- *Perfect Body*, by Roe Gallo
- *Rational Fasting*, by Arnold Ehret

You can begin to detoxify your body immediately by eliminating consumption of unhealthful foods, and beginning to eat raw plant foods.

Wolfe's book, *The Sunfood Diet Success System*, includes specific, simple recipes that will help to detoxify the body, and that consist of ingredients such as citrus fruits; avocados; cold-pressed flax seed oil, hemp seed oil and olive oil; figs; papaya; melons; all sorts of green vegetable juices; and salads, ginger, garlic, habanero pepper, fennel, broccoli, and berries. Other recipes can be found in the book, *Mucusless Diet Healing System*, by Arnold Ehret. The list of detox and fasting books above may also be helpful.

The less your diet and lifestyle consist of cooked and other processed foods along with sedentary activities, and the more your diet and lifestyle includes a variety and responsible quantity of healing raw plant foods along with adequate movement and exercise, the healthier your body will be.

Things you should immediately eliminate from your diet are white foods. These include potatoes, rice, pasta, breads, lard, mayonnaise, shortening, milk and milk products, eggs and egg products, processed sugar, foods with added processed sugar; foods containing MSG; and foods containing processed salt (instead of processed salt, use Celtic sea salt, Himalayan pink salt, powdered dulse, or powdered kelp).

Avoid corn oil, corn sweetener, and cooked corn. Fresh, raw, organic corn is okay.

Also avoid any food that contains artificial dyes, flavorings, scents, and other chemicals that large food companies often add to their products.

This is very important for those who want to experience vibrant health: Avoid all heated oils, especially foods that have been fried. Only allow cold processed plant fats/oils into your system. The best oil is organically grown hempseed oil. (More about cooked oil later.) Some of the worst oils you can eat are trans fats, such as processed tropical oils. (The palm oil industry is also causing a huge amount of destruction in

Southeast Asia, and the major player in the endangerment of the last wild orangutans.)

Begin to eat organically grown raw vegetables, raw fruits, raw nuts, and raw and sprouted seeds.

Learn to make foods that consist entirely of raw plant substances. Access the raw vegan recipe books so that you know the varieties of foods you can make. There are many raw vegan recipe books listed in this book. Those and others can be found on Sunfood.Com. Also, try your local library.

Set up a raw vegan kitchen. (See Kitchen: What's in the Sunfoodist's Kitchen.)

Stop allowing yourself to be influenced by the food advertising you see in pop culture and mass media.

Along with the constant push from food companies, restaurants, and supermarkets for people to buy mass-marketed food come a slew of substances that land in the tissues of the body. Especially when people are eating an unhealthful diet they are exposed to an enormous assortment of food ingredients. These substances are not good for the body and often end up as residues within the body cells, where they subsequently degrade health.

Together with eating habits that often include way too many calories than a person needs, the result of eating commercial foods is obesity. Within the deposits of fat are an unknown number of toxins, or at least substances that the body does not need.

Those following a typical American diet essentially become a toxic waste dump. Their health begins to falter, their senses dull, their thinking becomes clouded. The body becomes distorted as they become physically inactive because they don't have the energy or the feelings to exercise – or even to get physically intimate. Food becomes a focus, and this is prodded by hearing and seeing food advertised everywhere. Eating becomes the only glory time of their day. Meals are larger than they need to be and are made up of foods that are of a low nutritional quality. Money, time, resources, and health are wasted in the pursuit of unhealthful food.

"The major diseases and illnesses are diet-related. Detoxification through a raw vegan diet is a physical path back to radiant health. If diet is ignored, the maximum benefit of other therapies will not be achieved."
— David Wolfe

If you have been eating the unhealthful standard American diet, you should consider the process of detoxifying your body from accumulated residues and energies left from damaging, denatured foods.

One way to speed up the process of detoxifying the body is to "fast." This involves abstaining from food to allow the body to use its natural cleansing abilities to focus on what is already in the body, rather than dealing with a constant onslaught of new foods and other substances included in them.

People go through stages of fasting every day. When you sleep you are away from food for a third of your day, or more. This is beneficial to your system as it allows the body to push out what is not needed, and to revitalize the tissues through rest. When you eat the first meal of your day, it is called "breakfast." You are breaking, or ending, the "fast" that you were on throughout your night.

> "There are health conditions which do not react well to fasting. For instance, a fast is not recommended for diabetics who have taken insulin for more than two years.
> Those taking certain medication can have an adverse reaction to fasting.
> Those [with a history of] taking recreational drugs should also not fast – until they have stopped taking drugs, and detoxified their body of toxic chemicals to a point over several months by following a pure, raw-food diet consisting of organically grown foods – and especially of green-leafed vegetables. Otherwise fasting may cause too much of the residues from the drugs to flow out of the tissues and into the lymph and blood systems too quickly."
> — **David Wolfe**

Those who are taking certain medications and/or who have certain serious health conditions may have to reconsider a traditional fast that involves little to no food, and instead eat a diet that consists purely of healthful foods. A reduction in the food intake while limiting it to foods of the highest quality is key. By losing weight over a period of time, eating high-quality foods, and following a daily exercise regimen, those on medications may find their need for the medication is reduced. Some have found that their need for the medication goes away as they ridded themselves of their unhealthful diet and lifestyle.

Those who are pregnant or breastfeeding should follow a healthful diet of high-quality foods free of synthetic food additives, processed sugars, processed salts, and heated oils. It isn't their time to fast.

Those with diabetes should be cautious about attempting any sort of fast. However, it will benefit them to eliminate any junk foods from their diet, and to follow a diet made up of highly nutritious foods free of synthetic additives, processed salts, processed sugars, and heated oils. People with diabetes have experienced great improvements in their condition by following a strict, well-rounded, raw vegan food diet that consists of a variety of foods. Daily exercise is important for those with diabetes and blood sugar issues (and everyone else!).

When you fast, your blood and lymph fluids become thinner. Your body cells can then release waste products more easily. Undigested stores of fuel are used up and eliminated. Residues of toxic foods are worked out of the tissues. The entire system – from the skin to the brain – cleans house.

If you have essentially been eating a healthful diet, and not ingesting chemical drugs, and don't fall into any of the categories detailed in the above paragraphs, you could undergo a fast to help purify and maintain the function of your system. However, if you have been eating a very unhealthful diet, and/or have been taking chemical drugs over a period of time, it may be best to transition into a more healthful diet and lifestyle before undergoing an extended fast of more than two days.

Following a raw food diet that includes adequate amounts of quality water along with a variety of organically grown green-leafed vegetables will slowly detox your body, and will build a healthy base of amino acids, enzymes, essential fatty acids, and trace nutrients.

Including a green powder supplement in your diet can assist in detoxifying your body slowly before you undergo a long fast.

"Arrange to fast when the seasons change, or on a full moon; as these are times when the body cleanses the strongest. During each change of the seasons, Nature does its housecleaning by expelling poisons; this is why people experience the flu (which is often a detoxifying process) during the seasonal changes. When the moon is full, the tidal energies are pulled, and this lunar position also triggers the detoxifying process in the body – which, like the oceans that are affected by a full moon, is mostly water."
– David Wolfe

There are many types of fasts and cleanses that people can undergo to detox their system. Some involve staying away from all food, and only drinking water for a period of a day or more. Others may involve allowing in only certain types of foods that will assist the body in ridding itself of residues, plaque, and general waste from the cells.

One popular fasting program involves water, lemon juice, and cayenne pepper. Citrus juices help to clear toxins from the tissues, while also providing some nutrients. Lemon is a low-sugar fruit, and works well for a fast as it keeps the blood sugar low. Some people include a bit of powdered dulse or kelp in their juice.

Fasts may also involve initially abstaining from food for a day or more, then subsisting on limited quantities of juices made from high-quality raw vegetable and fruit for a number of days or weeks.

A juice fast that is done right, and that includes the right amount of quality nutrients from organically grown sources, can be of great benefit to a person's health.

A juice fast may involve juicing organically grown lemons and green vegetables, and blending the liquid with a small amount of high-quality oil, such as organically grown flax oil, hemp oil, grapeseed oil, or pumpkin seed oil. Some people may also include a little bit of high-quality organic green powder and/or grass juices. Kelp or dulse powder adds minerals to this fast.

> "Chlorophyll and the alkaline compounds in green-leafed vegetables combine with heavy metals and foreign chemicals in the body to form salts, allowing the body to eliminate them from the system."
> — **David Wolfe**

To end a fast, you may want to start by introducing a juice, such as water from a raw coconut, or a juiced cucumber or other raw green vegetables blended with high-quality raw green nutritious powder, such as VitaMineral Green (made by HealthForce). However, fresh greens are a better choice than processed green powder. Fresh greens and green powder are beneficial because they alkalinize the system, and the electricity increases the solubility of the blood. This allows for the suspension, metabolization, or removal of misappropriated minerals.

The amount of time you choose to remain on your fast should be in sync with the needs of your body, mind, and activities. Fasts may go on for several days, or for more than a week.

Fasts should be done in a way that is beneficial. If you are new to fasting, take care in undergoing a fast that will advance your well-being, which may mean a fast that lasts only one or two days of pure water.

Depending on your situation and goal, your fast may involve a day or more of water only. Then adding something like lemon juice to the water for a day or more. Then cucumber juice mixed with a little hemp seed oil, and water for a day or more. Introduce a green powder to the liquid, perhaps mixing it with freshly squeezed apple juice and/or rejuvelac.

An alternative would be water mixed with wild blue green algae, freshly squeezed lemon juice, and a teaspoon of hemp seed oil. Eventually you will be able to work up to longer fasts. Fasting becomes easier the more you practice and learn about it – and especially the more you understand, feel, and experience the benefits of it.

For solid food intake after a fast, start with something very gentle, such as raw papaya, avocado, or raw spinach and/or other green-leafed vegetables sprinkled with a little Celtic sea salt and/or kelp or dulse powder. Add a little of either raw olive oil, raw hemp oil, raw grapeseed oil, raw pumpkin seed oil, raw walnut oil, or raw flax oil.

Before fully breaking a fast and adding solid foods, you may also consider low-sugar juice fruits, such as grapefruit, and/or fresh figs (not dried), or cherries. After several hours, add a more substantial food, such as an avocado, or other simple food, such as spinach salad with vinegar and olive, hemp, or flax oil, and some walnuts or soaked sunflower seeds or pignolies. Later eat a piece of fruit. By doing this you will come out of your fast slowly over a period of days.

The quality of your fast will also be determined by the quality of foods that you introduce into your system as you come out of your fast. The longer you carry on your fast, the deeper the new foods will touch your system. Make special efforts to include organically grown foods.

As a water-based fast continues, and the stomach and intestines clear themselves of food through the natural digestion process, the body will then turn to sugar in the system. When that fuel source is depleted, the body turns to glycogen in the tissue cells as a fuel source. The body also starts to burn excess fat as a fuel source. This is the last stage anyone should go into during a fast, as the body will then start to break down protein as a fuel source.

Fasting should be used as a system cleansing process, and not as a weight control tool. Just because you still may be overweight is not a reason to continue a fast. Trying to lose excess weight too quickly is not only unhealthful, but can be dangerous. It is good to lose excess weight by following a healthful diet and reasonable exercise program over a period of months and years, and not to lose weight all at one time on a fast, which is clearly not healthful.

As you follow a water fast, the body keeps eliminating toxins. Digestive fluids are absorbed into the intestines and help to rid the body of unnecessary substances in the tissues. The blood and lymph keep carrying waste products out of the tissues, and the waste is eventually put out of the body through the eliminatory organs. For this reason it is beneficial to undergo colon hydrotherapy as part of the fasting process as colon hydrotherapy greatly assists in eliminating toxins from the body.

The amount of water you take into your body during a fast depends on what you are physically doing during the fast. If your fast includes intensive yoga sessions, and/or other physical activity, as well as reasonable use of a steam room or sauna, you will obviously need more water. If you are thirsty, listen to your body and drink a reasonable amount of water. Drinking water will help provide hydration for the blood and lymph systems, and this will assist in the diffusion of toxins to take place as the cells that are thick with toxins will push the toxins into the blood and lymph.

There are important physical, as well as mental and spiritual benefits to fasting.

Everyone has experienced times when he or she simply needs to rest, sleep, and rejuvenate. The constant bombardment of life can sometimes cause too much stimulation to the point of stress and irritation. People sometimes need a rest from the constant interaction with food, elements, people, and information. Resting from these can help heal stress-related issues and ailments. But also, fasting with someone with whom you are close can strengthen your bonds and improve your relationship.

Often what may be ailing you does not need attention. What it may need is no attention, no substances, no stimulation, and no manipulation. There are benefits in simply resting, being in a calm space, and stopping the input of anything into your system other than water and air and motivational thoughts. During this time, work your body daily with an hour or more of yoga, swimming, walking, or riding a bike. As you do this, your system keeps eliminating substances that are not needed in your system.

Fasting is similar to opening the windows of a smoky room and allowing the smoke to dissipate.

"Isn't it interesting that the major religions of the world teach the benefits of fasting? This is because the journey into fasting is about becoming a finely tuned spiritual instrument. Fasting on water is a spiritual practice. Undertaking a fast measures self-discipline and self-control. Fasting tests the will."
— David Wolfe

Fasting is more effective when you do it with purpose and intention, while distancing yourself from such things as entertainment and the daily grind. When you rest from the stimulation of your regular day, your mind naturally begins to realign and focus on the essence of your being and to tune into your current state of life.

Fasting from food and stimulation has a cleansing effect on all areas. It clears the tissues and the mind while lightening the body and enlightening the intellect. After a successful fast, a person's mind will work better because the body tissues are working better. With fewer toxic residues clogging the tissues, the electrical currents, talents, energies, and spiritual frequencies become more crystalline.

Besides yoga and colon hydrotherapy, fasts may also involve intensive physical as well as mental conditioning, such as massage, intentional study, and meditation. This can be particularly helpful if one can unplug from a busy schedule for a number of days, and focus on fine-tuning the physical, mental, and spiritual bodies. Doing so in a calm and natural environment, such as in a forest, can be particularly healing, energizing, and nurturing.

Fasting also shows us how little food our bodies need. I think that maybe if Nature were to provide us with little to no food during a certain part of the year, this would be a sign that we should not eat as much food during this time. The closest we have to this situation is the middle of winter when there is less food being produced by Nature in a large part of the hemisphere (February in the Northern Hemisphere, and August in the Southern Hemisphere). Even Nature seems to take a rest during the middle of winter. It is also a time when we use less energy as the cold naturally makes us less active. Perhaps this is a time when we should eat little, and consider an extended fast of some sort to clean and rest our systems. The fast may last for a few days, or more than a week. Some people advocate fasting for more than a month, but that is something that I question, unless it includes some form of nourishment and other factors are right. Do what is right and responsible for you.

A body that has subsisted on unhealthful foods likely shows particular evidence of toxins in the skin, eyes, hair, and nails. It is also evident in the weight, texture, smell, function, shape, and limited capabilities of the body.

These toxins include an accumulation of low-quality and cooked oils, foreign proteins, and various chemicals found in common unhealthful foods that prevent the system from radiating health. This is because the billions of cells of the body, which strive to eliminate improper material, are not able to keep up with the toxins they are being exposed to.

The mucous membrane of the digestive tract works to push out food residues toward areas of less concentration, up into the mouth and sinuses, and down toward the colon. This is so that the toxins can leave the system. This process works around the clock, and it functions better when a person is eating a healthful diet. Signs of this process working during the sleeping hours are evident in what people refer to as "morning breath" as the mouth and sinuses become coated with what the system has been eliminating. On the other end it is evident as the system has the urge to defecate soon after waking. The way this process works is one reason for diagnosing a person's health by looking at the coloration of the tongue, and by a colon exam. Those two areas of the body can give indications as to what is going on in the rest of the system.

Detoxifying the body frees cells to rebound into health, to generate healthy cells, and to function with a cleaner, brighter, and lighter energy.

> "Success philosopher and author, Og Mandino, taught that 'You are not a human being, you are a human becoming.'
> You are constantly becoming something different. Remember that the human body is constantly recreating itself out of the air, water, food, and energy you ingest as well as the thoughts you entertain. In just a few years you can completely reconstruct your entire body from totally brand new high-quality materials. It is never too late to start on the pathway to better health."
> **— David Wolfe**

Stopping the consumption of impure and unhealthful foods allows the body to stop spending energy on cleaning out the bad foods, and instead allows it to work on generating health. By beginning a pure diet, the rubbish of an unhealthful diet will no longer make the cells perform at a slothful level. Those people will have more energy, will likely require less sleep, and will be more mentally clear and aware. They will become more in tune with the energy of Nature. Their instincts will beckon them to do what is natural for them in the form of their talents and abilities. They will look and feel better. They will be driven to accomplish more and to work toward improving all areas of their life.

None of the good things that the body can naturally do can be done to the person's full potential if he or she is bogged down with a body that is saturated with residues from unhealthful food choices. The substances in those foods spread throughout the body and cause a sedation of the senses, intuition, and instincts. By detoxifying the body, the sedation wears off and the person becomes more alive as the deadness of the toxins leaves the body.

> **"Surgeons know that the blood is almost immediately thickened by eating heavy foods, making it dangerous to perform surgery. This is one of the reasons why they will perform surgery only after a patient has fasted on water for at least eight hours. Eating raw plant food thins the blood, as does fasting."**
> **— David Wolfe**

The two main fluids of the body are blood and lymph. There is more lymph fluid than there is blood in the body. The lymph fluid bathes every cell. The blood feeds the lymph system, and also carries waste away from it. When the blood is cleaned of toxicity by way of a healthful diet, it can then draw toxins out of the body at a faster rate.

> **"As the lymph unburdens itself of undigested proteins, toxins, chemicals, and other undesirable elements, the substances flow into the bloodstream. Instantly a poison may be all over the circulatory system before it is filtered out as waste. This is why some of those who begin a fast may have sudden cold or hot flashes, fevers, diarrhea, rashes, desires for poor foods, tastes of old medicines, mucus discharges, and other symptoms, while detoxifying. These physical eliminations may also carry with them a variety of emotional releases, such as anxiety, depression, and other imbalances. These are good signs – you want those poisonous substances and emotions out of your body. Don't worry about them, but embrace them as part of the detoxification process. Other detoxification symptoms may include bad breath, coughs, cold symptoms, drowsiness, headaches, momentary aches, nausea, unclear thinking, and/or weight loss."**
> **— David Wolfe**

In addition to the urinary tract (kidneys, bladder, etc.) and colon, the body eliminates toxins through the lungs, sinuses, mouth, and skin. Those going through a detox may notice that their skin becomes clammy – making them feel dirty. This detoxification process can be helped along if the person has access to a steam or dry sauna. Drinking reasonable amounts of high-quality water can assist this process of sweating and breathing out toxins. Freshly squeezed lemons, and small amounts of warming or stimulating foods, such as garlic, onions, red peppers, and ginger, can also assist the system in eliminating toxins.

If you introduce unhealthful food to your system during a fast, the body's process of detoxification slows. The detoxification process may have made you feel temporarily sickly, with more mucus, thicker and/or smellier sweat, etc., as the tissues released toxins into the blood and lymph to be eliminated. If that process stops or slows down when you begin to eat cooked or other unhealthful foods, it is not an indication that the detox was unhealthful. What happens is that the introduction of heavy foods slows down the detoxification process, making you feel as if you had become healthier. This is not the case, because the body didn't finish carrying out the detox. This is because the reintroduction of unhealthful food halted the major detox process, and the body went back to doing minimal detoxification, as it had to refocus energy onto dealing with all of the new substances being introduced in unhealthful foods.

The key to carrying out a detox program is to get past the stage where the body is eliminating the abundance of toxins, and get to the point where the body has detoxed and starts to operate at a higher and healthier level.

While those who have followed an unhealthful diet for years cannot expect to completely detoxify their body through a simple three- to seven-day detox program, they can expect to jolt their system into detox mode to begin to rid itself of garbage. Then, as the person follows a Sunfood diet the body will continue to detox. The longer the body stays on the raw vegan path, the cleaner and healthier the system will become.

In addition to eating a healthful raw vegan diet, one can assist the body in detoxifying by engaging in regular exercise, such as yoga or swimming and cardiovascular exercise; by getting therapeutic massage to help drain the lymph system; and by drinking high-quality water.

Wolfe talks about the process, or law, of diffusion. This involves the movement of particles from an area of greater concentration to that of lesser concentration. Elements take the path of least resistance. It is a process of diffusion.

Within the body, if the blood and lymph systems are slowed down by eating highly concentrated foods, such as those that are cooked, or that consist largely of heavy protein (meat, milk, eggs), the particles that would normally be flushed out of the cells as waste products stay in the cells. As a person continues eating an unhealthful diet, the cells become heavy with waste products, as the cells cannot dispose of the waste – because the blood and lymph are too thick with the substances of an unhealthful diet. When a person stops eating, such as during a fast, or goes into a period of eating healthful foods, the blood and lymph become more fluid. This allows the cells to dispose of waste products into the blood and lymph, allowing the body to rid itself of accumulated toxins and unhealthful fats.

This illustrates the law of diffusion. Eventually the tissues release the bulk of the toxins stored there; then, as the blood and lymph continue to push out toxins, they become lighter and the whole system functions better. The major detox session comes to an end.

Those who change their way of eating to a more healthful pattern, and the body detoxifies, they may notice changes in the color and texture of their skin, hair, and nails, and in the vibrancy and clarity of their eyes. They may also start to smell, taste, feel, see, hear, and think more clearly as their senses become more alive and free of toxins that deadened them. Essentially they become stronger, more alive, and aware. This is part of the magic process of the detoxification and health-infusion that happens while living the Sunfoodist diet.

As your body detoxifies and becomes healthier, it also utilizes nutrients better. This is because the very sensitive membrane that lines the digestive tract is constantly being restored. Within weeks of eating a raw vegan diet the mucous lining of the digestive tract, which becomes irritated on a cooked food diet, heals and begins to function as it should. Together with a healthy amount of intestinal flora (the bacteria that live in your intestines and help to digest your food), you will be on your way to not only better nutrition, but you will also be able to better absorb the nutrients that you do eat.

Dissection Dissent

"Though hundreds of alternatives are available, two million animals are killed and dissected in U.S. classrooms each year."
— A Voice for Animals, 2006

If your child is being told he or she needs to dissect a frog or other living thing in the classroom as part of getting a good grade, then the parents must voice their objection to the teacher. No child has to participate in the killing of or dissection of a frog or other living thing.

Students also do not need to participate in a dissection through observing other students conducting one. For more information on this topic, contact:

Physicians Committee for Responsible Medicine, 202-686-2210; PCRM.Org

Duck and Geese Torture:
Foie Gras (Fatty Liver)

"Foie gras, which is French for 'fatty liver,' is made from the grotesquely enlarged livers of male ducks and geese. Kept in tiny wire cages, the birds have pipes repeatedly shoved down their throats and up to four pounds of grain and fat pumped into their stomachs every day. This cruel procedure often causes severe injuries or death. Those who survive the force-feeding suffer from a painful illness that causes their livers to swell to up to 10 times their normal size. Many birds become too sick to stand. When the birds are slaughtered, their livers are sold for foie gras."
   — GoVeg.Com/Feat/Foie, 2006

"A farm worker grabs each duck and, one by one, thrusts a metal pipe down each throat so that a mixture of corn can be forced directly into the gullet. In just a matter of weeks the ducks become grossly overweight and their livers expand up to ten times their normal size."
   — NoFoisGras.Org, 2006

"Ducks and geese are social animals who suffer when confined in individual cages. The confinement also can lead to lesions of the sternum and bone fractures, as well as foot injuries from the cage floors. Ducks and geese also suffer when they're not allowed enough water to swim and preen, which they do naturally in the wild.
   Originally, all foie gras came from France, but now the United States has gotten into this cruel niche industry. Next time you go into a store or restaurant that sells foie gras, please let them know that a product that comes from force-feeding ducks and geese is more than you can stomach."
   — The Humane Society of the United States

"Sonoma Foie Gras is responsible for the production of 20 percent of the United States' foie gras, and the confinement, forced-feeding, and slaughter of over 100,000 ducks a year. At a very young age the ducks

are put into crowded pens in filthy sheds. The floor is covered with feces and vomit. The farm is so unsanitary that rats run freely. Investigators witnessed and documented a rat eating two ducks alive."
 — GourmetCruelty.Com, 2006

In the summer of 2006 Chicago became the first city to ban foie gras. Let us all work to spread this law across the continent!

All-Creatures.Org/sof/Plate-FoieGras.html

GourmetCruelty.Com
  Produced a movie about foie gras production titled *Delicacy of Despair*.

GoVeg.Com/Feat/Foie/

The Humane Society of the United States.
HSUS.Org/Farm_Animals/Factory_Farms/Foie_Gras.html

JewishVeg.Com/Media03.html

NoFoieGras.Org

Electronics Recycling

Book:
* *High Tech Trash: Digital Devices, Hidden Toxics, and Human Health*, by Elizabeth Grossman

Cell phones and other electronics contain toxic chemicals. Do you know that electronics that are thrown away often end up in landfills, or are shipped to other countries, where they end up in landfills, or are burned? In any of these scenarios the toxic chemicals end up in the environment, where they can lead to cancer, birth defects, miscarriages, and brain disorders in both humans and wildlife.

"The electronic waste (e-waste) crisis that our society has created is the result of the volume and toxicity of the offending materials, as well as our failure to take responsibility for managing these materials appropriately. Studies have estimated that between 1997 and 2007, more than 500 million computers will become obsolete in the U.S. alone. The toxics that we have effectively stored within these computers include approximately six billion pounds of plastic, 1.5 billion pounds

of lead, three million pounds of cadmium, two million pounds of chromium, and 600,000 pounds of mercury... Much of the electronic waste produced in the U.S. is shipped to developing countries such as China, India, and Nigeria."
    — **Building Toxic Waste Pipelines to Africa, by Richard Gutierrez,** *Earth First Journal*; July-August 2006

In 2006 it was estimated that about two billion people had cell phones and that over 700 million would be sold during that year. In California, and probably most everywhere cell phones are used, the life of a cell phone averages 18 months. In California that means that about 14 million cell phones had been disposed of during 2006.

Do you have cell phones, computers, radios, pagers, and other electronics that you don't use? Do not put them in the trash. If the retailer where you purchased the product, or bought a new one, doesn't have a recycle program, check with your local community recycling program, or check:

Basel Action Network, BAN.Org

Computer TakeBack Campaign, ComputerTakeBack.Com

EBay's ReThink program, Ebay.EZTradeIn.Com

FreeGeek.Org

PlanetGreenInc.Com

The Silicone Valley Toxics Coalition, SVTC.Org

Environmental Protection

Also see:
- Hemp Farming: Work to Legalize It
- Off-Road Vehicles: The Plague of the Wildlands
- Trees and Plants
- Waterlife Protection

Books:
- *Clearcut: The Tragedy of Industrial Forestry*, by Bill Devall
- *From the Redwood Forest, Ancient Trees and the Bottom Line: A Headwaters Journey,*

by Joan Dunning with photographs by Doug Thron

- *Heal the Ocean: Solutions for Saving Our Seas*, by Rod Fujita
- *The Key to Sustainable Cities: Meeting Human Needs, Transforming Community Systems*, by Gwendolyn Hallsmith
- *Igniting a Revolution: Voices in Defense of the Earth*, by Steven Best and Anthony J. Nocella II
- *The Last Stand: The War Between Wall Street and Main Street over California's Ancient Redwoods*, by David Harris
- *Lost Mountain: A Year in the Vanishing Wilderness: Radical Strip Mining and the Devastation of Appalachia*, by Eric Reece
- *Salmon Nation: People and Fish at the Edge*, Edited by Edward C. Wolf and Seth Zuckerman
- *Totem Salmon*, by Freeman House

"Polite conservationists leave no mark save the scars upon the Earth that could have been prevented had they stood their ground."
— **David Brower, first executive director of the Sierra Club; founder of Friends of the Earth; founder of Earth Island Institute; father of the modern environmental movement**

"The more clearly we can focus our attention on the wonders and realities of the universe about us, the less taste we shall have for destruction."
— **Rachel Carson**

"The human mind is a product of the Pleistocene age, shaped by wildness that has all but disappeared. If we complete the destruction of nature, we will have succeeded in cutting ourselves off from the source of sanity itself."
— **David Orr**

"If future generations are to remember us with gratitude rather than contempt, we must leave them something more than the miracles of technology. We must leave them a glimpse of the world as it was in the beginning, not just after we got through with it."
— **Lyndon B. Johnson**

"Nobody made a greater mistake than he who did nothing because he could do only a little."
— **Edmund Burke**

"How you imagine the world determines how you live in it."
— **David Suzuki**

"We have got to share this planet with the other living creatures, and sharing means not merely preserving them in zoos or National Parks, but setting aside huge areas. Whole regions perhaps that will be free of human interference. Ideally, I would like to see certain large areas of the planet set off-limits to human entry of any kind, even aerial over flights."

— Edward Abbey, *Deep Ecology for the 21st Century: The Natural Wonder: An Ecocentric World View*

Conservation of Nature should be part of everyone's life. The word *conservation* derives from the Latin word *conservare*, which means *to keep guard*. The following can help you be a guard to Nature.

100Fires.Com
  Sells books, CDs, DVDs, videos, cassettes, periodicals, and other items relating to the environment, peace, ecology, etc.

Act Against Cigarette Butt Litter; CigaretteLitter.Org

Action for Community and Ecology in the Rainforests of Central America; POB 57, Burlington, VT 05402; 802-863-0571; ACERCA.Org

Allegheny Defense Project, AlleghenyDefense.Org

Alliance for Sustainable Jobs and Environment, 1125 SE Madison, Portland, OR 97214; 503-736-9777; ASJE.Org

Appalachian Trail Conservancy, AppalachianTrail.Org

Australian Bush Heritage Fund, BushHeritage.Org

BAGHEERA - Endangered Species Web site, Bagheera.Com

Bristol Bay Alliance, PO Box 231985, Anchorage, AK 99523-1985; 907-276-7605; BristolBayAlliance.Com

Carbon-Info.Org

Care for the Wild International, CareForTheWild.Org

Caribbean Conservation Corporation, 4424 NW 13th St. Ste. A1, Gainesville, FL 32609; 352-373-6441; CCCTurtle.Org

Cascadia Rising EcoDefense, POB 12583, Portland, OR 97212; CascadiaRising.Org

Cascadia Wild, 1417 SE 34th Ave., Portland, OR 97214; 503-235-9533; CascadiaWild.Org

Cascadia Wildlands Project, POB 10455, Eugene, OR 97440; 541-434-1460; CascWild.Org

Center for Native Ecosystems, 2260 Baseline Rd., Ste. 205, Boulder, CO 80302; 303-247-0998; NativeEcoSystems.Org

Center for Science in Public Participation, 224 N. Church Ave., Bozeman, MT 59715; CSP2.Org

Circle of Life Foundation, POB 3764, Oakland, CA 94609; 510-601-9790; CircleOfLifeFoundation.Org
    Founded by Julia Butterfly Hill who lived near the top of a California redwood tree for two years and brought international attention to the horrors of the lumber industry and the state of the environment. Hill authored a book titled *The Legacy of Luna*.

ClimateArk, EcologicalInternet.Org

ClimateCrisis.Net

Communities for a Better Environment, CBECal.Org

Community Environment Legal Defense Fund, 2859 Scotland Rd., Chambersburg, PA 17201; CELDF.Org

Deep Ecology, Deep-Ecology.Net

Earth Communications Office, OneEarth.Org

Earth First!, Direct Action Fund, POB 210; Canyon, CA 91516; EarthFirstJournal.Org

Earth First!, POB 1415; Eugene, OR 97440; 541-741-9191; EnviroLink.Org/Orgs/EF

Earth Island Institute, 300 Broadway, Ste. 28, San Francisco, CA 94133; 415-788-3666; EarthIsland.Org

Earth Justice Legal Defense Fund, 180 Montgomery St., Ste. 1400, San Francisco, CA 94104; 415-627-6700; EarthJustice.Org/Support

Earth911.Org

Earth Share, IGC.Org/EarthShare

EarthWatch.Org

EarthWorksAction.Org

EcoEarth.Info

EcologyCenter.Org

Ecology Project International, EcologyProject.Org

Eco-Now.Net

EcoTrust Canada, EcoTrustCan.Org

EdwardGoldsmith.Com
Founder of *The Ecologist* magazine. Web site provides abundant writings on issues relating to ecology.

Endangered Earth: Center for Biological Diversity, BiologicalDiversity.Org

Environmental Defense Canada, EnvironmentalDefence.CA

Environmental Protection Information Center, POB 397, Garberville, CA 95542; WildCalifornia.Org

Environmental Working Group, EWG.Org

EnvironmentNow.Org

EverGreen Canada, EverGreen.CA/En/

Fondo Per La Terra Earth Fund, Italy, FondoPerLaTerra.Org

Friends of Clayoquot Sound, FOCS.Ca

Friends of the Earth, 1025 Vermont Ave., NW, Washington, DC 20005; 202-783-7400; FOE.Org

Friends of the Earth, England, FOE.Org.UK

Fund for Wild Nature, POB 42523, Portland, OR 97242; FundForWildNature.Org

Gifford Pinchot Task Force, POB 11427, Olympia, WA 98508; 360-753-4185; GPTaskForce.Org

Global Eco-Village Network, Findhorn, Scotland; EcoVillage.Org

Global Environmental Facility, GEFWeb.Org

GlobalGreen.Org

Global Resource Action Center for the Environment, 15 E. 26th St., Rm. 915, New York, NY 10010; 212-726-9161; GraceLinks.Org

Global Response, Environmental Action & Education Network, POB 7490, Boulder, CO 80306; GlobalResponse.Org

GRACE Factory Farm Project, 145 Spruce St., Lititz, PA 17543; 717-627-0410; FactoryFarm.Org

Granby Wilderness Society, POB 2532, Grand Forks, B.C. V0H 1H0 Canada; 250-442-2125; GranbyWilderness.Org

GrandCanyonTrust.Org

Green Anarchy, POB 11331, Eugene, OR 97440; GreenAnarchy.Org

Greenpeace, 702 H St., NW, Ste. 300, Washington, DC 20001; 202-462-1177; Greenpeace.Org

Green Power, Hong Kong, China, GreenPower.Org.HK

GreenVolunteers.Com

GrownUpGreen.Org.UK

HabitatWork.Org

Honor The Earth, HonorEarth.Org

Hydrosphere, Hydrosphere-Expedition.Com

International Forum on Globalization, IFG.Org

The International POPs (Persistent Organic Pollutants) Elimination Network, IPEN.ECN.CZ

Kahea: The Hawaiian Environmental Alliance, Kahea.Org
   Works with citizens organizing to protect sensitive shorelines and culturally significant sites from inappropriate development and to prevent the conversion of agricultural lands to gated communities, golf courses, and malls. Also works to protect Hawai'i's threatened biodiversity and endangered species of the land and water.

Kentucky Conservation Committee, POB 1152, Frankfort, KY 40602; 502-875-0909; Kentucky.SierraClub.Org/KCC/BillSummary.asp

298 SUNFOOD LIVING

Working to stop mountaintop removal coal mining operations in the Appalachian mountains.

KyotoUSA.Org,
Provides information on how you and your city or town can become more environmentally friendly by greatly reducing greenhouse gasses.

League of Conservation Voters, 1920 L. St. NW, Ste. 800, Washington, DC 20036; 202-785-8683; LCV.Org

The Leonardo DiCaprio Foundation, LeonardoDiCaprio.Org

Mayors for Climate Change, 436 14th St., Ste. 1520, Oakland, CA 94612; CoolMayors.Org

Mendocino Environmental Center, MECGrassroots.Org
Helpful list of links to environmental organizations, groups, societies, etc.

Mindfully.Org/Air

Mothers and Others for a Livable Planet, 40 W. 20th St., New York, NY 10011-4211; Mothers.Org

Mountain Justice Summer, MountainJusticeSummer.Org
Focused on the ecological disaster being caused by mountain top removal mining in the Appalachian mountains of Tennessee, Virginia, West Virginia, and Kentucky.

Natural Resources Defense Council, Natural Resources Defense Council, 40 W. 20th St., New York, NY 10011; NRDC.Org

The Natural Step, POB 29372, San Francisco, CA 94129-0372; 415-561-3344; NaturalStep.Org

Nature Foundation of South Australia, NatureFoundation.Org.AU

NatureInTheCity.Org

Northwest Ecosystems Alliance, 1208 Bay St., Ste. 201, Bellingham, WA 98225; Ecosystem.Org

Nova Scotia Nature Trust, NSNT.CA

Potomac Conservancy, Potomac.Org

Redefining Progress, 1904 Franklin St., 6th Fl., Oakland, CA 94612; 510-444-3041; RProgress.Org

Remineralize the Earth, Remineralize.Org

Resurgence.Org

Rising Tide Climate Justice Network, RisingTide.NL

Romanian Mine Accidents: Environmental Disasters in Central Europe, ZPOK.HU/Cyanide/Baiamare

Ruckus Society, 2054 University Ave., Ste. 204, Berkeley, CA 94704; 510-848-9565; Ruckus.Org
 Helps environmental and human rights organizations develop skills in civil disobedience.

Sathirakoses-Nagapradeepa Foundation, Sulak-Sivaraksa.Org/

SaveHappyValley.Org.NZ

Shenandoah Ecosystem Defense Group, POB 1891, Charlottesville, VA 22903; 804-971-1553; AlleghenyDefense.Org

Siskiyou Project, 917 SW Oak, Ste. 407, Portland, OR 97205; Siskiyou.Org

SkyTruth.Org
 Uses remote sensing and digital mapping to educate the public and policymakers about the environmental consequences of human activities.

Society for Ecological Restoration International, SER.Org

SkyIslandAlliance.Org

StopGlobalWarming.Org

Student Environmental Action Coalition, POB 31909, Philadelphia, PA 19104; SEAC.Org

Sustainable Development Institute, SusDev.Org

Taiwan Nature Trail Society, NatureT.NGO.Org.TW/NatureT2/

Tasmanian Wilderness Society, Wilderness.Org.AU/Regions/Tas/

Tidepool, Tidepool.Org
 Environmental news.

Union of Concerned Scientists, 2 Brattle Sq., Cambridge MA 02238; 617-547-5552; UCSUSA.Org

UnitedMountainDefense.Org

Western Mining Action Network, WMAN-Info.Org

Wild Earth, POB 455, Richmond, VT 05477; 802-434-4077; Wild-Earth.Org

Wilderness Society, Wilderness.Org.AU
Works to protect Australian wildlands, including the tallest hardwood trees in the world.

Wildlands Center for Preventing Roads, Missoula Office: POB 7516, Missoula, MT 59807; 406-543-9551; Colorado Office: POB 2353, Boulder, CO 80306; 303-247-0998; WildlandsCPR.Org

The Wildlands Project, WildlandsProjectRevealed.Org

"The only hope of the Earth is to withdraw huge areas as inviolate natural sanctuaries from the depredations of modern industry and technology. Move out the people and cars. Reclaim the roads and the plowed lands."
— Dave Foreman, *Confessions of an Eco-Warrior*

Worldwatch Institute, 1776 Massachusetts Ave., NW, Washington, DC 20036; 202-452-1999; WorldWatch.Org

Yellowstone to Yukon Conservation Initiative
114 West Pine, Missoula, MT 59802; 406-327-8512; Y2Y.Net

Enzymes

"Enzymes are substances that make life possible. They are needed for every chemical reaction that takes place in the human body. No mineral, vitamin, or hormone can do any work without enzymes. Our bodies, all our organs, tissues, and cells are run by metabolic enzymes."
— Dr. Edward Howell, *Enzyme Nutrition*

"Through years of research Dr. Ann Wigmore discovered that all the enzymes, vitamins, and minerals that the body needs are found within the foods we eat – IF these foods are prepared in such a way as to maintain or unlock their life-giving nutrients."
— Creative Health Institute, CreativeHealthUSA.Com/LivingFoods.htm.

The standard American diet (often referred to as the "SAD" diet) is lacking in quality enzymes. This is because heating and intense processing of food kills enzymes. Enzymes are necessary for life. The better the quality of enzymes that your body is supplied with, the better health you can experience.

All living things contain enzymes. There are more than 2,500 different types of enzymes in the body. They are protein molecules that are paramount to all chemical reactions within the body. They act along with minerals, fats, carbohydrates, vitamins, minerals, amino acids, and all other necessary elements of the body tissues to produce living functions throughout the body. Enzymes are central to the formation, repair, restoration, and revitalization of all tissues.

If you do not have a healthy bank of enzymes within your body, your health suffers.

People who consistently consume raw plant matter have a better store of enzymes in their bodies than those who eat a diet that is all or partially made up of cooked food.

There are three classes of enzymes: metabolic enzymes, digestive enzymes, and food enzymes.

The first class, metabolic enzymes, are within the cells of the body tissues. They are essential to all cellular activity, including breathing, healing, and movement.

The second class, digestive enzymes, are produced by all areas of the alimentary tract, from the mouth to the colon. Amylase enzymes are essential to the digestion of carbohydrates. Lipase enzymes are essential to the digestion of fats. Protease enzymes are essential to the digestion of proteins.

The third class, which are essential to the formation of both metabolic and digestive enzymes, are food enzymes. These are supplied to the body through raw plant substances.

Living enzymes exist in all plant life. They are essential to the ripening of food. There are some plants that survive in areas where temperatures get above 120 degrees, such as some types of cactus, but in large measure, most plants die (because their enzymes are greatly damaged or are killed) at temperatures above 120 degrees. Freezing food may damage most enzymes, and can kill them. Also, there are some plants that exist in areas where temperatures drop well below freezing, but again, most plants on the planet die when temperatures drop below freezing.

Because fermenting of raw foods, such as in raw sauerkraut, kimchi, and seed cheeses, increases enzymatic activity, some people encourage the use of fermented foods for healing of the body. Dr. Ann Wigmore, a raw-food enthusiast and author of several books, advocated the use of fermented foods in healing the body.

When people follow a diet that is lacking in high-quality plant enzymes, their cellular activity begins to vibrate at a lower frequency, and their health degenerates into *dis-ease*.

When a person is lacking in high-quality food enzymes, the digestive enzymes degrade and begin to draw on the metabolic enzymes. This series of events weakens the body, causes sluggishness, and paves the way for illness to set in. The standard American diet, therefore, is responsible for a human who is not living a quality life. The body is alive, but the system is breaking down, and eventually is susceptible to limited physical and mental abilities, to unhealthful and damaged body tissues, to all sorts of illness, and to premature death.

You can weaken your enzyme potential permanently if you follow an unhealthful diet. Just as a houseplant may show damage from a time that it was neglected, the body may also be permanently damaged in its ability to produce and manage enzymes. But, just as a plant can regain vigor when it is supplied with the right nutrients, so too can the human body.

Foods that damage enzymatic activity within the body include meat, milk, eggs, and products made with them. They also included all cooked, baked, and fried foods, foods that contain artificial dyes and flavors, as well as other artificial ingredients and/or those that have been overly processed. Eating these deadened foods drains the system of health and puts the body out of tune with Nature.

The good news is that a system that has been damaged by unhealthful eating can be made healthier by cutting out deadened foods, and by eating a healthful, vibrant diet. Because the biological factory that exists within the body is designed to function in a certain way, it will always work better if it is given the proper fuel.

Your body cannot function at its highest level if you are not feeding it what it needs to function at that level. You can change that now, today, with your food choices. Make a conscious decision to select and eat food that is high quality, and preferably consisting of raw, organically grown fruits, vegetables, herbs, berries, nuts, seeds, and water vegetables.

Essential Fatty Acids

Quality fat sources (all **MUST** be eaten raw to get the best quality fats undamaged by heat):

Seeds can be ground in a coffee grinder and used in dressings, smoothies, dips, and other foods. They can also be sprouted and used in salads or as garnishes.

- **Coconut**, fresh, or cold-processed coconut oil
- **Grapeseed oil**, cold-processed
- **Green-leafed vegetables**
- **Flax seeds**, or cold-processed flax oil
- **Hemp seeds**, or cold-processed hemp seed oil
- **Olives**, or cold-processed olive oil
- **Pumpkin seeds**, or raw pumpkin seed butter
- **Soybeans**, raw, uncooked, fresh
- **Sunflower seeds**, or cold-processed sunflower seed oil
- **Walnuts**, raw, or cold-processed walnut oil
- **Other unheated, organically grown edible plant oils**

Wolfe points out that since fat is an insulator, it is something the body craves when it needs insulation. Those living in heavily populated cities may desire more fatty foods as insulation against the elements of the city. Those who are in abusive relationships, neglected relationships, or unsatisfying relationships, or who are not dealing well with life issues, often binge on fatty foods.

Eliminating unhealthful fats and strictly limiting quality fats improves health in more ways than one. It helps the body get to an ideal weight, removes the physio-emotional shield a person may have been brandishing to avoid facing troubles or issues in life, and allows people to focus more clearly on those things in their life that need their attention.

We all need fat. How's that for a diet plan? If you don't get quality fats in your diet, your health suffers.

While some may tell you that you can get quality fats by eating salmon, or from cod liver oil, what they may be overlooking is that you also get a whole slew of other things when you rely on fish as a source of quality oils. Fish are constantly taking in water, just as we take in air. Fish work as filters as they are filtering all sorts of toxins from whatever water they are in. Unfortunately, even the distant seas are now polluted with substances like mercury, farming chemicals, military and cruise ship pollution, industrial and city runoff, and toxins absorbed in the oceans from airplanes and from air pollution drifting from distant cities. Pollutants tend to accumulate in fat. If you choose to eat salmon or cod liver oil, or other fatty fish, or any sea creature, what you are getting is a collection of any toxins in the water where that creature lived. Since many of the sea creatures that humans tend to eat are also creatures that eat smaller creatures, the larger fish are consuming the toxins that exist in the smaller fish, and on up the food chain, one concentrating the toxins of the other. It all accumulates in the fat of the fish.

Cod liver oil is also not good to consume. The liver is the detoxification center of the body. All toxins pass through the liver. If you choose to consume cod liver oil you are getting the most concentrated amount of toxins that exist within that fish.

Fish are not healthful to eat. Besides the toxins in their fats, they may also be harboring parasites that make people sick. They also contain cholesterol and saturated fat. Fish do not contain fiber, carbohydrates, vitamin C, or many nutrients that are what the human body needs.

You can exist on fish, and do so for years at a time. But your bones will suffer. At this stage in the industrialization of the world, when you eat fish you may be poisoning yourself with pollutants that can cause neurological disorders, birth defects, miscarriages, hormonal imbalances, and cancers. If you are a pregnant or nursing mother, that means that your child can be harmed if you are consuming fish.

The best sources of essential fatty acids are raw plant substances.

The way food is prepared affects the quality of the fat. Heating fat degrades it, and turns it into something that can be damaging to health – rather than healthful.

Fats are important in the digestion of sugars because fats surround sugars, slowing down their absorption into the digestive tract. This allows for a more even flow of energy obtained by the sugars.

Fats also are important because they lubricate the tissues; insulate the nerve tissues; play a part in transporting nutrients to the tissues, including minerals to the bones; and feed the fat cells that pad and support the organs.

High-quality fats from raw plant sources help to reverse cell damage from the consumption of cooked fats that leads to obesity, organ diseases, and heart issues. This is because the lipase enzyme that is present in raw plant fats helps to metabolize the cooked fats that clog the blood and lymph systems. Within the membrane of cells the quality raw fats replace the trans-fatty acids that hinder the respiration of the cells.

High-quality fats from raw plant sources stabilize and ground the body and provide fuel. In comparison, cooked and low-quality fats destabilize the body, collect and prevent the release of toxins from the body, clog and slow down the body systems, weaken the immune system, and pave the way for illness to set in.

The source of the fat is one factor that determines its quality. Because fats collect toxins, fruits and vegetables that are grown with the use of toxic farming chemicals contain traces of the chemicals. Therefore, organically grown fruits, nuts, seeds, and vegetables are a better source for fat.

Fat is made up of glycerin and fatty acids. The type and number of fatty acids that are attached to the glycerin molecule are what determine the type of fat.

Because the body cannot manufacture certain types of fats called linoleic and linolenic, these fats are called "essential fatty acids." These fats, grouped into omega 3 and omega 6 fatty acids, exist in many types of fatty plants, such as avocados, olives, nuts, seeds, and young coconuts. Raw hemp seeds and flax seeds contain high-quality fats (these seeds can be easily ground into a powder in a coffee grinder and added to juices, smoothies, dressings, and salads). Raw walnuts are also a high-quality fat source. The best balance of essential fatty acids is contained in raw hemp seeds, and fresh, cold-processed hemp seed oil.

> "I recommend adding flaxseed to your diet regularly. Flaxseeds have a tough outer coating and should be freshly ground in order to receive the most nutritional benefit. You can grind whole seeds with a coffee grinder or in a VitaMix blender dry container. I recommend adding one or two tablespoons of ground flax meal to your salads, soups, or smoothies. Flaxseed is also a good source of omega-3 fatty acids, and it is by far nature's richest source of plant lignin, an important anti-cancer phytonutrient."
> — **Victoria Boutenko in her book** *Green for Life*; **RawFamily.Com**

> "On the walls of the intestines we find villi. These are small, hair-like tissue structures containing blood capillaries. The villi absorb carbohydrates and amino acids. The villi of the small intestine contain lacteals (lymph channels) that absorb fats into the lymphatic system. The fat is conducted through the lymphatic vessels to the liver, where the fat is prepared for distribution throughout the body."
> — **David Wolfe**

Fats from animals are of low-quality, are damaging to cell walls, and should be avoided. They contain residues of all the toxic chemicals the animal was exposed to, as well as the chemistry of the animal it came from.

One environmental toxin that accumulates in animal fat is dioxin. This is a long-lasting, hormonal-disrupting compound that has been linked to cancer, birth defects, and developmental problems. Dioxin is commonly found in all animal products that are sold as food, including meat of all varieties (including seafood and birds), eggs, and dairy. Foods likely to contain dioxin residues should especially be avoided by women planning on becoming pregnant, by those who are pregnant, and by nursing mothers.

Animal fats are rarely eaten raw because milk products are usually heated, and meat is usually cooked in some manner. The heating of the animal oil destroys most of what could be considered to be the beneficial dietary qualities of the oil, and turns it into a substance that is harsh on the human system. (I don't advocate eating meat or milk in any form, raw or cooked. But, if you do choose to consume milk, it is much better to get it from an organic dairy where the cows graze in open fields, and to consume that milk raw, and not pasteurized. Milk from cows that graze in open fields and that are not treated with common drugs has much higher levels of beneficial essential fatty acids, including omega-3 and the omega-6 conjugated linoleic acid.)

Another problem with oils from animal flesh is that it is saturated and contains cholesterol. The consumption of saturated fat in the human body triggers the production of cholesterol. This leads to the scenario of heart disease, gallstones, strokes, and many degenerative conditions, including vision problems.

Those who are experiencing heart disease, who have had a stroke, or have been told their arteries are clogged, would be very wise to remove all animal products from their diet, as well as heated oils, all fried food, and all foods containing processed salt, corn syrup, sweetener, and all synthetic dyes, flavors, and preservatives. They should transition to a raw vegan diet consisting of a variety of high-quality, organically grown foods. Then the body can go about the process of removing the accumulation of cholesterol in the system.

Although the process of ridding the body of cholesterol plaque from the tissues can take years, benefits can be seen within days of eliminating all milk, egg, and meat products from the diet.

Plant oils do not contain cholesterol. Although cholesterol is needed in the human body, it does not need to be obtained from food. The body creates the cholesterol that it needs. Any additional cholesterol that is introduced into the body through the consumption of meat and dairy products is not needed, and becomes a problem for the body to eliminate.

The only people who need cholesterol in their diets are infants and babies, who need it for proper brain formation. Ideally they get their cholesterol from their mother's milk.

As mentioned earlier, fats play a part in the distribution of nutrients throughout the body, including minerals to the bones and tissues. As Wolfe points out in *The Sunfood Diet Success System*, raw plant fats also effectively increase the electric tension on cell membranes, making the cells more permeable to oxygen and nutrients. Unhealthful fats damage the cell walls, allow toxins to enter, and limit the cells' ability to rid itself of waste products and to maintain health.

Eating foods containing cooked fat, especially foods that have been cooked at high temperatures, is damaging to the body. These are the undesirable trans-fatty acids. They clog the system; slow the blood and lymph systems; irritate the alimentary tract; and interfere with the function of the power generators of every cell within the body.

Those power-generating structures within the cells are called the mitochondria. They become less effective in the cells of a person eating a junk diet, and especially of a diet containing cooked fat.

All fats that have been heated to high temperatures, hydrogenated, pasteurized, or oxidized should be avoided. They are damaging to health, and cause the body to accumulate toxins. They lead to obesity and degenerative diseases.

Oils from raw plants are much less likely to lead to the accumulation of toxins in the system. This is because the cells accommodate, work with, and need the essential fatty acids of raw plants.

Eliminating all cooked fats and animal fats from the diet and allowing in only raw plant fats actually leads to weight loss when a person is overweight. This is because the toxic fats will begin to be eliminated, and the cells will also be able to release the toxins that were contained in those unhealthful fats. Then the cells can begin to work more efficiently.

Raw plant fats contain lipase enzymes, which play a part in the "burning" of fats for body fuel. This fat-splitting enzyme is typically lacking in the bodies of overweight people, and in the bodies of those who subsist on unhealthful diets. The enzymes help the body metabolize collections of cooked fat residue in the bodies of cooked-food eaters.

As people transition into a raw vegan diet from that of a cooked diet

— and especially from a diet that contained meat and dairy — they may mistake the empty feeling they have for a lack of protein. Some may try to fill this feeling with cooked vegetables, or cooked starches. What they typically do have is a lack of high-quality raw plant fats.

The body desires fat, and quality fat is what it really needs. Eating a good selection of raw fruits and vegetables will provide an abundance of the amino acids the body needs to form protein.

Nothing can make up for a lack of high-quality essential fatty acids. For this reason you should be sure to include fatty plants in your diet.

Nuts are a fatty food more than they are a protein food. They (almonds, cashews, hazelnuts, macadamias, pecans, pine nuts, walnuts, etc.) should be eaten raw, and never heated, roasted, sautéed, toasted, or microwaved.

Eating too many nuts can be a bit harsh on the digestive tract; they carry a lot of calories; are acid-forming in large quantities; and, because they are acidic, eating too many can trigger mucus formation as the body works to be alkaline.

The consumption of nuts should be balanced by raw greens and fruits. In fact, nuts are excellent in both green salad and fruit salad.

The consumption of greens with nuts counteracts the acid of the nuts, and prevents a mucus-forming reaction, as greens are an alkaline food.

Soaking raw nuts for several hours in water can reduce the enzyme inhibitors that exist in them and that work to prevent their growth into a plant.

Adding raw plant oils to the diet — such as in homemade salad dressings — is a good way to get quality essential fatty acids into the system.

Quality oils from raw, organically grown plant sources are available at many natural foods markets. These oils should be purchased in dark bottles, and kept out of direct light. To prevent rancidity, oils should be kept in a very cool place or refrigerated.

Many seeds contain more fat than protein, and are considered to be fat-dominant. Raw seeds that are fat-dominant and have high-quality fats are the previously mentioned flax, hemp, pumpkin, grapeseed, and sesame. Many people do not consider a coconut to be a seed, but it is, and raw coconut is a fat-dominant seed that is of a high quality (when it is raw).

Plant fats contain all three types of fats: saturated, monounsaturated, and polyunsaturated. All three, when obtained from raw plants, are beneficial to health. Only when plant fats are heated are they damaging to health. Otherwise, raw plant fats are good for the body. Coconuts have saturated fat. Avocados, and raw olives, olive oil, and nuts contain monounsaturated fat. Polyunsaturated fat is found in walnuts, and in sunflower, flax, hemp, sesame, and other seeds.

> "Polyunsaturated fatty acids have a horseshoe shape. Their strong electrical nature allows them to split easily, enabling them to bind with and carry toxins out of the system. Because of their ability to bind with toxins, raw polyunsaturated fats are the most healing fats for the body. They are also highly sensitive and are the most subject to structural derangement through heating, hydrogenation, and oxidation.
> Damaged polyunsaturated fats are the most damaging fats for the body, and should be totally avoided."
> — David Wolfe

Raw plant fats contain antioxidants and help to prevent free radicals from damaging the tissues. Free radicals are electron-deficient molecules that are produced by oxygen and cooked fats in the body. Free radicals damage amino acids, enzymes, and other elements of the cells by taking electrons.

Raw plant fats have long-chain fatty acids and carry an abundance of electrons, and this allows for free radicals to obtain the electron from the fat without robbing the cell.

Fats that have been cooked both allow for, and cause, free radical damage. But raw plant fats, especially those that are in the polyunsaturated fat class, prevent free radical damage. This is because raw plant fats contain nutrients, such as vitamins C and E, as well as carotene and selenium. In addition, various other raw foods contain antioxidants, such as bioflavonoids in citrus and beta-carotene in certain vegetables. So the abundance of electrons provided by the raw plant fats saturates the body with spare electrons, and this essentially deactivates free radicals, allowing the cells of the body to remain healthier.

Some people think that they are eating healthfully if they are staying away from cooked foods that contain animal oils, and instead, eating cooked foods that contain plant fats, such as sunflower, canola, palm, or safflower oils. While eating plant fats is better than eating fats from animals, cooking any kind of fat damages nutrients and changes the chemistry of the fat, making it into something that is not wholly good for the body.

As mentioned earlier, fats from animals carry environmental and farm toxins the animals were exposed to; are saturated and cause the production of cholesterol in the body; contain cholesterol from the animals that overloads the human system, causing plaque to form within the blood passageways; contain the hormonal chemistry of the animals; and carry energy and hormones that are not good to put into the human body. Animal fats are toxic to the human system, lead to fat buildup, contain toxic residues, and result in compromised health.

Those who consume milk are also exposing themselves to the toxins, cholesterol, and unhealthful energy of the animal. While milk fat is a healthier animal fat than the fat from the meat of the animal, it does not carry the health benefits many people believe it has. Raw milk fat is also better than cooked milk fat. Milk from animals that are raised eating organic foods where they graze in open fields, and raised in a way that does not expose them to toxic farming chemicals and drugs, is much healthier than milk from factory farms where the animals are fed unnatural diets; exposed to unhealthful conditions that cause stress and disease; treated with growth hormones and other drugs; and exposed to various chemicals.

Goat milk is also likely to be more healthful than cow milk. But if goat milk is consumed, it should be from an organic farm source, and consumed raw, not pasteurized.

It may surprise those who have lived in a milk-consuming society that people in many parts of the world frown on drinking milk and on eating cheese, and think of consuming animal milk in any form as disgusting.

About the only time that I can imagine advising anyone to eat dairy products would be if there were no access to raw greens. If that is the case, and they also cannot obtain some quality green powder nutritional supplement, the ideal would be raw, organic milk that has not been pasteurized, and that is from cows that freely graze in an open field. Also, if you consume butter or cheese, it should also be organic and raw, and from cows that graze in open fields, and not cows confined to barns or factory farms.

Pasteurization of milk is a heating process, which damages the fats and creates a product that leads to degenerative conditions in the human body, such as heart disease. The casein protein in milk can also cause mood swings, depression, and anxiety. Those who experience depression would be wise to avoid milk, processed sugar and salt, cooked oils, and cooked grains, and increase the ratio of raw green vegetables and raw plant oils in their diet.

Raw dairy may provide some substances beneficial to establishing a base of healthy intestinal flora. But if dairy is consumed, it should be minimally. Ideally one would obtain minerals and flora from raw plant sources and not depend on dairy, which is mucus forming, acidifying, can leach minerals from the system, and most always carries a negative energy into the system. (For more information about the negative impact dairy products have on human health, and the health of the environment, read the books *Diet for a New America* and *The Food Revolution*, by John Robbins.)

BanTransFats.Com

Omega Nutrition, 6515 Aldrich Rd., Bellingham, WA 98226; 800-661-3529; OmegaNutrition.Com

Sunfood Nutrition, 11655 Riverside Drive, Lakeside, CA 92040; 800-205-2350; 888-RAW-FOOD; International: +001-619-596-7979; Sunfood.Com

Fair Trade

"There is no shame in not knowing; the shame lies in not finding out."
— Russian proverb

"Fair Trade is an innovative, market-based approach to sustainable development. Fair Trade helps family farmers in developing countries to gain direct access to international markets, as well as to develop the business capacity necessary to compete in the global marketplace. By learning how to market their own harvests, Fair Trade farmers are able to bootstrap their own businesses and receive a fair price for their products. This leads to higher family living standards, thriving communities and more sustainable farming practices. Fair Trade empowers farming families to take care of themselves – without developing dependency on foreign aid.

Most Fair Trade Certified coffee, tea, and chocolate in the U.S. is certified organic and shade grown. This means that the products you buy maintain biodiversity. Growing coffee and cocoa under the shade of a natural forest canopy preserves crucial habitats and shelter for a diverse array of plants, animals, insects, and migratory birds – helping to reduce global warming.

Fair Trade guarantees that farmers use eco-friendly practices. Fair Trade encourages farmers to use sustainable post-harvest processing. For example, many Fair Trade cooperatives compost coffee pulp rather than dumping it into local waterways. Some cooperatives have also invested in new environmentally friendly processing mills that greatly reduce resource use.

Nearly all Fair Trade Certified™ coffee in the U.S. carries organic certification. Even nonorganic Fair Trade farmers are required to use integrated pest management systems, which emphasize alternatives to chemical use.

By keeping traditional small-scale coffee and cocoa farmers in business, Fair Trade helps maintain diverse forested ecosystems – one of the most threatened environments in the world. Farmers who participate in Fair Trade implement additional soil and water conservation measures such as composting, terracing, and reforestation.

The result is responsibly grown products that are healthy for you and for the world we live in."
— **TransFairUSA.Org**

Although Fair Trade isn't perfect, it does provide for a better way to do business than what has typically been done. Please, if you purchase coffee or chocolate, seek out organically grown, Fair Trade products.

FairTrade.Net

TransFairUSA.Org

Farmers' Markets

Farmers' markets, where farmers sell their produce directly to the public, are becoming more popular as a source for getting organic food. To find a farmers' market near you, check out the following sites:

AMS.USDA.GOV/FarmersMarkets

FarmDirectCoOp.Org

FoodRoutes.Org
Provides information on Community Supported Agriculture

National Sustainable Agriculture Information Service, Local Food Directories, ATTRA.NCAT.Org/ATTRA-Pub/LocalFood_Dir.php

Local Harvest, 831-475-8150; LocalHarvest.Org
Site lists farmers' markets, family farms, and sources for food grown locally in your

area.

National Farmers' Retail & Markets Association (FARMA), FarmShopping.com
Farmers' markets in England.

North American Farmers Direct Marketing Association, NAFDMA.Com

Fasting

Also see:
• Detox and Fasting

Book:
• *The Fasting Handbook: Dining from An Empty Bowl*, by Jeremy Safron

Flowers to Eat & Flowers to Avoid

Also see:
• Gardening and Farming

Edible flowers contain an amazing selection of vitamins, minerals and other nutrients, including riboflavinoids, beta carotene, pectin, and various other antioxidants. They also provide more variety in and on food as they can be used in food as garnishes, color, flavor, and aroma. They can be used in salads, floated on drinks, and used to flavor drinks, as well as in salad dressings, and to garnish food. Certain flowers can also be used with or without herbs, lemon, and/or shaved ginger root to make Sun tea. This is done by soaking flowers in a bottle of water set for a few hours in direct Sun light.

It is important to know which flowers are edible, and which ones may cause stomach upset, allergies, and worse.

Even some of the most common edible flowers may cause allergic reactions.

Most flowers are used in such small portions, such as to garnish salads, that they are not likely to cause an adverse reaction. But each person reacts differently, so take precautions to know which flowers are okay to eat, and which are not.

Introducing flowers into your diet should be done one at a time, and sparingly to see if you experience any adverse reactions.

The flowers of most culinary herbs, such as basil and oregano, are commonly used in foods.

It is important to eat flowers that have been grown organically, and not those that have been grown using chemical fertilizers, herbicides, fungicides, pesticides, and other toxic chemicals. Flowers that are sold at floral shops, garden centers, and nurseries are not good to eat, as they are most certainly chemically grown and sprayed.

If you grow flowers to eat, use seeds bought from good sources, or those you have gathered from wild pollinated flowers. Use a mulch to keep weeds down, and to prevent water from splashing too much dirt during watering and heavy rainstorms; many flowers are delicate and hard to clean without damaging. Use a drip-hose system to water as that will help protect against mold on the plant. Do not use chemical sprays or fertilizers, even if they have been approved for use on fruits and vegetables. Flowers grow differently, and chemicals approved for use on other foods are not tested on flowers. Besides, it is best to grow organically, and not rely on toxic chemicals.

Use the flowers at their peak, as that is when the nutrients are at their strongest, and their flavor is full. All culinary flowers should be used fresh. Long-stemmed flowers should be kept in water. Stemless flowers may be kept in a bag with a damp towel to maintain humidity, and kept in a cool area. Some flowers may be kept in refrigerated bottles of olive oil and vinegar to use at a later date as salad dressing. Some flowers can be dried for later use when they can be sprinkled over food to add color and/or flavor.

When using flowers in food, add the flowers just before serving. Unless of course you are making Sun tea, or using the flowers to flavor vinegars or olive, hemp, flax, or other oils.

Don't toss flowers into salad mixed with dressing as the dressing will wilt and discolor the flowers. First toss the salad with the dressing, and then place the flowers on top. Or first put the salad on the serving plate, then garnish with flowers.

When using flowers to garnish desserts, add the flowers just before serving.

Avoid flowers that are wilted as their flavor fades and may become bitter as they age.

When selecting culinary flowers, keep an eye out for bugs, because like people, bugs are attracted to flowers. To clean flowers, rinse in water, and place between two soft towels and refrigerate them until you are ready to use them. Flower petals will last longer if you keep them attached to the stem until you are ready to use them.

The stems, stamens, pistils, and anthers of the flower may add a bitter taste, so these should be removed. The white base ("heel") area of the petals on many flowers is bitter, and should be removed (chrysanthemums, dianthus, marigolds, and roses). This may also reduce the chance of an allergic reaction in those who suffer from hay fever.

Common edible flowers include (must be organically grown to be safely edible):
- **African marigold**
- **Allums**
- **Alpine strawberry**
- **Angelica**: May cause skin reaction in some people.
- **Anise hyssop**
- **Apple and crabapple blossoms**: Avoid the seeds. The flowers should also be eaten in moderation as they may contain cyanide precursors.
- **Artichoke**: Artichokes are actually the immature flower of the artichoke plant.
- **Arugula blossoms/rocket flowers**: Once the plant has flowered, the leaves of the plant are usually too bitter to use as an herb.
- **Bachelor's button**: Only use the petals. Dispose of the calyx, as it is bitter.
- **Banana**: The whole flower is edible.
- **Basil/tulsi**: The flowers correspond to the type of basil they come from, such as lemon basil, mint basil, anise basil, cinnamon basil, etc.
- **Bee balm**
- **Bellis/English daisy**
- **Bergamot (similar to oswego) and bee balm (monarda)**: Native Americans used it to treat headaches, backaches, colds, stomach issues, and the flu. Bee balm is particularly rich in antioxidants.
- **Borage**
- **Broccoli**: Green. Yes, broccoli is a flower.
- **Burnet**
- **Calendula/pot marigold**: This is a composite flower. Only the petals should be eaten. Those with asthma, issues with ragweed, and who experience hay fever may have adverse reactions to ingesting composite flowers, which carry pollen that is allergenic.
- **Carnation**: The bases are bitter.
- **Cauliflower**: Yes, cauliflower is also a flower.

- **Chamomile/English chamomile:** May lead to drowsiness, so consume no more than one cup of tea per day, or equal amount when using as garnish. This is a composite flower. Only the petals should be eaten. Those with asthma, issues with ragweed, and who experience hay fever may have adverse reactions to ingesting composite flowers, which carry pollen that is allergenic.
- **Chervil**
- **Chicory:** This is a composite flower. Only the petals should be eaten. Those with asthma, issues with ragweed, and who experience hay fever may have adverse reactions to ingesting composite flowers, which carry pollen that is allergenic.
- **Chive blossoms**
- **Chrysanthemum and Shungiku (Asian chrysanthemum):** This is a composite flower. Only the petals should be eaten. Those with asthma, issues with ragweed, and who experience hay fever may have adverse reactions to ingesting composite flowers, which carry pollen that is allergenic.
- **Clover:** Although they are edible, they may be difficult for some people to digest. Use sparingly.
- **Columbine**
- **Coriander/Cilantro**
- **Cornflower:** This is a composite flower. Only the petals should be eaten. Those with asthma, issues with ragweed, and who experience hay fever may have adverse reactions to ingesting composite flowers, which carry pollen that is allergenic.
- **Daisy**
- **Dandelion:** This is a composite flower. Only the petals should be eaten. Those with asthma, issues with ragweed, and who experience hay fever may have adverse reactions to ingesting composite flowers, which carry pollen that is allergenic.
- **Daylily:** May have a laxative effect if too many are eaten, so use sparingly. Be careful not to confuse them with other types of lilies, which may contain alkaloids, and make you ill.
- **Dianthus/pinks:** Remove the white base of each petal, as that area of the petal is bitter.
- **Dill**
- **Elderberry**
- **English daisy:** This is a composite flower. Only the petals should be eaten. Those with asthma, issues with ragweed, and who experience hay fever may have adverse reactions to ingesting composite flowers, which

carry pollen that is allergenic.

- Fava bean
- Fennel
- Freesia
- Fuchsia
- Gardenia
- Garden sage
- Garland chrysanthemum /shungiku
- Garlic chive blossoms
- Geranium
- Gladiola: This is a composite flower. Only the petals should be eaten. Those with asthma, issues with ragweed, and who experience hay fever may have adverse reactions to ingesting composite flowers, which carry pollen that is allergenic.
- Grape hyacinth
- Guava/ pineapple guava
- Hibiscus/China rose
- Hollyhock
- Honeysuckle: The berries are poisonous.
- Hosta
- Hyssop: Bitter, tonic-like flavor. These flowers are used to flavor chartreuse liqueur. Expectant mothers, and individuals with epilepsy and hypertension as well as those who experience sleepwalking should avoid these.
- Iceland poppy
- Impatiens
- Jasmine (Arabian)
- Johnny jump-up: Use sparingly as they contain saponins and can be toxic in large amounts. A few petals to garnish a salad are fine.
- Lavender: Use sparingly. The oil from the plant may be poisonous.
- Lemon balm
- Lemon blossoms
- Lemon verbena
- Lilac
- Linden: Use very sparingly. Frequent consumption of this flower can cause heart damage.

- Lovage
- Mallow
- Marigold (signet)
- Marjoram
- Mint
- Mustard: Some people may have an allergy to this flower causing red patches on the skin. There are many varieties of mustard plants.
- Nasturtium
- Okra
- Orange blossoms
- Oregano blossoms
- Pansy: Use sparingly as they contain saponins and can be toxic in large amounts. A few petals to garnish a salad are fine.
- Passionflower: Avoid these during pregnancy.
- Pea vegetable blossoms: Don't eat ornamental sweet pea blossoms, as they are poisonous.
- Pineapple guava
- Pineapple sage
- Plum blossoms
- Primrose: May cause dermatitis.
- Queen Anne's lace: Avoid these during pregnancy.
- Radish flowers
- Redbud: Pink flowers. Mildly sweet tart apple to bean-like flavor.
- Red clover blossoms: Not easily digestible.
- Rose: The white portion of the petals may be more bitter, and are best removed before putting into food. The base of the flower, the rose "hips," is also edible (some people call them "rose berries"), and a good source of vitamin C as well as bioflavonoids, beta-carotene, pectin, and other nutrients. Rose hips can be harvested and eaten throughout winter. They can be crushed and soaked in water with mint and lemon and/or honey for flavored water.
- Rosemary
- Rose-of-Sharon
- Runner bean
- Safflower: This is a composite flower. Only the petals should be eaten. Those with asthma, issues with ragweed, and who experience hay fever

may have adverse reactions to ingesting composite flowers, which carry pollen that is allergenic.

- Sage
- Savory
- Scarlet runner bean
- Scented geranium
- Scotch broom
- Signet marigold: Use sparingly as large amounts can make you sick.
- Snapdragon
- Society garlic
- Squash or pumpkin blossoms
- Sunflower: This is a composite flower. Only the petals should be eaten. Those with asthma, issues with ragweed, and who experience hay fever may have adverse reactions to ingesting composite flowers, which carry pollen that is allergenic.
- Sweet woodruff: Consuming large amounts can have a blood-thinning effect.
- Tarragon
- Thyme
- Tiger lily
- Tuberous begonia: The oxalic acid of the flowers and stems is not good for those who suffer from kidney stones, gout, or rheumatoid arthritis. Use the flowers sparingly. Some say that only the hybrid varieties are edible.
- Tulip: Only the petals are edible. Use them to create little finger foods stuffed with hummus and diced vegetables. Make sure they are organically grown.
- Violet
- Yucca blossoms: Use sparingly. The petals are edible; the other parts of the plant contain saponin, which is poisonous to humans. The center part of the flower is particularly bitter. Use the petals.

Sunfood Nutrition, 11655 Riverside Drive, Lakeside, CA 92040; 800-205-2350; 888-RAW-FOOD; International: +001-619-596-7979; Sunfood.Com
Sells a chart detailing a variety of edible flowers.

Food Irradiation: A Growing Threat

"A chest x-ray gives about 0.01 rad of energy. The average dose of radiation from background radiation (radiation due to cosmic rays and natural radioactivity such as radon in rocks) annually is 0.1 rad. On the other hand, the dose of radiation from gamma rays applied to food during irradiation is 100,000 to 1 million rads (1-10 kGy). The amount of radiation being applied to food during irradiation is therefore massive, 10 million to 100 million times the dose of a chest x-ray... Food irradiation creates nuclear waste just like a nuclear power plant."
— Citizen.Org/CMEP/FoodSafety/International/Canada/Articles.cfm?ID=9532

Irradiation of food is a form of pasteurization. It uses high doses of radiation to kill microbes in food. Not only does it kill what may or may not be something that can cause human illness, it also kills enzymes, and damages some other nutrients. It also exposes food to, you guessed it, radiation. It is a technology developed by the U.S. Department of Energy's Byproduct Utilization Program. The word "byproduct" in this case refers to leftovers of the nuclear industry. In this case, cesium 37 and cobalt 60.

Lots of food products sold in markets and distributed in school lunch programs are irradiated, or "cold-pasteurized." Foods that have been imported, and foods being exported are also irradiated. This is done even though it is known that irradiation creates free radicals and radiolytic substances in the foods.

Do you really want to be eating foods exposed to radiation, which accumulates in tissues? I don't.

Irradiated foods are not labeled as such.

Two ways you can prevent irradiated foods from entering into your diet is to eat organically and locally grown foods, and to grow your own food.

FactoryFarm.Or/Topics/Irradiation/

FoodCom.Org.UK/Irradiation_Probs.Htm

FoodIrradiationInfo.Org

FoodIrradiation.Org

Irradiation.Info

Nocobalt-4-Food.Org

SafeLunch.Org

Funerals and Burial

Did you know that many people are now buried after their bodies have been embalmed with very toxic, environmentally damaging chemicals that release dioxin and mercury into the soil? Often the chemicals used include formaldehyde and mercuric chloride. In addition, many people are now buried in caskets that don't degrade for thousands of years. Whatever happened to returning to Earth? Why must we be so disrespectful of Earth at every stage of our existence?

Embalming is not required by law. The Jewish religion is one that prohibits embalming and requires that the casket be a plain wood box, which degrades into the soil.

Arrange for your remains, and those of your loved ones, to be treated in a way that doesn't destroy Nature.

I used to loathe the site of graveyards. Not because I get spooked, but because of how much land they take up that could be wildland if people would be cremated instead. I changed my mine when I spent a day with friends making a movie in Los Angeles. We filmed at an old, broken-down graveyard that was the only green space in the neighborhood. There were butterflies and birds and signs of larger animals. After that experience I didn't think of graveyards as negatively because they may at least be preserving land in areas that would otherwise be turned into parking lots, industrial zones, tract housing, and supermarkets. In some countries where food is scarce the people have planted food gardens in the graveyards.

There are a growing number of graveyards with set rules requiring people to be buried in natural wood caskets, or in shrouds that degrade into the soil. They don't allow embalmed bodies to be buried there, and they allow only flat gravestones, or trees or bushes to be planted as grave markers.

The following companies provide alternatives to embalming and burial services.

Fernwood, 415-383-7100; ForeverFernwood.com

Eternal Reefs, 888-423-7333; EternalReefs.Com

Fur: Extreme Cruelty

"Eighty-five percent of the fur industry's skins come from animals kept captive and slaughtered on fur farms.

No U.S. federal laws regulate how animals on fur farms are housed, cared for, or killed.

As many as 85 percent of the animals in fur farms develop psychological and behavioral abnormalities from captivity.

Approximately 90 percent of today's farm-raised fox is used for fur trim.

Between four and five million animals are trapped and killed annually in the United States for the commercial fur trade.

By more than a four-to-one margin, U.S. consumers prefer to shop at stores that do not sell fur, and 77 percent of Americans polled think fur products are unacceptable."
    — **A Voice for Animals, VoiceForAnimals.Org; 2005**

The fur industry is disgusting and terrible and causes extreme pain and suffering to animals who are killed so that their skins can be used for clothing, furniture, car seats, key chains, doll dresses, and stuffed toy animals.

"Mink, which are naturally aquatic and fiercely territorial, with a range of more than ten miles when free, are forced to spend their short lives in cages 16 by 20 inches. For fox, also natural roamers, cells tend to be three by four feet, if they're lucky. Bobcats and lynx are forced into a wire box five feet square.

Techniques used to kill fox and mink include anal electrocution, neck-breaking, carbon dioxide gassing and crushing. Bobcats and lynx are either shot in the head at point-blank range with a .22 caliber short bullet or darted using a blowgun with an overdose of drugs."
    — **Freedom for Fur Farm Prisoners, Rod Coronado, *Earth First! Journal*, December-January 2002**

Please help put an end to the grotesque and horrible fur industry. Get involved in letter-writing campaigns and protests. Get the word out to clothing manufacturers, designers, stores, and models and celebrities who use, sell, or wear fur, that fur products are the result of torture and murder.

"Humans – who enslave, castrate, experiment on, and fillet other animals – have had an understandable penchant for pretending animals do not feel pain. A sharp distinction between humans and 'animals' is essential if we are to bend them to our will, make them work for us, wear them, eat them – without any disquieting tinges of guilt or regret.

It is unseemly of us, who often behave so unfeelingly toward other animals, to contend that only humans can suffer. The behavior of other animals renders such pretensions specious. They are just too much like us."

— Dr. Carl Sagan and Dr. Ann Druyan, *Shadows of Forgotten Ancestors*, 1992

As I write this I am thinking of the nauseating "fashion" choices of actress/singer/clothing designer/producer Jennifer Lopez, and of actress/singer/clothing designer Beyoncé. These wealthy women blatantly use fur in their clothing lines. Lopez has been known to use fur eyelash extensions. These "fashion icons" should know better. Maybe one day they will realize how repulsive they look wearing those fur coats, and how much pain and cruelty their business decisions have caused the animals of this planet.

"F*** animals."

— British clothing designer Julien Mcdonald, as quoted in London's *Daily Mail*, Fur Is Alive on the Catwalk, by fashion writer Liz Jones; October 2006

"I watched the PETA video – the one Beyoncé, when sent it, refused even to look at – and there is footage of a fox being skinned. When it has been reduced to a bloody pulp, you can see its heart still beating, its long lashes blinking in shock at what has happened."

— Fashion writer Liz Jones, Fur Is Alive on the Catwalk, London's *Daily Mail*; October 2006

"To make a 40-inch fur coat it takes between 30 and 200 chinchilla, or 60 mink, 50 sables, 50 muskrats, 45 opossums, 40 raccoons, 35 rabbits, 20 foxes, 20 otters, 18 lynx, 16 coyotes, 15 beavers or 8 seals.

Eighty-five percent of the fur industry's skins come from animals living captive on fur factory farms. Life on a fur farm is short and painful. Animals such as foxes, who would naturally roam hundreds of miles, live miserable existences on fur farms in cramped cages. They are killed by the cheapest methods available, including anal electrocution, injection of insecticide, hanging, gassing, and suffocation.

Ten to 20 million raccoons, coyotes, wolves, bobcats, opossums, nutria, beavers, otters, and other fur-bearing animals are trapped every year for their fur. For every targeted animal, two nontarget animals, which trappers call 'trash animals,' are also killed."

— DawnWatch.Com/Clothing.htm

> "For me, it is a principle. I just don't understand why these beautiful creatures have to die for someone's coat. It is both medieval and barbaric, and I think there are plenty of alternatives out there. Comfy? Warm? The very idea leaves me cold."
> — **Clothing designer Stella McCartney, 2006**

There have been many instances where imported fur toys and clothing have been found to be the fur of cats and dogs. This dog and cat fur is imported from countries (usually Asian) where the factories agree to put any label on the fur that the clothing company wants. Not that other animals should be valued less, but to help make people consider the disgusting fur industry for what it is: deplorable and repulsive.

AnimalLiberation.Net

BontVoorDieren.NL

Coalition to Abolish the Fur Trade, CAFT.Org.UK

Compassion over Killing, NeimanCarcass.Com

The Fund for Animals anti-fur campaign, FundForAnimals.Org/Fur/
This Web site explains why the fur trade is so vile. Fur comes from animals who are either trapped in the wild or raised in cages in fur factories – often referred to as "fur farms" or "ranches."
Altogether, roughly 40 million animals are killed for the fur trade each year. Millions of additional animals, including dogs, cats, and endangered species, are accidentally caught in traps each year.

Fur Free Alliance, InFurmation.Com

FurKills.Org

PETA's anti-fur campaign, FurIsDead.Com

RespectForAnimals.Org

Tribe of Heart, POB 149, Ithaca, NY 14851; 607-275-0806; TribeOfHeart.Org
Created an anti-fur documentary titled *Witness*.

WorldAnimal.Net

Gardening and Farming

Also see:
• Seeds

Books:
• *American Green: The Obsessive Quest for the Perfect Lawn*, by Ted Steinberg
• *The Edible Flower Garden*, by Rosalind Creasy
• *Edible Gardens: From Garden to Palate*, by Cathy Wilkonson
• *Edible Forest Gardens Volume 1 & 2*, by Dave Jacke with Eric Toensmeier
• *Food Not Lawns: How to Turn Your Yard into a Garden and Your Neighborhood into a Community*, by Cascadia Food Not Lawns co-founder Heather Coburn Flores
• *Gaia's Garden: A Guide to Home-Scale Permaculture*, by Toby Hemenway
• *Gardening Without Digging*, by A. Guest
• *How to Grow More Vegetables*, by John Jeavons
• *Natural Pest Control: Alternatives to Chemicals for the Home and Garden*, by Andrew Lopez
• *The One-Straw Revolution: An Introduction to Natural Farming*, by Masanobu Fukuoka
• *Organic Pest Control for Home and Garden*, by Tom Roberts
• *Organic Gardening*, by Maria Rodale
• *A Patch of Eden: America's Inner-City Gardeners*, by Patricia Hynes
• *Raising Less Corn, More Hell: The Case for the Independent Farm and Against Food*, by George Pyle
• *Square Foot Gardening*, by Mel Bartholomew
• *Superbia: 31 Ways to Create Sustainable Neighborhoods*, by Dan Chiras and Dave Wann
• *Tangled Routes: Women, Work, and Globalization on the Tomato Trail*, by Deborah Barndt
• *This Land is Their Land: How Corporate Farms Threaten the World*, by Evaggelos Vallianatos

Documentaries:
• *My Father's Garden*, MirandaProductions.Com/Garden/Index.htm
• *The Future of Food*, TheFutureOfFood.Com
• *Troublesome Creek*, WestCityFilms.Com/TC.html

"Let's not dissect the evils of corporate food – let's feed ourselves! The creation of a garden is as simple as you make it. Be it a barren patch of Earth newly liberated from the smothering embrace of con-

crete, a rooftop or a porch smattering of five-gallon buckets, it can take any form you desire. Be resourceful! Imagination can manifest square-foot primitive horticulture just about anywhere... Free yourself from wage slavery by eliminating the need to buy some or most of what you eat. Grow enough to feed the nomads among us. Ingesting fresh, native, seasonal plants gives us vibrant health. And how delicious it is to sink our fangs into a succulent squash that we first knew as a seed!"
   — **The Moment is Ripe, Aleksandra,** *Earth First! Journal*, **December-January 2002**

"Today, 58 million Americans spend approximately $30 billion every year to maintain over 23 million acres of lawn. That's an average of over a third of an acre and $517 each. The same-size plot of land could still have a small lawn for recreation, plus produce all the vegetables needed to feed a family of six. The lawns in the United States consume around 270 billion gallons of water a week – enough to water 81 million acres of organic vegetables all summer long.

Lawns use ten times as many chemicals per acre as industrial farmland. These pesticides, fertilizers, and herbicides run off into our groundwater and evaporate into our air, causing widespread pollution and global warming, and greatly increasing our risk of cancer, heart disease, and birth defects. In addition, the pollution emitted from a power mower in just one hour is equal to the amount from a car being driven 350 miles. In fact, lawns use more equipment, labor, fuel, and agricultural toxins than industrial farming, making lawns the largest agricultural sector in the United States. But it's not just the residential lawns that are wasted on grass. There are around 700,000 athletic grounds and 14,500 golf courses in the United States, many of which used to be fertile, productive farmland that was lost to developers when the local markets bottomed out.

Turf is big business: $45 billion-a-year big. The University of Georgia has seven turf researchers studying genetics, soil science, plant pathology, nutrient uptake, and insect management. They issue undergraduate degrees in Turf. The turf industry is responsible for a large sector of the biotech (GMO) industry, and much of the genetic modification that is happening in laboratories across the nation is in the name of an eternally green, slow-growing, moss-free lawn."
   — **Heather Coburn, author of** *Food Not Lawns: How to Turn Your Yard into a Garden and Your Neighborhood into a Community*; **FoodNotLawns.Org**

In addition to wild foods, the best way to get fresh food bursting with nutrients is to grow your own organic food garden.

Growing a food garden is good for the soul, for the mind, for the body, and for your life. Growing and harvesting your own food gives you exercise; connects you with Nature; tunes you into the seasons; adjusts your frequency to a higher level; bonds you with your environment; and provides you with the freshest food you can possibly have.

If you live in nearly any town or city you are living on land that was once farmland of some sort. Cities now cover most of the ancient farmland. This is because people originally settled on land that was good for growing food. As the settlements grew into towns and cities, houses, stores, schools, churches, jails, office buildings, streets, and parking lots covered the farmland. By planting food gardens in your area you are bringing back an ancient culture of growing and harvesting food.

"Growing our own food decreases pollution because we reduce our participation in the pollution incurred by shipping, packaging, advertising, and selling of commercially grown food."
— David Wolfe

By maintaining your own organic garden you can feel assured that there are no toxic farming chemicals on your food. Not only will you experience the benefit of getting food as fresh as possible, you will also benefit from food that is nutritionally and energetically stronger than food available at the store.

Chemically grown food is weaker in electrical frequency and has diminished nutritional properties. Studies have shown that organically grown food has a denser reserve of vitamins, minerals, and other nutrients than food that has been grown chemically. Perhaps this is because the organically grown plants have to fend for themselves, and don't rely on chemical fertilizers for nutrients, or depend on chemicals to protect them. Like people who become weak when they are pampered, plants also can become weak if they are grown in an atmosphere where too much is done for them.

In America today about 35 percent of all household water goes to tend lawns. Because there are so many lawns, including those on school campuses, golf courses, cemeteries, around government buildings, office buildings, and even prisons, the number-one crop being produced in the U.S., and many other countries, is landscape clippings.

It is amazing how much time, energy, money, and water is spent in the U.S. and other wealthy countries to try to keep home lawns green. The people get nothing out of it but a green lawn. They don't have food gardens, even though they have the land to grow them, but instead buy all their food at grocery stores, snack shops, and restaurants. This scenario has helped create the situation that exists today where, on average, the typical meal in the U.S. has traveled 1,250 miles from farm to consumer. This is a terrific waste of resources and causes enormous amounts of pollution.

According to Ted Steinberg, author of *American Green: The Obsessive Quest for the Perfect Lawn*, there are 25 million acres of lawn in America, more land than what is used to grow cotton. To care for those lawns, there are more than 35 million gas-powered lawn mowers, and over 25 million leaf blowers. And all this produces things like landscape clippings, air pollution, and polluted soil and water.

Think of how much better people would be if, instead of spending time, energy, water, and money, and using toxic fertilizers and weed killers to try to keep their lawns green with perfectly trimmed hedges, they would plant organic food gardens, including fruiting trees – and let the rest of the land grow wild and free. Not only would they not spend money and time on landscaping, they would save money on food as well. They would pollute less: A typical lawnmower can use enough gas in an hour to operate a small car for over 50 miles.

The chemicals commonly used to keep a residential lawn green and weed-free contain many toxic chemicals. Glyphosate, a chemical in weed killer, which is poisonous to a variety of plants and wildlife, has been linked to non-Hodgkin's lymphoma, a cancer that is becoming more common. Other lawn chemicals are known to cause breast cancer, birth deformities, and learning disabilities. Lawn chemicals also cause health problems in pets and wildlife. Ironically, the companies that manufacture these toxic chemicals are often the same companies that manufacture cancer drugs.

When used as a well-organized food garden, a small plot of land the size of a common lawn can produce more food in a season than a family of four can consume. The result would be that people would be sharing their food with neighbors, family, and friends. The people, their environment, and their community would be healthier.

Growing your own food may be a new concept for those who have lived their lives relying on commercial and restaurant food. It isn't new to a large percentage of the world's population that has always grown some or all their own food. Some countries that have relied on commercial food are now encouraging their citizens to grow more food gardens. Venezuela and Cuba are two countries that have been promoting self-sufficiency through home food gardens. The U.S. hasn't been involved in this type of program since the 1940s. At that time the government encouraged its citizens to grow "victory gardens."

Even if you don't grow part, or all, of your own food, you can at least get involved with purchasing foods that have been grown locally. You can find these at your nearest farmers' markets.

You may also obtain locally grown food through "community supported agriculture" (CSA) co-ops that prepay local farmers for produce. This is an idea that began in the 1970s, and has been growing in popularity in Europe, the U.S., and other regions of the world.

Some people have the idea of moving the CSA and organic farming movement into the restaurant food sector. They want to gather people to gather the finances to open co-op vegetarian restaurants that use locally grown produce.

If you live in a city you may find that growing a garden in an abandoned lot to be an awarding experience. Many people have done this throughout the years and it has spurred activism to create and maintain food gardens in the largest cities. The city or other government department may own the land, or it may be privately owned. Many communities have grown food on such land for many years without any problem from the landowner.

When New York's Mayor Giuliani announced that more than 100 city-owned lots where gardens had been planted were to be auctioned off to land developers in the Spring of 1999, a citizen's campaign was organized to save the gardens. It was only a last minute arrangement by entertainer Bette Midler and some others that the gardens were saved as they were purchased by the Trust for Public Land.

In Los Angeles a plot of land that contained garden plots maintained by hundreds of families was bulldozed in 2006. The South Central Community Farm was planted with an enormous variety of food and medicinal plants and trees. It came into existence after the riots that took place after the 1992 Rodney King verdict. Originally purchased by the city through the eminent domain process, the city had planned to build trash incinerators on the site. The local community spoke out against this plan. The Concerned Citizens of South Central organized protests and the city eventually canceled their plan to build the incinerators. After the riots the city offered the land as space for community gardens. Many of the farmers were people who had moved to Los Angeles from Central and South America. As the years went by the farming gardens became a center of community with generations of families involved in planting and maintaining their gardens. Then, the person who originally owned the land wanted it back. In 2003 the land was transferred back to the original owner, who had plans to build warehouses on the property. As time passed, lawsuits were filed and the community organized protests. By the Spring of 2006 the future of the farm was dismal. Community activists gathered to maintain a 24/7 presence. Julia Butterfly Hill, who once lived in a redwood tree for two years, joined Darryl Hannah and other activists who camped in the farm. Finally, on a June morning hundreds of riot police were brought in to evict the protestors. Some, including Darryl Hannah, who were camping in a tree, were handcuffed and taken away. In the end the land owner won, bulldozing the gardens and placing people back in line at the supermarkets to purchase their food.

Wherever you are, get involved in growing some of your own food. If you don't have land, borrow some, or use pots, a roof, or window boxes. Be sure to plant some native flower species so that your garden attracts native bees and other helpful insects.

When you look for plants and seeds to plant in your garden, seek out those that have been organically grown, and that have not been genetically altered. You also may want to try "open pollinated" "heirloom" seeds, which have not been hybridized, and that can provide a better variety of food plants. Look into planting some food plants that you have never heard of. See the Seeds section of this book for more information on this topic.

There are many organizations involved in getting people to grow their own food. From the Slow Food movement that started in Italy when McDonald's opened at Rome's Spanish Steps in 1986 to city farming activists, there is likely an organization that is near you and/or can help you get into growing food.

Acres: The Voice for Eco-Agriculture, Austin, TX, 78709; 512-892-4400; AcresUSA.Com
   Sells books on organic gardening and farming.

Alternative Farming Systems Information Center, Community Supported Agriculture, NAL.USDA.Gov/AFSIC/CSA/

American Community Gardening Association, Council on the Environment, 51 Chambers St., Ste. 228; New York, NY 10007; CommunityGarden.Org

American Farmland Trust, 1200 18th St., NW, Washington, DC 20036; Farmland.Org

AppleLuscious Organic Orchards, AppleLuscious.Com

Avant-Gardening.Com

BarefootFarmer.Com

BigBarn.Co.UK

Bio-Integral Resource Center, IGC.Org

Black Farmers and Agriculturists Association, POB 61, Tillery, NC 27887; BFAA-US.Org

Bountiful Gardens, 18001 Shafer Ranch Rd., Willits, CA 95490-9626; 707-459-6410; BountifulGardens.Org

California Certified Organic Farmers, POB 8136, Santa Cruz, CA 95061; CCOF.Org

California Rare Fruit Growers, CRFG.Org

Canadian Organic Growers, COG.Ca

Cascadia Food Not Lawns; SeedGeek@Yahoo.Com

Center for Food and Justice, 323-341-5099; Departments.Oxy.Edu/UEPI/CFJ

Center for Informed Food Choices, InformedEating.Org

Center for Rural Affairs, POB 136, Lyons, NE 68038-0136; CFRA.Org

Center for Vegan Organic Education, POB 13217, Burton, WA 98013; 206-463-4520; VeganOrganicEd.Org

City Farmer, Canada's Office of Urban Agriculture, Box 74561, Kitsilano RPO, Vancouver, BC V6K 4P4; Canada; CityFarmer.Org

City Repair Project, POB 42615, Portland, OR 97242; CityRepair.Org

Coalition of Immokalee Workers, POB 603, Immokalee, FL 34143; CIW-Online.Org

Common Ground Garden Program, CELosAngeles.UCDavis.Edu/Garden

Community Farm Alliance, 614 Shelby St., Frankfurt, KY 40601; CommunityFarmAlliance.Org

Community Food Security Coalition, Venice, CA; FoodSecurity.Org
    Site contains listings of community gardening and urban farming resources.

The Cornucopia Institute, POB 126, Cornucopia, WI 54827; Cornucopia.Org

DesertHarversters.Org

EatGrub.Org

Earth Works Gardens, 1820 Mount Elliot, Detroit, MI 48207; Earth-Works.Org

Eat the View, England, Countryside.Gov.UK/LAR/Landscape/ETV/Index.asp

Ecological Farming Association, Watsonville, CA; Eco-Farm.Org

Edible Estates Initiative,
FritzHaeg.Com/Garden/Initiatives/EdibleEstates/Main.html

EdibleForestGardens.Com

EdibleSchoolyard.Org

Environmental Working Group, 1436 U Street NW, Ste. 100, Washington DC 20009; EWG.Org

Fair Trade Resource Network, POB 33772, Washington, DC 20033-3772; FairTradeResource.Org

Family Farm Defenders, POB 1772, Madison, WI 53701; FamilyFarmDefenders.Org

Farm Aid, 11 Ward St., Ste. 200, Somerville, MA 02143; FarmAid.Org

Farmers' Legal Action Group, 360 N. Robert St., Ste. 500, St. Paul, MN 55101; FLAGInc.Org

FarmingSolutions.Org

Farm Labor Organizing Committee, 1221 Broadway St., Toledo, OH 43609; FLOC.Com

Farm Worker Justice Fund, 1010 Vermont Ave., NW, Ste. 915, Washington, DC 20005; FWJustice.Org

Food First, Institute for Food and Development Policy, 398 60th St., Oakland, CA; FoodFirst.Org

Food Not Bombs, POB 744, Tucson, AZ 85702; 800-884-1136; FoodNotBombs.Net

Food Not Lawns, POB 42174, Eugene, OR 97404; FoodNotLawns.Org

The Food Project, POB 705, Lincoln, MA 01773; TheFoodProject.Org

TheFutureOfFood.Com

GardenProject.Org

GardenValleySeedTrust.Org

Global Exchange, 2017 Mission St., #303, San Francisco, CA 94110; GlobalExchange.Org

GoingOrganic.Com

Green Guerillas, New York, NY; GreenGuerillas.Org
Helping establish community gardens.

GreenPeople.Org
Site contains a list of companies that sell organic seeds.

Growing Gardens, 2003 NE 42nd Ave., #3, Portland, OR 97213; Growing-Gardens.Org

Growing Power, 5500 W. Silver Spring Rd., Milwaukee, WI 53218; GrowingPower.Org

GuerrillaGardening.Org
A group of people in London who have late night planting parties to enliven previously neglected small plots of city land.

Heirloom Gardening Newsletter, 203-354-8756; HeirloomGardening.Com

HomeOrchardSociety.Org

Institute for Community Economics, 57 School St., Springfield, MA 01105; ICECLT.Org

International Confederation of Autonomous Chapters of the American Indian Movement, AmericanIndianMovement.Org

International Culinary Tourism Association, 4110 SE Hawthorne Blvd., #440, Portland, OR 97214; CulinaryTourism.Org

International Society for Ecology & Culture, ISEC.Org.UK

The Land Institute, 2440 E. Water Well Rd., Salina, KS 67401; LandInstitute.ORg

Land Stewardship Project, 2200 4th St., White Bear Lake, MN 55110; LandStewardshipProject.Org

Land Trust Alliance, 1331 H St., NW, Ste. 400, Washington, DC 20005; LTA.Org

Local Harvest, Santa Cruz; CALocalHarvest.Org
Searchable database of farmers' markets, small farms, and related groups and businesses.

Leopold Center for Sustainable Agriculture, Iowa State University; Leopold.IAState.Edu

Linking Environment and Farming, England; LeafMarque.Com/LEAF/

LocalHarvest.Org

Lost Valley Educational Center, LostValley.Org

Maine Organic Farmers and Gardeners Association, POB 170, Unity, ME 04988; MOFGA.Org

Mindfully.Org/Farm

Mindfully.Org/Food

More Gardens Coalition, 376 E. 162nd St., #2, Bronx, NY 10451; MoreGardens.Org

Mountain Gardens, Burnsville, NC; MountainGardensHerbs.Com
   A botanical garden featuring the largest collection of native Appalachian and Chinese medicinal herbs in the eastern U.S.

Mycorrhizal Applications, Mycorrhizae.Com
   Information on beneficial fungi that improves soil health, plant health, and crop yields.

National Coalition for Pesticide-Free Lawns,
BeyondPesticides.Org/PesticideFreeLawns/DoorHanger/Index.htm
   This organization offers door tags you can put on your neighborhood doors encouraging people to stop using pesticides on their lawns. The first 50 are free, and they ask only for a donation to handle the postage. You can also purchase more.

National Family Farm Coalition, 110 Maryland Ave., NE, Ste. 307; Washington,

DC 20002; NFFC.Net

National Farm to School Program, Center for Food and Justice, Occidental College, Los Angeles, CA; FarmToSchool.Org

National Farm Transition Network, FarmTransition.Org

National Immigrant Farming Initiative, 88 Atlantic Ave., #8, Brooklyn, NY 11201; ImmigrantFarming.Org

NativeSeeds.Org

New England Small Farm Institute, 275 Jackson St., Belchertown, MA 01007; SmallFarm.Org

NewFarm.Org
Sponsored by the Rodale Institute. Community Supported Agriculture information.

New World Publishing, Auburn, CA 95602; NWPub.Net
Books on small-scale farming.

North American Fruit Explorers, NAFEX.Org

North American Native Plant Society, NANPS.Org

Northeast Organic Farming Association, Barre, MA; NOFA.Org

Northern Nut Growers Association, ICSERV.Com/NNGA/Index.html

OrganicVolunteers.Org

Oregon Tilth, Tilth.Org

Organic Gardening magazine, OrganicGardening.Com

Osborn International Seed Co., OsbornSeed.Com

Pennsylvania Association for Sustainable Agriculture, POB 419, Millheim, PA 16854; PASAFarming.Org

Permaculture Institute, PortlandPermaculture.Com

Pesticide Action Network, San Francisco, CA; PANNA.Org

Planet Natural, 1612 Gold Ave., Bozeman, MT 59715; 800-289-6656; 406-587-5891; PlanetNatural.Com

PlanOrganic.Com

Plants for a Future, 1 Lerryn View, Cornwall, United Kingdom; PFAF.Org

Portland City Repair Project, CityRepair.Org

Portland Permaculture Institute, PortlandPermaculture.Com

ProActiveEcology.Org

Real Goods, 966 Mazzoni St., Ukiah, CA 95482; 800-762-7325; RealGoods.Com

Resource Centres on Urban Agriculture and Food Security, RUAF.Org

Robin Van En Center for Community Supported Agriculture; Center for Sustainable Living, Wilson College, Chambersburg, PA; CSACenter.Org

SacredEarthInstitute.Org

SafeFoodAndFertilizer.Org

SaltSpringsSeeds.Com

San Francisco League of Urban Gardeners (SLUG), Grass-Roots.Org/USA/Slug.shtml

SeasonalChef.Com

Seattle Tilth Association, 4649 Sunnyside Ave. North, Rm. 120, Seattle, WA 98103; SeattleTilth.Org

Seeds of Change, POB 15700, Santa Fe, NM 15700; 888-762-7333; SeedsOfChange.Com

Seeds of Diversity, Seeds.CA/EN.php

Seedsaving and Seedsavers' Resources, Homepage.Eircom.Net/%7Emerlyn/SeedSaving.html

Seed Savers Exchange, SeedSavers.Org

Seed Savers Network, Australia; SeedSavers.Net

The School of Self Reliance, Los Angeles, CA; Self-Reliance.Net

SFGreenSchool.Org

SlowFood.Com

SlowFoodUSA.Org

Small Farm Association, England, Small-Farms-Association.CO.UK

Snow Seed Organic, 831-758-9869; SnowSeedCo.Com

Soil and Health Library, SoilAndHealth.Org

Soil Food Web, Inc., SoildFoodWeb.Com

South Central Farmers, SouthCentralFarmers.Com

Sow Organic Seed, POB 527, Williams, OR 97544; 888-709-7333; OrganicSeed.Com

Spiral Gardens Community Food Security Project, 2880 Sacramento, St., Berkeley, CA 94702; SpiralGardens.Org

SunBowFarm.Org

Sunfood Nutrition, 11653 Riverside Dr., Lakeside, CA 92040; 800-205-2350; 888-RAW-FOOD; International: +001-619-596-7979; Sunfood.Com

SustainableFood.Com

Sustainable Table, New York, NY; SustainableTable.Org

Sustain: The Alliance for Better Farming and Food, London, UK; SustainWeb.Org

ToledoGarden.Org

True Food Now Campaign, Greenpeace USA, TrueFoodNow.Org

Trust for Public Land, 116 New Montgomery St., 4th Flr., San Francisco, CA 94105; TPL.Org

United Plant Savers, UnitedPlantSavers.Org

ViaCampesina.Org

Virginia Association for Biological Farming, Lexington, VA, VABF.Org

Virginia Independent Consumers and Farmers Association, POB 915,

Charlottesville, VA 22902; VICFA.Net

Washington State University's Organic Agriculture Program, 888-468-6978; World-Class.WSU.Edu/2006/Organic/Index.html
  In 2006 Washington State University became the first university in the U.S. to offer a major in organic agriculture.

White Earth Land Recovery Project, 32033 E. Round Lake Rd., Ponsford, MN 54575; NativeHarvest.Com

WildFoodAdventures.Com

Willing Workers on Organic Farms, OrganicVolunteers.Org

Women, Food, and Agriculture Network, 59624 Chicago Rd., Atlantic, IA 50022; WFAN.Org

World Social Forum, Rua General Jardin, 660, 8th Flr., Sao Paulo, SP 01223-010; Brazil; WorldSocialForum.Org

Worldwide Opportunities on Organic Farms, WWOOF.Org

Worm Digest, POB 2654, Grants Pass, OR 97528; WormDigest.Org

ZengerFarm.Org

Genetic Engineering and Food Safety

Also see:
- Gardening
- Organic Foods

Books:
- *Against the Grain: Biotechnology and the Corporate Takeover of Your Food*, by Mark Lappe, Ph.D., and Britt Bailey
- *Seeds of Deception: Exposing industry and government lies about the safety of the genetically engineered foods you're eating*, by Jeffrey M. Smith

Documentaries:
- *The Future of Food*, TheFutureOfFood.Com
- *A Silent Forest: The Growing Threat, Genetically Engineered Trees*, narrated by Dr. David Suzuki

"I don't think we evolved to eat white flour. Frankly, I don't think we evolved to eat factory farmed animal products. I don't think we evolved

to eat genetically engineered food. But today two thirds of the foods in our supermarkets contain genetically engineered ingredients already. And they are not labeled."
— **John Robbins, author of the books** *The Food Revolution, Diet for a New America, May All be Fed,* **and** *Reclaiming Our Health*

S tudy up on biotechnology and what these companies are doing to the food plants of the world. Work to educate others about it.

Alliance for Bio-Integrity, 406 W. Depot Ave., Fairfield, IA 52556; 515-472-5554; Bio-Integrity.Org

Ban Terminator Campaign, 431 Gilmour St., 2nd Flr., Ottawa, ON K2P OR5, Canada; BanTerminator.Org

Californians for GE-Free Agriculture, CalGEFree.Org

The Campaign to Label GE Foods, POB 55699, Seattle, WA 98155; 425-771-4049; TheCampaign.Org

Center for Ethics and Toxics, POB 673, 39141 S. Highway One, Gualala, CA 95445; 707-884-1700; CETOS.Org

The Center for Food Safety, 666 Pennsylvania Ave., SE, Ste. 302, Washington DC, 20003; 202-547-9359; CenterForFoodSafety.Org

Center for Science in the Public Interest, 1875 Connecticut Ave., NW, Ste. 300, Washington, DC 20009; 202-332-9110; CSPINet.Org

Citizens for Health, POB 2260, Boulder, CO 80306; 800-357-2211; Citizens.Org

CorpWatch, 1611 Telegraph Ave., #702, Oakland, CA 94612

The Council for Responsible Genetics, 5 Upland Rd., Ste. 3, Cambridge, MA 02140; 617-868-0870; Gene-Watch.Org

GE Fee Maine, POB 7805, Portland, ME 04112; GEFreeMaine.Org

Gene.CH

GENET, GENet-Info.Org

Genetically Engineered Food Alert, 1200 18th St., NW, 5th Flr., Washington, DC 20036; 800-390-3373; 3435 Wilshire Blvd., #380, Los Angeles, CA 90010; 213-251-3680; GEFoodAlert.Org

Genetic Engineering Network, GeneticsAction.Org.UK

Genetic Resources International, Girona 25, Pral., E-08010; Barcelona, Spain; Grain.Org

Indigenous Peoples Council on Biocolonialism, POB, Nixon, NV 89424; IPCB.Org

Institute for Responsible Technology, POB 469; Fairfield, IA 52556; ResponibleTechnology.Org

Mindfully.Org/GE

MonsantoWatch.Org

Mothers for Natural Law, Safe-Food.Org

National Family Farm Coalition, NFFC.Net

Network of Concerned Farmers, Non-GM-Farmers.Com

Northwest Resistance Against Genetic Engineering, POB 15289, Portland, OR 97293; 503-239-6841; NWRage.Org

The Organic Consumers Association, 6101 Cliff Estate Rd., Little Marais, MN 55614; 218-226-4164; Purefood.Org; OrganicConsumers.Org
  Sells a documentary titled *The Future of Food*. It tells about the dangers of genetic engineering of food plants, and the lies being told by the companies producing GE foods. Get a copy of the documentary, and show it to your friends and neighbors.

Physicians Committee for Responsible Medicine, 5100 Wisconsin Ave., NW, Ste. 404, Washington, DC 20016; 202-686-2210; PCRM.Org

Public Citizen, 1600 20th St. NW; Washington, D.C. 20009; 202-588-1000; Citizen.Org

Public Citizen Stop Food Irradiation Project, 215 Pennsylvania Ave., SE, Washington, D.C. 20003; Citizen.Org/CMEP

Resistance Against Genetic Engineering, POB 15289, Portland, OR 97293; 503-239-6841; NWRAGE.Org/NWRAGE.html

Rural Advancement Foundation International, POB 640, Pittsboro, NC 27312; 919-542-1396; RAFIUSA.Org

Safe Tables Our Priority, POB 46522, Chicago, IL 60646-0522; Media and business 312-957-0284; Victims and victims' families 800-350-STOP; Stop-USA.Org

SeedsOfDeception.Com

StopGETrees.Org

The True Food Network, TrueFoodNow.Org

United Kingdom Agricultural Biodiversity Coalition; UKABC.Org

Union of Concerned Scientists, 2 Brattle Square, Cambridge, MA 02238; UCSUSA.Org

World Social Forum, Rua General Jardim, 660, 8th Flr., Sao Paulo, SP 01223-010, Brazil; WorldSocialForum.Org

Girl Pollution: The Plethora of Plastic Tampon Applicators

"An average woman throws away 250 to 300 pounds of tampons, pads and applicators in her lifetime. The great majority of these end up in landfills, or as something the sewage treatment plants must deal with.

Plastic tampon applicators from sewage outfalls are among the most common forms of trash on beaches.

For building owners, pads and tampons that are flushed down the toilet are the most common cause of plumbing problems.

A March-April 2001 *E Magazine* article states that, according to the Center for Marine Conservation, over 170,000 tampon applicators were collected along U.S. coastal areas between 1998 and 1999."
— TheKeeper.Com

One day I found myself standing on Green Beach, which is near the southernmost tip of the Big Island of Hawaii. It is in the middle of the Pacific Ocean, far away from the continents and large cities. Spread over the beach were a variety of plastics that had floated across the ocean from various places on the Pacific Rim, from North America, Central America, South America, Australia, Asia, and various islands in the Pacific. Some of this plastic pollution was likely also the result of trash thrown off cruise ships, yachts, military craft, and industrial ships. Standing there I could see broken plastic toy pieces, foam cups, broken surfboard chunks, brightly colored plastic holiday doodads. But by far the most common type of plastic I saw on that beach on that island in the middle of the Pacific Ocean was that of tampon applicators. Dozens of them. It occurred to me that there must be billions of these applicators on the planet. It is simple math, and not hard to figure, and unfortunately true. There are billions of plastic tampon applicators that will take thousands of years to decompose.

Throughout girl history, various items have been used to absorb the periods of the billions of women who have lived. But in recent history women have begun to use nonbiodegradable applicators. In addition to the applicators there are other plastics used in the products that are mass-marketed to both women and men for their personal care. The products marketed to males that contribute most to this are disposable razors.

How to solve this plastic pollution? What can be done? How can we go to the beaches of the most isolated parts of Earth and not think about this type of pollution when we find them sitting at our feet?

Seventh Generation, the maker of biodegradable, biocompatible cleaning and personal care products has started a discussion board on this topic. The site also encourages people to tell their stories about the topic of menstruation. Anything from serious to comical to poetry is apparently welcome there.

The companies below produce organic cotton, rayon-free, chlorine-free, hydrogen peroxide-whitened, nonsynthetic, non-GMO, biodegradable feminine care products.

GladRags.Com

InOtherWords.Org
Women's books and resources.

The Keeper, Keeper.Com
The Keeper is a reusable rubber menstrual cup. It is made from the same type of rubber used to make baby bottle nipples.

NatraCare.Com

Nature Boy & Girl, Gamlavärmdövägen 10, 13137 Nacka, Sweden; +46-8-6449696; NatY.SE/

OrganicCottonPlus.Com

PandoraPads.Com

PerfectPads.Net

Sckoon.Com

Seventh Generation, SeventhGeneration.Com; TamponTification.Com

Golf Courses: Destroying Ecosystems, Polluting Water, Damaging the Environment

"If you scraped a golf green and tested it, you'd have to cart it away to a hazardous waste facility."
— **Ted Steinberg, quoting a biologist, *American Green: The Obsessive Quest for the Perfect Lawn***

To build a golf course land has to be prepared to provide large stretches of fields. Often this destroys not only the natural structure of the land that took many thousands of years for Nature to form, but also kills off native species of trees, bushes, wildflowers, and other plants. Often native animals are killed, or at least have their habitat degraded or reduced by the construction of golf courses. Non-native varieties of grass and plants are put in, and wildlife is kept off. Toxic chemicals are used to grow the grass, kill the weeds, kill the bugs, and to poison wildlife that may damage the turf. Some of the grasses being planted on golf courses are genetically altered to be resistant to drought and weed growth. This makes the whole course not only unnatural for the region, but also out of tune with Nature, and essentially a field of poison.

In June 2006, developers in Pebble Beach, California, were planning a golf course resort that would require the removal of 17,000 trees, and require redesigning the landscape in a way that would result in damage to wetlands. The trees they were planning to remove would have decimated one of the largest remaining forests of Monterey pine. The plan received so much scrutiny by the public, the California Coastal Commission, and by environmental groups such as the Sierra Club, that the company withdrew the plan so that they could revise it.

Unfortunately most golf course companies don't get scrutinized the way the Pebble Beach Company did. As golfing and golf tourism has increased in popularity around the world, golf courses are being built at a rapid pace, especially in Southeast Asia and the Caribbean. This has degraded coastal environments, damaged wildlife populations, poisoned water tables, and reduced farmland. As I write this there is a company working to develop a golf course and resort on land that wild Elephants use as a passageway next to Zambia's Victoria Falls.

Often golf courses are put onto land that was being used as farmland, other times they are built on land that had never been touched by land developers.

Golf courses require about 3,000 cubic meters of water per day. A typical 150-acre golf course can use more water than is used by a town of over 10,000 people. Often this water is pumped from wells, depleting water tables and causing saline intrusion. Some golf courses existing near the oceans have built desalination plants to provide fresh water for their greens.

In the southwestern United States, where a dwindling water supply is often an issue because a large portion of it has to be piped in or brought in through aqueducts, golf courses continue to be built. There are nearly 500 golf courses in Southern California.

The lush green lawns of golf courses are a common site in and around southwestern desert communities such as Las Vegas, Palm Springs, and Phoenix. It is in those areas that golf courses appear so alien. It is obvious that the golf courses would not exist there if it were not for a tremendous amount of water being pumped in from someplace outside of the region. And it is in those regions that golf courses contribute to the drought and deplete underground water tables. It is estimated that golf courses in Coachella Valley, home of Palm Springs, use about 35 billion gallons of water per year.

Golf course chemical runoff is often mentioned in water pollution studies. Golf courses have become a major threat to coastal environments around the world.

When a golf course is being built, the bulldozing and land reconstruction often lead to sediment runoff into water tables and surrounding water bodies, which kills water life and damages the populations of wildlife that relies on the water and the life in it for survival.

Larger golf courses often have their own gas station where underground storage containers are installed to prevent exposure to heat, fire, and extreme weather. These storage containers sometimes leak the petroleum products into the underground water tables, contaminating what the surrounding community uses as its own water source.

To keep the grass green, toxic chemical fertilizers, pesticides, fungicides, biocides, and miticides are applied. To keep them weed-free, more toxic chemicals in the form of "weed killer" herbicides are sprayed onto the greens. These chemicals pollute groundwater as well as nearby ponds, lakes, streams, rivers, and oceans. The chemicals also evaporate, adding to air pollution.

Many of the chemicals typically used on golf courses are in the category of persistent organic pollutants (POPs) that cause birth defects, learning disabilities, cancers, and hormonal and immune disorders in both humans and wildlife.

In addition to being POPs, the fertilizers used on golf courses lead to nitrate and phosphorus contamination that cause algae blooms in ponds, rivers, lakes, and oceans that reduce oxygen levels, killing fish and sea life, and reducing food sources for birds and other wildlife.

Where golf courses have been built on tropical and subtropical islands (such as Hawaii), the fertilizer runoff has caused algae blooms that have choked off and killed coral reefs and damaged many varieties of marine life.

Some golf course companies say they work to prevent the chemicals they use from entering the surrounding environment. They do this by planting a buffer zone of foliage meant to absorb pollutants. That is a good thing. But it works only partially. The chemicals they use also evaporate into the air, and seep into water tables, polluting them. The chemicals most commonly used on golf courses do not degrade in the environment for many years, and may remain problematic for decades, centuries, or even longer.

Many golf courses also use toxic chemicals to kill off land mammals. When birds and snakes feed off the mice, shrews, rabbits, gophers, squirrels, groundhogs, and other animals that have been poisoned, the poison in the flesh can poison and/or kill the predators.

Some land developers market their plans to build a golf course by claiming it will be beneficial to the community while being environmentally friendly. But it is easy to see why the typical golf course is anything but beneficial, and is more of a detriment on many levels.

Golf courses may be easy to manage in some regions of the world where the grass is native and the rain is sufficient. But golf courses are not natural and damage habitat in regions where the water has to be pumped in; where the grass is not native and has to be kept alive with chemical treatments; and where the course can exist only with great alteration of the natural landscape.

Since golf courses are often the only open space free from structures in a community, it would be nice if they could be built and maintained in a way that is safe for the native plants, for wildlife, for water, and for the environment.

It is true that many golf courses provide habitat for wildlife that otherwise would have been destroyed by other violations of the land. And golf course shrubs, bushes, and turf cool the air while providing oxygen and absorbing air pollutants, such as ozone, carbon dioxide, and hydrogen fluoride. But the damage that most golf courses cause to the environment doesn't offset the good.

There are a small number of golf courses working to clean up their act by using organic, non-POP chemicals; using bugs and soil organisms to improve the soil; reducing turf areas; designating no-mow areas; planting native vegetation on their grounds; inviting school children to plant wildflowers; and leaving wildlife alone to the point of becoming havens for them. Some of these golf courses specifically work to provide nesting areas for native bird species, as well as for bats, bees, and butterflies, amphibians, turtles and other wildlife.

But those golf courses that are working to be environmentally friendlier are few. The great majority of them continue to wreak havoc on the environment.

Golf courses take up hundreds of thousands of acres of land on each continent. In 2005 there were over 16,000 golf courses in the U.S. Some have recently gone under, being sold to developers of malls, condos, and car lots. But many more golf courses are being built.

Communities should rise up and require existing golf courses to become more environmentally friendly. Any golf courses that are in the planning stages should be required to follow standards that provide for protection of wildlife, plant, land, soil organisms, and water. Or the land should be left as wildlife habitat.

Grains

Grains are in the seed family. Common grains include oats, rye, barley, wheat, rice, millet, and quinoa.

When cooked grains are eaten they are especially problematic as their starchiness clogs the system, slows the blood and lymph systems, and creates a sugar rush.

Some people have allergies to gluten, which is a protein found in certain grains. This includes people who become depressed, irritable, or experience anxiety after eating wheat, oats, rye, and barley (eggs and dairy can also trigger these maladies, as can deficiencies in certain vitamins, such as the B vitamins, and a diet lacking in the enzymes and essential fatty acids found in raw plant substances). This allergy can mistakenly be diagnosed under the label of "manic depression," or "bipolar disorder" for which the patient is prescribed various chemical drugs.

Some people do not have mood, energy, or personality reactions to grains that have been sprouted before use.

Raw grains can be beneficial in adding fiber to the diet. It is best to use them whole, uncrushed, and to soak them in water, or even fruit juice, for a few hours before eating them. (A raw vegan breakfast may consist of soaked quinoa mixed with berries or fruit and/or nuts, or nut milk.)

Healing Retreats

The following offer retreats to detoxify and heal the body and soul with living foods. Yoga and massage is often part of the program. Styles, menus, cost, and daily programs vary according to the philosophy, accommodations, and location of each center. Accommodations may be in a house, hotel, yurt, tent, or in the open wilds. Research the retreat that most fits your needs, comfort level, and style.

<u>World-Wide:</u>

Kerrie Cushing, DancingButterfly.Net
Kerrie runs retreats in connection with Eden Retreats.

Eden Retreats, Sunfood Nutrition, POB 900202, San Diego, CA 92190; 888-729-3663; Sunfood.Com
 - Conducts several Sunfoodist retreats per year, including in Hawaii, California, upstate New York, Arizona, Georgia, England, Bali, Peru, and Central America.

<u>The United States:</u>

The Assembly of Yahweh Wellness Center, 7881 Columbia Hwy., Eaton Rapids, MI 48827; 517-663-1637; AssemblyOfYahweh.Com

Dr. Ralph Cinque, 305 Verdin Dr., Buda, TX 78610; 512-295-4256; DrCinque.Com

The Center for Healing with Nature, 593 Poipu Dr., Honolulu, HI 96825; 808-394-6240; HealingWithNature@Hawaii.RR.Com

The Creative Health Institute, 112 W. Union City Rd., Union City, MI 49094; 517-278-6260; CreativeHealthInstitute.US

Hippocrates Health Institute, 1443 Palmdale Ct., West Palm Beach, FL 33411; 800-842-2125; HippocratesInst.Com

Living Foods Institute, 1530 Dekalb Ave., NE, Ste. E, Atlanta, GA 30307; LivingFoodsInstitute.Com

Nature's Raw Energy, 640 15th Ave., East Moline, IL 61244; 309-755-0200; NaturesRawEnergy.Com

Optimum Health Institute, 6970 Central Ave., Lemon Grove, CA 91945; 619-589-4098; OptimumHealth.Org

Optimum Health Institute, Rural Rte. 1, Box 339-J, Cedar Creek, TX 98612; 512-303-4817; OptimumHealth.Org

Oxygen Life Spa and Raw Superfood Store, 609 N. Locust, Denton, TX 76201; 944-384-7946; OxygenLifeSpa.Com

Rainbow Gathering, WelcomeHome.Org

This is a free gathering of people who camp for about two or three weeks. There are Rainbow Gatherings on every continent (many take place during different parts of the year).

The gathering in the U.S. takes place in a different National Forest every year. It begins around June 20th and continues into the first week of July. July 4th is the main day of the U.S. gathering, with silence until 12 noon with a focus on meditating on world peace. The silence ends with a parade of children festively entering into the main meadow, which then turns into a massive drum circle with dancing and people from various camps handing out food.

Most people find out about the location of the annual Rainbow either by word-of-mouth or by searching the Internet on or about June 20th.

There are usually more than 15,000 people who gather to camp at the U.S. annual Rainbow. There is every type of person, including all age groups, races, gender and religions. The gathering is often compared to a Native American gathering of tribes where all peace-loving people are welcome.

There are often more than 20 different camps with their own kitchen operations. Most are vegan, but a few of them are not. Some are run by people who follow a certain religious belief, and other camps are run by regional groups who are not associated with a particular religion. At least one camp has several yoga sessions every day. Another is a massage camp where volunteer massage therapists give massages. Another only serves tea. One serves soup to anyone who wants it. One is set up as a library of books to read. And medical professionals who volunteer to take care of those who may need assistance staff another. There is usually at least one baby born at the gathering every year.

Raw vegans often gather at the "Sprout Kitchen." But you can stay in any camp where you feel comfortable.

One camp, "Granola Funk," creates a stage out of fallen wood and rope and puts on theatrical presentations. The stage is also used by other groups for talks and non-electric "unplugged" music concerts.

If you go, bring water (most kitchens are continuously boiling stream water for drinking), food to share, especially ingredients to donate to the kitchen where you stay; a tent and sleeping pad, blankets and pillows; warm clothing (temperatures in the mountains at night can dip quite low); Sun protection; an umbrella; biodegradable, plant-based soaps; a hammock (with towels to wrap the rope so you don't damage the tree bark); drums and acoustic, string, and wind instruments; dancing feet; hugging arms; kindness; gracious manners; a good book or two; a journal; a drawing pad; non-petroleum candles; eating utensils; and a willingness to work for about two or more hours per day to help run the camp.

Do not bring any drugs, alcohol, weaponry, or fireworks to a Rainbow gathering. They are not welcome.

Do not bring electric music, electric instruments, boom boxes, or radios to a Rainbow gathering. Unplug from society and live free of electricity.

Photography is discouraged. Respect the wishes of those who gather free from the intrusion of cameras and electronic devices. Only take memories.

Before you leave, help clean up, help carry out trash, and leave the forest in better condition than when you arrived.

Rest Of Your Life Health Retreat, POB 102, Barksdale, TX 78828; 830-234-3488; ROYLRetreat.Com

River Canyon Retreat, 18262 Slide Mine Rd., N. San Juan, CA 95960; 530-292-0171; RiverCanyonRetreat.Com

Sprout Raw Food Learning Center, 1085 Lake Charles Dr., Roswell, GA 30075; 770-992-9218; SproutRawFood.Com

Tree of Life Rejuvenation Center, Dr. Gabriel Cousens, 686 Harshaw Rd., Patagonia, AZ 85624; 520-394-2520; TreeOfLife.NU

Vitality Health Center, Dr. Rick Dina, 4340 Redwood Hwy, Ste. 414, San Rafael, CA 94903; VitalityHealthMarin.Com

Ann Wigmore Foundation, POB 399, San Sidel, NM 87049; 505-552-0595; Wigmore.Org

Wild Food Adventures, John Kallas, Ph.D., Director, 5036 Southeast Mitchell St., Portland, OR 97206; WildFoodAdventures.Com

Yoga Oasis, POB 1935, Pahoa, HI 96778; 808-965-8460; YogaOasis.Org

<u>Australia:</u>

Hippocrates Health Center of Australia, Elaine Ave., Mudgeeraba 4213, Gold Coast Queensland, Australia; 07-5530-2860; Hippocrates.Com.AU

<u>Canada:</u>

New Life Retreat, RR4, 453 Dobbie Rd., Lanark, Ontario, KoG 1Ko, Canada; 613-259-3337; NewLifeRetreat.Com

Nonpareil Natural Health Retreat, RR#3, Stirling, Ontario, KoK 3Eo, Canada; 613-395-6332; NonpareilHolistic.Com

Costa Rica:

Cascada Verde, Apdo 888, 8000 San Isidro PZ, Costa Rica; CascadaVerde@Hotmail.Com

Spirit of the Earth, 5871 Bells Rd., London, Ontario, N6P 1P3, Canada; 519-652-9109
   Canadian address, but retreats are held in Costa Rica.

Pacha Mama, Nicoya Peninsula, Costa Rica; 506-289-7081; Pacha-Mama.Org

England:

Detox Your World Retreats, Cambridgeshire, England, UK; 44-(0)8700 113 119; DetoxYourWorld.Com

Heartspring, Hill House, Llansteffan, Carmarthen, Wales SA33 5JG; HeartSpring.Co.UK

Karuna Detox Retreats, 42 Corn Park, South Brent, Devon, TQ10 9DG; KarunaRetreats.Com

The UK Centre for Living Foods, Holmleigh, Gravel Hill, Ludlow SY8 1QS; LivingFoods.Co.UK

Indonesia:

Ubud Sari Health Resort, 35 Jl. Kajeng, Ubud, Bali 80571; UbudSari.Com

Mexico:

Sanoviv Medical Institute, 2602-C Transportation Ave., National City, CA 91950; 800-SANOVIV (726-6848); Sanoviv.Com
   California address, but retreat is held in Baja, Mexico.

Philippines:

The Farm at San Benito, Isle of Luzon, Philippines, Hippocrates Health Resort of Asia, The Farm at San Benito Manila Office, Mandarin Hotel, Makati Ave., Makati City; 632-751-3498; TheFarm.Com.PH

Puerto Rico:

Ann Wigmore Institute, POB 429, Rincon, Puerto Rico 00677 USA; 787-868-6307; AnnWigmore.Org

South Africa:

The Hydro at Stellenbosch, 7600 Western Cape; TheHydro.Co.ZA

The Natural Hygiene Clinic, Dr. Karalis, Hermanus, Western Cape, South Africa; DrKaralis.Net

Spain:

Comunidad de Alimentacion, Cruda Internacional, "Frinca Cruda," Revista NaturalezaCruda, Arroyo del Viejo-Alpujata, 29110 Monda, Malaga, Costa del Sol, Spain; 952 119929, 619 78 85 70; BaltaCrudo@Yahoo.ES; ComunidadCruda.Com/Contact.php?lang=es

Ecoforest, Apdo. Correos 29, 29100 Coin, Malaga; EcoForest.Org

Thailand:

ProCynergy, 120/51 Palm Springs Pl., Ciang Mai, 500000, Thailand; 053 241 249; JuliaJus.Com

Rainbow Community, Thailand, Com.To/Apamada

Trinidad:

Otas Holistic Health Center, 461 Circular Dr., Lange Prk, Chaguanas, Trinidad, West Indies; Sat@Carib-Link.Net

Heart Disease? Become a Vegan

McDougall Wellness Center, POB 14039, Santa Rosa, CA 95402; 800-941-7111; 707-538-8609; DrMcDougall.Com

Dr. Michael Greger, DrGreger.Org

Dr. Michael Klaper, VegSource.Com/Klaper

Preventive Medicine Research Institute, 900 Bridgeway, Sausalito, CA 94965; 415-332-2525; PMRI.Org
Therapies based on comprehensive lifestyle changes that begin to reverse even severe coronary heart disease, without drugs or surgery.

"The progression of even severe coronary heart disease can be stopped or reversed simply by making comprehensive changes in one's diet and lifestyle."
— **Dr. Dean Ornish, M.D.**, Founder and President, **Preventive Research Institute**

Hemp Farming: Work to Legalize It

Also see:
• Bamboo
• Cotton: Seek Organic

Books:
• *Demons, Discriminations & Dollars: A Brief History of the Origins of American Drug Policy,* by David Bearman, M.D.
• *The Emperor Wears No Clothes: The Authoritative Historical Record of Cannabis and the Conspiracy Against Marijuana,* by Jack Herer, JackHerer.Com
• *The Great Book of Hemp: The Complete Guide to the Environmental, Commercial, and Medicinal Uses of the World's Most Extraordinary Plant,* by Rowan Robinson
• *Hemp for Health: The Medicinal and Nutritional Uses of Cannabis*, by Chris Conrad
• *Hemp Horizons: The Comeback of the World's Most Promising Plant*, by John W. Roulac
• *Hemp: Lifeline to the Future: The Unexpected Answer for Our Environmental and Economic Recovery,* by Chris Conrad
• *Hemp Masters – Getting Knotty: More Ancient Hippie Secrets for Knotting Hip Hemp Jewelry,* by Max Lunger
• *The Hemp Manifesto: 101 Ways That Hemp Can Save Our World*, by Rowan Robinson
• *Hemp: What the World Needs Now,* by John McCabe
• *Human Rights and the U.S. Drug War,* by Chris Conrad, Mikki Norris, and Virginia Resner
• *Marijuana: The First Twelve Thousand Years,* by Ernest L. Abel
• *Shattered Lives: Portraits from America's Drug War,* by Mikki Norris, Chris Conrad, and Virginia Resner
• *Smoke and Mirrors: The War on Drugs and the Politics of Failure,* by Dan Baum
• *Substituting Agricultural Materials for Petroleum-Based Industrial Products,* Institute for Local Self-Reliance

Documentary:
• *The Emperor of Hemp,* directed by Jeff Jones, narrated by Peter Coyote. Tells the story of Jack Herer and the history of hemp. The DVD includes the U.S. govern-

ment's 1943 film for farmers, *Hemp for Victory*. JackHerer.Com

In addition to all the benefits of hemp in the areas of fuel, construction, cleaning the air, improving soil quality, reducing the use of toxic farm chemicals, protecting forests, and providing material for clothing, it is an excellent source of nutrition.

Hemp seeds do not contain tetrahydrocannabinol (THC), the psychoactive properties of the adult marijuana plant. There is often some very small amount of THC residue on the seed hulls from the flowers. But this is a minimal amount that would not contribute to a person getting high from consuming hemp seeds or hemp oil.

Raw hemp seeds contain enzymes, which are essential to life.

Hemp seeds contain amino acids and essential fatty acids that are exactly what a human body needs to maintain health.

The amino acids in hemp seeds are of the highest quality.

Amino acids are the building blocks of protein. The human body needs a constant supply of quality amino acids, and hemp seeds and the oil extracted from the seeds provides these.

A body fed with a diet rich in quality amino acids is able to maintain the best quality of health. Collagen protein is the most abundant protein in the body and is largely dependant on a constant supply of amino acids. Collagen is often cited as the protein that provides for skin health, strength, elasticity, and beauty. Collagen actually plays a part in the health of all body tissues, from the bones and teeth to the hair and nails. It also is present in the corneas and lenses of the eyes. Those who follow a diet that is lacking in quality amino acids and essential fatty acids exhibit this in a less vibrant physical appearance, including in the skin, hair, nails, and eyes. Hemp seed provides the essential fatty acid and amino acid nutrients in the best form and at the best ratio for the body to maintain vibrant, strong, elastic, and healthy tissues.

Hemp oil also provides for the health of our blood. It provides nutrients to maintain the collagen protein in the blood vessels, and also helps to maintain a healthy cholesterol level. The essential fatty acids in hemp oil assists in the transference of fat-soluble nutrients throughout the body. The globule edestins protein found in hemp is similar to the globuline of blood plasma that are essential to the formation of antibodies that fight of disease.

"Hemp seed oil appears to be one of nature's most perfectly balanced EFA oils. It contains both EFAs in the right proportion for long-

term use, and also contains gamma-linolenic acid (GLA). It is the only vegetable oil with this combination."
— **Udo Erasmus,** *Fats that Heal, Fats that Kill*; **UdoErasmus.Com**

The gamma-linoleic acid (GLA) nutrient in hemp seeds is also found in mother's milk as well as black currant oil, borage oil, and primrose oil. GLA is good for the skin, hair, and nails, tissue growth, and reduces inflammation. Along with all the other stellar quality nutrients in raw hemp seeds, the GLA in milk made from raw hemp seeds is excellent for babies.

"Hemp seeds contain up to 24 percent protein. A handful of seed provides the minimum daily requirement of protein for adults."
— **Ed Rosenthal,** *Hemp Today*, **page 101**

Hemp seeds are also a high-quality source of calcium, phosphorus, potassium, vitamin A, vitamin E, and trace minerals including iron, manganese, and magnesium.

"You can basically divide (hemp seed nutrition) roughly into three components. There are essential fatty acids in the oil – omega-6, omega-3, omega-9 – and also minor fatty acids like gamma linolenic acid and stearidonic acid. So that's one-third of its composition. Another one-third consists mostly of fiber, both soluble and insoluble. And it's also one-third protein.
... There are some oils on the market – hemp oil, crushed from the hemp seed. Again, that has the same ratio of omega-6 to omega-3 – which it's most known for – as well as the other omegas that I described, and we can talk more about that. So there are oils. People also take the entire seed and shell it – that is, take the shell off the inside and you then just have the soft interior. So you're removing a lot of the carbs and leaving primarily protein and oil. Then you can make protein powders from them by removing the oil and milling the rest into something like flour, then sifting it to remove more of the carbs so that you're left with a higher protein fraction. I make all those products and I make them certified-organic. In addition to that, I incorporate hemp seeds into more commonly used foods, like energy bars and salad dressings."
— **Ruth Shamai, RuthsHempFoods.Com; in interview with Mike Adams, Health Benefits of Hemp Foods, NewsTarget.Com; August 23, 2005**

Hemp oil contains more of the essential fatty acids than any food oil. No food oil provides the balance that hemp seeds provide. With a minimal 35 percent oil content, hemp seed oil is only 8 percent saturated fatty acid, plus 55 percent linoleic acid (Omega-6), 25 percent alphalinolenic acid (Omega-3), and 1.7 percent gamma linoleic acid (GLA: Super Omega-6). These oils are essential to the human body in building a strong immune system. The linoleic acids found in hemp seeds are vital to the transfer of nutrients and oxygen throughout the body, to the health of cell membranes, and to the removal of toxins. They also lower cholesterol, improve brain function, keep the joints healthy, and maintain nerve health.

According to research detailed in the book *Fats That Heal, Fats That Kill* by Udo Erasmus, deficiencies in essential fatty acids play a role in a variety of health problems, including allergies, arthritis, bone depletion, cancer, cardiovascular disease, depression, diabetes, glandular atrophy, hair and nail problems, liver disease, multiple sclerosis, poor wound healing, premenstrual syndrome, skin issues, sleep disorders, slowed brain function, sterility, stress, weakened immune system, and weight problems.

Currently it is illegal to have raw, alive hemp seeds in the U.S. All seeds that are brought into the country must be heated or fumigated to kill them so that they can't sprout. This damages the nutrients of the seed, greatly lowering the quality of some of the nutrients, and killing others.

When a person purchases hemp seed oil at a natural foods store or other venue in the U.S., that oil has either been brought into the U.S. in oil form after the raw seeds have been pressed, or the oil is from seeds that were killed before they were brought into the country and then crushed for their oil.

It is better to have hemp seed oil that was taken from living seeds, and the fresher the oil the better. The oil is fragile and breaks down easily when exposed to heat or light.

If hemp were legal to grow in the U.S. the nutritional value of the oil would be higher and the price would be lower.

Americans for Safe Access, SafeAccessNow.Org

AngelJustice.Org

Artists Helping End Marijuana Prohibition, AHEMP.Org

Boston Hemp Fest, BostonHempFest.Com

Business Alliance for Commerce in Hemp,
EqualRights4All.Org/BACH/BACHCore.html

Campaign for the Restoration and Regulation of Hemp, CRRH.Org

Cannabis Culture **magazine,** CannabisCulture.Com

CannabisNews.Com

ChangeTheClimate.Org
   Founded by parents and business professionals to educate the public about the tremendous waste of tax dollars for the "war on marijuana" and the increasing threat to our basic civil liberties.

Common Sense for Drug Policy, CSDP.Org

CompassionateMoms.Org

ChrisConrad.Com

Conscious Clothing; 505-982-7506; GetConscious.Com
   Creates hemp/tencel blend wedding dresses. Tencel is made from wood pulp and is biodegradable.

California Cannabis Research Medical Group, CCRMG.Org

Campaign for the Restoration and Regulation of Hemp, CRRH.Org

Cannabis.Com

CannabisNews.Com

CannaBusiness.Com

The Canadian Hemp Trade Alliance, HempTrade.CA

Common Sense for Drug Policy, CommonSenseDrugPolicy.Org

DrBronner.Com
   Produces hemp-based soaps and foods. They donate a portion of their profits to work to make hemp farming and hemp products legal. Their site contains interesting information about hemp and the government's unfair and unwise treatment of, and concern about, hemp.

Drug Policy Alliance, DrugPolicy.Org; DPF.Org

Drug Reform Coordination Network, DRCNet.Org

DrugSense.Org

Drug Truth Network, DrugTruth.Net

DrugWarFacts.Org

Educators for Sensible Drug Policy, EFSP.Org

Dr. William Eidelman, DrEidelman.Com

EmperorOfHemp.Com

4Hemp.Org

GlobalHemp.Com

GlobalHempStore.Com

GlobalRevolutions.Com

GreenTherapy.Com

HempAdvocates.Org

HempCar.Org

Hempest.Com

HempExpo.Com

HempFabric.Com

Hemp for Health, EqualRights4All.Org/Books/Health.html

Hemp4Fuel.Com

HempGuide.Com

Hemphasis.Net

The Hemp Industries Association, TheHIA.Org

HempIndustries.Org

HempLobby.Org

HempMagazine.Com

HempMasters.Com

HempNation.Com

Hemp.Net

The Hemp Party, HempEmbassy.Net/hp2/Index.html

HempStores.Com

HempTimes.Com

The Industrial Hemp Network, POB 1716 Sebastopol, CA 95473; HempTech.Com

International Hemp Association, POB 75007, Eugene OR 97401; HempReport.Com/IHA

International Hemp Association, Postbus 75007, 1070 AA Amsterdam, the Netherlands

International Hemp Fair, CannaTrade.CH

JackHerer.Com
    Web site of the author of *The Emperor Wears No Clothes: The Authoritative Historical Record of Cannabis and the Conspiracy Against Marijuana*. When you buy a copy of the book, you help support the fight to legalize hemp. He is also the subject of the documentary, *The Emperor of Hemp*, narrated by Peter Coyote.

The Journal of the International Hemp Association, The International Hemp Association (IHA), Postbus 75007, 1070 AA Amsterdam, The Netherlands; +31 20 6188758; IHA@EuroNet.NL

Kentucky Hemp Growers' Cooperative Association, POB 8395 Lexington, KY 40533; 606-252-8954

Kentucky Hemp Museum, POB 8551; Lexington, Kentucky 40533; 606-873-8957; KyHempMuse@AOL.Com; KentuckyHemp.Com

Law Enforcement Against Prohibition, LEAP.CC
LEAP is a 5,000-member organization created to: 1. Give voice to law enforcers who know the U.S. War on Drugs is a failed policy and 2. Support legalized regulation of drugs as an alternative that will lower incidence of death, disease, crime, and addiction while saving tax dollars.
LEAP produced a documentary giving voice to those who have worked in the drug war and who are now against the failed policies of the War on Drugs.

"Anyone concerned about the failure of our $69 billion-a-year War on Drugs should watch this 12-minute program. You will meet front-line, ranking police officers who give us a devastating report on why it cannot work. It is a must-see for any journalist or public official dealing with this issue."
— **Walter Cronkite**

LivingTreePaper.Com

Living Harvest Hemp Seed Nutrition, LivingHarvest.Com

Dr. Tod H. Mikuriya, Mikuriya.Com

MoreTreesHemp.Com
A percentage of their sales go to plant trees.

Multidisciplinary Association for Psychedelic Studies, MAPS.Org

National Organization for the Reform of Marijuana Laws, NORML.Org
This organization can't advertise on radio, TV, or in newspapers because it has the word "marijuana" in its name.

NaturalHighLifestyle.Com

New Democratic Party, Canada, EndProhibition.CA

North American Industrial Hemp Council, POB 259329, Madison, WI 53725-9329; NAIHC.Org

North Dakota's Proposed Industrial Hemp Rules of April 26, 2006, AgDepartment.Com/PDFFiles/ProposedIndustrialHempRules5-2006.pdf

The November Coalition, November.Org
Working to end the drug war.

Online Library of Drug Policy, DrugLibrary.Org

RuthsHempFoods.Com

"Hemp has been eaten for thousands of years in different parts of
the world. It's the seed that we eat, and its beneficial in terms of protein and essential fatty acids. People in Persia used to eat it, and they
still do, actually. I know Iranians who grew up eating toasted hemp
seeds. There's evidence that goes back thousands of years that it was
being eaten in China and in different places around the world for those
health benefits. Hemp has kind of had a renaissance starting in the
early 1990s. I was part of the lobby that helped to legalize or re-legalize
hemp in Canada, which we accomplished in 1998 for commercial
growth. Since then, I have been producing a line of hemp foods to
spread the news and the nourishment of hemp."
— **Ruth Shamai, 2005**

Saskatchewan Hemp Association, SaskHemp.Com

Seattle Hempfest, HempFest.Org, SeattleHempfest.Com

The Science of Medical Marijuana, MedMJScience.Org

Society of Cannabis Clinicians, CCRMG.Org.html
   Publishes O'Shaughnessy's *The Journal of Cannabis in Clinical Practice.*

Southern Humboldt Hemp Fest, 3Americas.Org/Hempfest/

StopTheDrugWar.Org

United Kingdom Cannabis Internet Activists, UKCIA.Org

VoteHemp.Com, POB 862, Bedford, MA 01730

VoiceYourself.Com

Washington Hemp Education Network, Hemp.Net/Vote

The Wo/Men's Alliance for Medical Marijuana, WAMM.Org

Women's Organization for National Prohibition Reform, WONPR.Org

Honey, Bee Pollen, Royal Jelly, and Propolis

Book:
• *The Forgotten Pollinators*, by Stephen Buchmann and Gary Nabhan

The consumption of bee products is the one thing that separates some Sunfoodists from those who call themselves vegan. I say "some" because not all Sunfoodists consume bee products.

Vegans believe that collecting honey and other bee products from bee nests is unfair and enslaves the bees. This is because the bees are gathering food for the bee colony. The bees have to work harder to forage for their needs after their honey, pollen, royal jelly, and propolis have been taken.

Some beekeepers protect the hives they manage by killing wildlife, such as bears. If you choose to consume bee products, please seek out the products from beekeepers that don't kill other wildlife.

For more on whether or not to consume bee products, do research that will help you make the right choice. Plenty of books have been written about bees and honey. Some of the first books published after the invention of the printing press were on the topic of bees and honey.

A spoonful of honey or an equal amount of grains of bee pollen requires a lot of work from honeybees. A teaspoon of either is the result of hundreds of foraging trips. A jar filled with honey requires tens of thousands of foraging trips.

Another concern is that bees are often killed in the process of harvesting of honey. Most beekeepers practice methods that are designed to protect the bees. Harvesting from the wild is more likely to cause damage to the bee colony.

To "control" the bees during the harvesting of the wax cells, smoke, butyric acid (found naturally in rancid butter), or pressurized air is passed over the hive to blow away the bees. This isn't done to harm the bees, but to calm them so the beekeeper can go about removing the shelves of honeycomb from the supers, the boxes on top of the main hive where the queen lives. Some people think that bees react to smoke by sticking close to the hive, or evacuating it, as a natural reaction to the smoke of forest fires.

Taking the wax cells, which are filled with honey, from the hive may also kill bee eggs and larvae. But modern beekeeping equipment uses "queen excluder" shields that prevent the queen bee from getting into the boxes from where the honey is "harvested." The queen excluder shields greatly reduce the chances of bee eggs and larvae being in the honey combs from which the honey is taken.

To separate the honey from the cells, the cells are either melted, crushed, or spun in a centrifuge. The most common is the centrifuge method where the frames/shelves containing the honeycomb filled with honey are removed from the hive/apiary. The frames are taken to a processing room, or a portable processing room on a truck. The cells are uncapped using a heated knife or a mechanical tool, and the frames are spun, pulling out the honey. The emptied honeycomb frames are taken back to the apiary and put back in their slots. The bees instantly begin the work of repairing the cells and filling them with honey or pollen. When a cell is filled, the bees cap it with wax, which protects the honey from moisture and contamination.

Humans have been keeping honeybees for thousands of years. Images of beekeeping have been found drawn on cave walls, illustrated on ancient pottery, and on architectural ruins. Ancient texts often mention bees, sweet honey, and bee pollen. Mud structures in Africa have been found with areas built into their walls for beehives. Apiaries were built into walls surrounding castles. Houses built in Europe in the last few hundred years feature coves on exterior walls for beehives to be kept. Bees provided honey for food and wax for candles. What we have today as cookies were originally sweetbreads made of grain and honey and that were a part of ancient ceremonies and celebrations.

In Africa there is a bird called the "honey bird" that seeks out honey. It can't get the honey out of the hives, but will chirp in a way to get the attention of an animal there called the "honey badger." The honey badger will follow the chirping bird to the hive, break open the hive, and enjoy the honey along with the bird. Humans have also depended on the honey bird to find beehives.

Bees that produce enough honey to make it worthwhile to keep apiaries compromise a small percentage of the types of bees that exist. Bees native to the North American continent didn't make enough honey for the settlements of Europeans who moved here. "Domesticated" European honeybees were brought to America by the seventeenth-century Spanish missionaries and by the colonists of Jamestown and Williamsburg. Within a hundred years after their introduction to the American continent honeybees had established colonies throughout much of North America. Bees brought to the U.S. from Italy in the 1800s quickly became the most common type of honeybee to keep because they tend to gather more honey than other types of bees.

I use the term "domesticated honeybees" because that is the term most often used to describe the bees kept by beekeepers. But bees aren't trainable, and can't be changed from their natural behavior. What can be done is provide bees with places to build their hives, and these hives can be kept by the beekeepers.

Some people who keep bees don't harvest the honey, but only keep the bees as a hobby or to help pollinate crops, and to help local flower species get pollinated so the people can then spread their seeds. These non-honey harvesting beekeepers refer to themselves as "beetenders." They don't necessarily keep honey bees, but may be involved in providing ideal living arrangements for any number of native species of bees.

Both wild and "domesticated" bees are only one form of wildlife that pollinate plants resulting in the crops that humans and animals eat and flowers that they enjoy. Other pollinators include butterflies, flies, moths, wasps, snails, snakes, worms, lizards, frogs, bats, and hummingbirds and other types of birds, as well as some animals that inadvertently spread pollen as they move from place to place. The wind and rain also spread certain types of pollen. Tragically, because the populations of so many types of wildlife have been damaged by human activity, there has been a worldwide decline of all types of "wild pollinators."

Some beekeepers transfer their colonies to different parts of the continent via highway, train, boat, and airplane. Transferring bee colonies from place to place to collect honey is not a new practice. The ancient Egyptians floated their bee apiaries up and down the Nile so their bees could forage from various types of flowers that came into season along the banks of the river.

Because of a worldwide shortage of honeybees, there are now bee colonies being sent around the world to pollinate farms. In America it is getting more common for bee colonies to be sent from Australia and New Zealand. Additionally, because some types of native bees have died off as a result of pesticides and urban sprawl, U.S. farmers purchase bees from other areas of the world.

Some people hold the opinion that foreign bees should never have been brought to North America from another continent because the bees are invasive. When non-native bees are introduced into an area they may crowd out native species of bees, reducing populations to dangerous levels – populations that may have already been damaged by the use of toxic farm chemicals and urban sprawl. This is because humans have disproportionately increased domesticated honeybee populations, and they may harvest pollen and nectar that native bee populations would otherwise survive on.

Bees typically gather nectar and pollen from an area within four miles of the hive. Their eyes can decipher movement about six times faster than humans can, which means it is harder for them to recognize slow movement. They also see ultraviolet colors. Both of these help bees to determine whether or not to stop at a flower to gather nectar, pollen, and even water.

Inside the nest different types of dances performed by the bees communicate what needs to be done, including sending out an announcement for others to gather. When a bee finds a good source of nectar, she returns to the nest and performs a dance to announce to the others that she has found a source, where the source is according to the angle of Sun, and the type of nectar it holds.

The foraging bees gather the nectar or water in their honey-stomach. They store pollen in little holding bags naturally formed on their hind legs. These harvested goods can be over twice the weight of the bee.

When bees fly, their bodies build static electricity. When they land on a flower the bee's vibrating body shakes pollen from the flower. The pollen showers and clings onto the bee because of the static. The bee uses her numerous comb-like legs to gather the pollen from her body and put it into the collection pouches on her hind legs.

On a single foraging trip bees will stick to one type of flower. As bees move from plant to plant, they inadvertently spread the pollen from the male to the female structures of the plants, which results in about 1/3 of the food in the form of produce that humans eat. On their return to the nest the foraging bees regurgitate the nectar or water, and unload the pollen.

The nectar is taken by the middle-aged bees who either distribute it as food, or process it into honey by regurgitating it and dehydrating it by fanning it with their wings. They then store it in the nest cells for food. One bee colony may process two pounds of honey per day.

The nurse bees use the water to dilute honey to feed the others, or use it to cool the hive by spreading water on the comb and allowing it to evaporate.

While nectar, after it is turned into honey, is the colony's source for carbohydrates, the pollen provides nutrients such as amino acids, fats, and vitamins. Some of the pollen is consumed by the bees as it is first gathered. The rest is stored in special pollen cells, which the nurse bees access to feed the larvae. During the winter the worker bees may eat over two pounds of honey per week.

Beeswax is synthesized from eating nectar honey. It is extracted from slits in the overlapping armorial bands on the bee's abdomen. It first appears as liquid, and then cools into flakes. It is a fatty substance consisting of hundreds of naturally formed chemicals, including esters and fatty acids. The bee will take the flakes from her abdomen, chew them into a malleable consistency, then uses this soft concoction in the sculpted creation of the hexagonal hive cells. Only the cell for the queen bee is made larger than the others. The wax cells are used to store honey, pollen, water, and the eggs that turn into larvae.

When a baby female bee emerges from her cell, she is fully grown and immediately gets to work helping in the business within the hive.

The male bees (drones) emerge and basically hang out until their sexual services are needed. They appear to serve no other purpose than to provide sperm for the queen bee. They aren't involved in gathering nectar and pollen, don't participate in making honey, don't help build the wax cells, and don't help take care of the eggs or larvae. Because they don't have stingers, the male bees can't even help defend the hive from intruders. These slovenly dudes defecate in the hive, leaving their droppings for the female bees to clean up.

Beeswax has been used throughout history to make candles, to plug bottles of wine and other drinks, to seal containers, and to preserve food of all types, such as cheese, by dipping cheese in wax. Beeswax has also been used to preserve wood and plaster, as an ingredient in cosmetics, as a fixative, as a base for drawing materials, and to plug small leaks in boats. It has also been used for centuries to waterproof tents and other structures. Clay molds were created by making a wax form of an object to be created out of metal. The form was coated with clay, which was fired. This both hardened the clay and melted the wax, creating a perfect mold. This is how many bronze statues were created. Wax is still used in the glazing process of pottery and ceramics. Some cultures have included beeswax in ceremonies and others have relied on it as a food source. Some ancient cultures covered their dead in beeswax, or in fabric coated in beeswax, which preserved the bodies. The Egyptians may have gotten this idea from bee colonies that will sting an invading mouse or bird to death, and then surround it in wax so that it doesn't spoil the hive.

A major threat to honeybees are pesticides. Bees are especially sensitive to these chemical poisons that are used on farms, around homes, on golf courses, and on the property of campuses and other public and private land. As mentioned in other areas of this book, pesticides are chemicals designed to poison living things. When pesticides are spread across farm fields, bees are particularly susceptible to poisoning because bees harvest from the flowers at the tops of plants, where the pesticides settle. When the bees unknowingly carry the poisons back to the hives, more bees, and their larvae, are poisoned, and many die.

When you support organic agriculture, and nongenetically engineered agriculture, you are protecting the bee populations of the world.

Nonstop urban sprawl and industrial agriculture has also damaged bee terrain. Huge amounts of land have been covered by buildings, homes, sidewalks, roads, freeways, and parking lots. This construction along with agriculture has wiped out many of the flowering plants the bees depend on. The situation now exists where the over 4,000 different species of bees (not honeybees) in America are in danger. Similar situations exist for the worldwide bee species that are estimated to be over 30,000. It is important to have a diverse population of bees because some bees will only pollinate certain plants.

Because the wild bee population has been on a dramatic decrease, farmers are depending more on beekeepers to pollinate their plants. Formerly beekeepers used to pay farmers to be able to place their hives in their fields, but now farmers are paying the beekeepers.

The bees kept by the beekeepers are not enough to make up for the loss in the native bee populations. In the 1940s there were an estimated 5 million bee colonies being kept by American beekeepers. By 2004, that figure had decreased by half.

Honeybees aren't the only type of bee needed. Some native bees harvest from plants that honeybees do not. Because of the reduction in wild bee populations farmers increasingly rely on bees brought in from other parts of the world. This bee importing increases the risk of transferring infectious diseases among bee populations. At least one native American bee species, *Bombus occidentalis*, has been devastated by an infection disease brought to North American soil by bees imported from Belgium.

In an attempt to bring back and preserve native bee populations, some farmers are planting parts of their fields with native blooming plants.

Because bees are so sensitive to pesticides, nobody knows how long some of the fields sprayed with pesticides will be poisonous to bees. Increased urban and government sprawl will continue to reduce bee habitat.

You can help the bee populations in your region by planting native flowering plants and trees, by protecting fields of native weeds, by stopping urban sprawl, and by never using pesticides.

Some honey processors heat their honey to break down the sugar crystals. If you purchase honey, make sure it says "raw" or "unheated" on the label. Otherwise you will likely be purchasing honey that has been heated, which damages the enzymes.

In addition to enzymes, raw honey contains vitamins (especially pantothenic acid, riboflavin, thiamin, and vitamin B6), minerals (calcium, copper, iron, magnesium, manganese, phosphorus, potassium, sodium, and zinc), amino acids (the building blocks of protein), antioxidants (especially pinocembrin), and other trace nutrients.

A teaspoon of raw honey mixed in water, or in rejuvelac, is helpful for reintroducing food to the stomach after a lengthy fast.

Honey is an inverted sugar, doesn't ferment in the digestive tract, and doesn't encourage bacterial growth. Raw honey has antibacterial substance called inhibine, as well as anti-inflammatory, antifungal, and anti-allergy properties.

The enzymes in honey aid in digestion. New Zealand researchers at the University of Waikato concluded that honey can stop the growth of the bacterium associated with gastric ulcers. Because it is antibacterial, eating large globs of raw honey can help relieve food poisoning.

Honey can also assist the body in healing skin wounds, including burns and cuts.

When you consume locally produced raw honey it will assist the body in building an immunobiological defense to pollens, dusts, and molds that can result in allergic reactions. In this way honey can help prevent hay fever and asthma.

Propolis, bee pollen, and royal jelly are three beneficial honey-related products.

Propolis mostly consists of resin or sap of vines and trees. The bees gather resin similarly to how they forage for nectar. They mix the resin with pollen and honey to make propolis. The bees use propolis as a glue to coat their nests and the doorway to the nest. They also use it to mend and partially build their hives. Beekeepers harvest propolis by placing screens into a hive. The bees work to plug the screen with propolis. Propolis mixed with royal jelly is commonly sold at natural foods stores. In addition to vitamins and amino acids, propolis contains antiviral and antibacterial properties. It has been used as an antihistamine as well as an anti-inflammatory. Propolis contains caffeic acids that help prevent cancers of the colon and skin. Some people believe a teaspoon a day on an empty stomach relieves heartburn. Ancient people have often used it for this reason, as well as a treatment for ulcers.

Bee pollen also contains an assortment of nutrients. Pollen is the male reproductive matter of plants. Because it is rich in amino acids, by weight, bee pollen contains about the same amount of protein as beef, but contains more potassium and calcium. Unlike beef, bee pollen contains a number of nutrients, such as A, niacin, nitrogen, riboflavin, and potassium. The Egyptians call bee pollen "bee bread." Ancient people often carried packs of bee pollen with them on long trips. They felt it gave them energy, and they were correct. Bee pollen has often been used by humans with the belief that it is an aphrodisiac and that it boosts male libido. Today athletes and body builders use bee pollen. Those with seasonal allergies may benefit from eating pollen to desensitize from the allergens.

Royal jelly is rich in amino acids. It is what the worker bees, who are all female and make up the large majority of the nest bees, exclusively feed to the queen bee. The food of the worker bees is about 10 percent sugar, and the food for the queen bee is made to be about 35 percent sugar.

The queen bee grows larger than all the other bees and lives to be about three years old, which is years longer than the other bees, which live for about six weeks in warmer months, and sometimes much longer than that in the winter months.

When it is time to replace the queen bee, the worker bees will feed royal jelly to some of the larvae. This will make the larvae grow into a queen bee. Knowing they are to grow a new queen, they make the cells for those larvae they are to feed with royal jelly larger than the other cells. The first queen to emerge from her cell will kill the other baby queen bees. She will also kill her mother, force her from the cell, or ban her to one part of the hive. Then the new queen will hang out for about a week until it is time to take her mating flight.

If there is some sort of incident that kills the queen, such as if her reign ends in a violent death when a bear or other wild animal breaks into the hive to steal some honey, the worker bees will immediately go about feeding royal jelly to some of the surviving larvae, creating a new queen bee.

When the queen mates, she does so with as many as 12 men to gather several million sperm. If that doesn't sound wild enough, consider that it is done while flying. When the couple is finished, the queen bee detaches from the male bee. Because his sex organs are pronged, detaching rips out the sex organs of the male bee (drone), killing him.

After the shameless queen is done with her slutty behavior, she returns to the hive, where she spends the rest of her life laying eggs and being cared for by the worker bees. Nearly all the eggs she lays will be female.

Because the queen only needs to mate one time during her life, the male bees are not needed after the queen has completed her public sex romp. The male bees soon find that they are kicked out of the hive. Those who refuse to leave are sometimes maimed, having their body parts ripped off by the female bees, and pushed out of the hive before winter starts. No male bees are allowed to remain in the honeybee hive over winter. Because drones have no foraging skills, they starve to death after being kicked out of the hive.

Chicago Honey Cooperative, 2000 West Carroll St., Ste. 301, Chicago, IL 60612; HoneyCoOp@GMail.Com

National Honey Board, Honey.Com/HoneyIndustry
Their HoneyLocator.Com provides contact information about a number of beekeepers and lists what types of honey they produce.

ReallyRawHoney.Com

Smiley Apiaries, FloridaTupeloHoney.Com
They promise that their honey is "raw" and has not been heated to the point of destroying the nutrients. Tupelo honey is supposed to be some of the best tasting honey in the world.

WeeBeeHoney.Net

Hospital Food

Hospital cafeterias typically serve the most unhealthful food a person can eat. If you ate nothing but what is served in the hospitals, you would come down with many of the very same diseases that the medical staff spend their careers "treating."

Hospitals would do good to get involved with serving organically grown produce, such as those in Oregon:

"The Oregon Center for Environmental Health's Healthy food in Healthcare initiative is bringing together a community committed to institutional change in healthcare food services. The principal goal of the project is to leverage the significant purchasing power and influence of hospitals to support regional markets for fresh, sustainable food to

model healthy food choices to the public. Representatives from seven major health systems in the region are involved. The initiative has also partnered with Oregon Tilth and organizations such as the Food Alliance, Physicians for Social Responsibility, Organically Grown Company, and the Portland/Multomah Food Policy Council to connect healthcare systems with established sustainable food networks and to connect this work to the larger community."
— **Cultivating Relationships, by Chris Schreiner, In Good Tilth, September/October 2006; Tilth.Org**

Hunger and Homelessness

Food First, Institute for Food and Development Policy, 398 60th St., Oakland, CA 94608; 510-654-4400; FoodFirst.Org

Food Not Bombs, POB 744, Tucson, AZ 85702; 800-884-1136; FoodNotBombs.Net

The Hunger Project, 15 E. 26th St., New York, NY 10010; 212-251-9100; THP.Org

National Coalition for the Homeless, 2201 P St. NW, Washington, DC 20037; 202-462-4822; NationalHomeless.Org

Infinite Intelligence

"Look within. The secret is inside you."
— **Hui Neng**

There are things that you know that nobody ever taught you. They are things that are natural to you that you cannot deny exist. These are natural things that have to do with your instinct, talents, essence, spirit, power, and intelligence. In his book *The Sunfood Diet Success System*, Wolfe calls these phenomena "infinite intelligence." He gives examples of spiders who always construct their webs in a certain way, and various types of birds who build their nests in a particular style.

Each being is connected to a spiritual side of life that provides infinite wisdom. The cleaner and more pure the being, the better its nerve system will be able to tune into the high frequency of this infinite wisdom that works as instinct in a living being.

When a person or animal maintains an unhealthful diet, is put into an unnatural environment filled with unhealthful air, violated land, and noise pollution; and their thought patterns are filled with negativity and doubt, then the individual will become less pure, less natural, and less attuned to his or her natural instincts. Their systems become frustrated. It clogs their ability to tap into the high frequency needed to access any basic and infinite wisdom, and subsequently not only limits potential, but also damages it.

> "Within you is a vast genetic library containing all the wisdom you need to accomplish everything you desire. The essence of your spirit has the capability to tap infinite intelligence, which is the ether, the storehouse of eternal knowledge."
> — David Wolfe

When you purify your body through a pure, raw, plant-based diet; clarify your physical structure through daily exercise, such as yoga; develop your talents through practice; expand your knowledge through study; focus your mind by planning an agenda of success; clear your thought patterns through meditative thought; fuel your actions with positive thinking; surround yourself with that which inspires you; and improve your communication with other people through respect, kindness, patience, forgiveness, and love, you are tuning your frequency to your instinct that is purely the work of infinite intelligence. It is then that you will begin to recognize your potential and power.

Infinite intelligence is what brings the intricate structures of all living beings to form into what they are. It is what drives us to desire that which is good, nurturing, and loving.

> "Infinite intelligence is the spiritual energy that turns seeds into plants and plants into flowers. It arcs flowers toward the lively face of Sun. Though it may be quiet and extremely subtle, infinite intelligence is there and it stays there, never to be underestimated."
> — David Wolfe

Living in a way that is tuned to Nature awakens your body cells, your mind, and your whole system to the thing that had been dormant because of wrong living, unhealthful diet, limited thinking, unhealthful atmosphere, and damaging concepts. Through living in tune with Nature your system begins to communicate with the frequency of infinite intelligence that can guide you toward health and happiness, success, and beauty.

Various religious teachers have some understanding of a concept of a power that exists throughout the world and universe. They teach that you can live your life better by paying attention to this power. They seem to have an idea of what paying attention to it means, in both actions and thoughts. Some have certain names for it. Some define it in a way that limits it to certain individuals or ways of living. Some say it is this thing, and others say it is that thing. But all seem to agree that it is there. Some call it a form of intelligence. Some call it spirit. Some call it soul.

Infinite intelligence exists in a realm that is both far beyond the façade of physical elements that are common to the worldly, but it is in a realm that is within all that exists. It is in all and through all. It is beyond the comprehension of the unnatural person, but saturates all the elements that everything consists of. It is tuned into the nurturing energy of love, which is the most powerful and pristine energy of all. It exists. It is there. It the sacred power that is throughout all.

You can put it to work for you in your life. You know that it is there because you can see that it has formed you, others, and the plants, animals, birds, fish, and all living things. You know that there are certain things you do that make you feel more comfortable with this energy. Respect for your life, as well as for the lives of others, and for the lives of animals, as well as living in a way that is in tune with Nature will help you to tune into the high frequency wavelength of this power and keep it working for you in your life.

Junk Mail and How to Stop It

"Each year, junk mail destroys about 80 million trees, wastes 28 billion gallons of water, and costs about $450,000,000 of your money to cart its promos, pleas, and promises to and from incinerators, garbage dumps and recycling centers. That equates to about 34 pounds of junk mail for every man, woman and child in the U.S. It's like stuffing a whole tree into our mailboxes every year."
— EcoCycle.Org, 2006

This junk mail ends up in the garbage, and hardly any of it is recycled. Work to stop this assault to the forests of the planet. See the Trees section of this book to learn how you can get involved in protecting the forests of the planet. Work to get industrial hemp farming made legal so that we can use hemp for paper instead of cutting down the world's forests.

EcoCycle.Org
   Click on the "stop junk mail" button and learn how to stop junk mail from cluttering your mailbox.

JunkBusters.Com

Kitchen Appliances, Supplies, and Specialty Raw Food Items

Kitchens can be interesting places. Gathering people and making food together for a feast is one way to create community. In fact, throughout human history this is often how food was made with neighbors, friends, and generations of families creating and sharing food. Eventually more and more single-family dwellings were built, each having a kitchen. With this change the communal eating events became much less common. Traditions in food making were lost and more people began to rely on manufactured food. Instead of dinners shared by many people it became common for people to eat alone.

Single kitchens are a stagnating force in human relations. It would be nice and less wasteful if more people shared their food and ate together.

Rich, poor, dark, light, old, young, bookish, artistic, diverse genders, or whatever, the one thing we have in common is that we need nourishment.

It is fun to invite people over and get busy creating food that may be for one meal, or that might last for several days, and that will bring groups of people together for sit-down social meals. I have either organized or been to many such feasts. No two have been alike and each brings the opportunity for building community, life-long friendships, healing to wounded relationships, and matching up of lovers.

Having access to a functional kitchen is key to creating many of the best foods. While sharing kitchens with others can be beneficial in many ways, creating a kitchen doesn't have to be expensive. Many kitchen tools, utensils, and serving doohickeys can be bought second-hand at garage sales, in secondhand shops, and through community bulletin boards.

Rather than having conformity in color and design, it can be more interesting to have plates, bowls, glasses, and eating utensils that are mismatched. Make the table look as diverse and eclectic as the people gathered to eat.

BestJuicers.Com

Creative Health Institute, 112 W. Union City Rd., Union City, MI 49094; 517-278-6260; CreativeHealthUSA.Com
Dr. Ann Wigmore Institute conducts seminars and sells books, kitchen supplies and equipment, and teaches the philosophies of the late doctor.

DiscountJuicers.Com

DiscountVegetarian.Com

Eden Foods, 701 Tecumseh Rd., Clinton, MI 49236; 888-441-3336; EdenFoods.Com

Frontier Natural Brands, POB 299, 3021 78th St., Norway, IA 52318; 800-669-3275; FrontierNaturalBGrands.Com

Gold Mine Natural Food Co., 7805 Arjons Dr., San Diego, CA 92126; 800-475-Food; GoldMineNaturalFood.Com

Govinda's, 2651 Ariane Dr., San Diego, CA 92117; 858-270-0691; Govinda-Foods.Com

Great Eastern Sun; 92 McIntosh Rd., Ashville, NC 28806; Great-Eastern-Sun.Com

HealthyHome.Com

Jaffe Brothers, 28560 Lilac Rd., Valley Center, CA 92082; OrganicFruitsAndNuts.Com

Lehmans, Lehmans.Com
Sells a blender that doesn't use electricity.

Living Light Culinary Arts Institute, 301-B N. Main St., Fort Bragg, CA 95437; 800-816-2319; 707-964-2420; RawFoodChef.Com
This is Cherie Soria's certified raw vegan chef school. She has been active in the raw community for many years, and is the author of *Angel Foods: Healthy Recipes for Heavenly Bodies, and The Raw Food Diet: Feast, Lose Weight, Gain Energy, Feel Younger!*

Both Dr. Ann Wigmore and Viktoras Kulvinskas, author of *Survival into the 21st Century*, recognized Soria's gift for creating amazing food, and encouraged her to share her talent. Her Living Light Center contains Living Light To Go, a deli offering organic raw vegan cuisine, juices and smoothies; and Living Light Marketplace, a retail store featuring kitchen equipment, supplies, recipe books, and specialty food items. The store products are also sold through the Internet site. They also run Living Light Events, which offers event planning and catering, chef placement services, and healthy retreats.

Living Tree Community Foods, POB 10082, Berkeley, CA 94709; 800-260-5534; 510-526-7106; LivingTreeCommunity.Com

Lydia's Organics, 81 Upland Ave., Mill Valley, CA 94941; 707-576-1330; LydiasOrganics.Com

Maine Seaweed Company, POB 57, Steuben, ME 04680; 707-546-2875

MarathonJuicer.Com

Pure Joy Living Foods, POB 460268; San Francisco, CA 94146; 415-558-1624; PureJoyLivingfoods.Com
   This is Elaine Love's site where she sells kitchen equipment, her recipe book, and raw food supplements. She also organizes and gives seminars and teaches raw food preparation classes.

Rawcreation Ltd. / Shazzie, POB 223, Belton, Great Yarmouth, NR31 9WX, England; 08700 113 119; +44 8700 113 119; Shazzie.Com
   Shazzie is an author and chef who conducts talks, workshops, consultations and demonstrations around the world. Through her site she provides kitchen equipment, recipe books, nutritional supplements, and food preparation videos. She is the author of *Detox Your World*. Along with David Wolfe, she wrote *Naked Chocolate*, which details the nutritional value as well as the colorful history of chocolate.

Raw Family & Victoria Boutenko, POB 172, Ashland, OR 97520; RawFamily.Com
   This is the inspirational Boutenko family. They teach food preparation classes, conduct seminars, write recipe books, and sell books and kitchen supplies.

The Raw Gourmet, RawGourmet.Com
   This is Nomi Shannon's site. She is the author of *The Raw Gourmet* recipe book. Through her site she provides recipes, sells gourmet instruction videos, arranges to teach raw food preparation classes, and sells kitchen supplies.

Rawlifeline.Com Shipped Raw Meals, Huntingdon Valley, PA 19006; 800-RAW-9197; RawLifeline.Com

RawOils.Com

Rejuvenative Foods, POB 8464, Santa Cruz, CA 95061; Rejuvenative.Com
Sells all raw food products, including nut butters, tahini, kimchi, sauerkraut, salsas, and chocolate.

Seeds of Change, POB 15700, Santa Fe, NM 87506; SeedsOfChange.Com
Organic seeds.

SproutHouse.Com

Sunfood Nutrition, 11653 Riverside Dr., Lakeside, CA 92040; 800-205-2350; 888-RAW-FOOD; International: +001-619-596-79798; Sunfood.Com
Stephen Arlin and David Wolfe founded this company. Their site has the largest selection of raw vegan-related items for sale on the Internet. They sell kitchen equipment, recipe books, specialty foods, and many other items. They also conduct seminars and retreats.

Sun Frost, 707-822-9095; SunFrost.Com
It is estimated that refrigerators use at least 7 percent of the electricity used in the U.S. Sun Frost manufactures refrigerators and freezers that use much less electricity than other models. They can be used with solar, hydro, or wind power. They also sell composters and composting toilets.

SunOrganic Farm, 411 S. Las Posas Rd., San Marcos, CA 92078; 888-269-9888; Outside U.S. 760-510-8077; SunOrganicFarm.Com

Vision Inc., POB N, Klamath Falls, OR 97601; 888-800-7070; 888-233-1441; International: 541-273-2212; E3Live.Com
This company sells E3Live™, a wild grown fresh water algae superfood.

WalnutAcres.Com

WildernessFamilyNaturals.Com

Kitchen: What's in the Sunfoodist Kitchen?

Book:
• *Living Cuisine: The Art and Spirit of Raw Foods*, by Renée Loux

Vegetables of all sorts, especially those that are seasonal, organically grown, and not genetically engineered. Some are home grown, especially green-leafed vegetables and weeds. Others are wild harvested.

Yes, I know, tomatoes are technically a fruit, as are squash, peppers, cucumbers, etc. But most people think of them as vegetables.

- **Artichoke:** Young artichokes may be soft enough to eat raw. Or steam them.
- **Arugula**
- **Asparagus**
- **Baby lettuces**
- **Beet greens:** You can grow beet greens by cutting the top off a beet and letting it stand in a bowl of water or a pot of moist soil on your windowsill.
- **Beets**
- **Bell peppers**
- **Bok choy**
- **Broccoli**
- **Brussels sprouts**
- **Burdock root**
- **Butternut:** Shred for use in soups and salads.
- **Cabbage**
- **Carrots**
- **Carrot greens**
- **Cauliflower**
- **Celery**
- **Celery root/celeriac**
- **Chard**
- **Chickweed**
- **Chicory/curly endive**
- **Chili peppers**
- **Chives**
- **Clover**
- **Cilantro**
- **Collards**
- **Corn:** Never cook it. Simply cut it off the cob and eat raw, or use in raw recipes. Try purple corn and other nonhybridized, heirloom corn.
- **Cucumber:** Officially a fruit.
- **Daikon radish**
- **Dandelion**
- **Eggplant:** Officially a fruit.
- **Endive**
- **Escarole**
- **Fennel**
- **Frisee**

- Garlic
- Garlic greens/scapes (preflowering stalk)
- Ginger root (fresh)
- Green onions
- Jerusalem artichoke: The root of a plant.
- Jicama
- Kale of all varieties: May contain more antioxidants than any of the common vegetables. It contains calcium and vitamin K, which are good for the bones, and is rich in the cancer-fighting phytochemicals called indoles.
- Lambsquarters
- Leeks
- Lettuce
- Mache/lamb's lettuce/field salad
- Malva
- Miner's lettuce
- Mizuna
- Mustard greens
- Okra: Officially a fruit.
- Onion greens
- Onions
- Parsley
- Pepper: Officially a fruit.
- Pumpkin
- Purslane
- Radicchio
- Radish
- Radish greens
- Red leaf lettuce
- Romaine lettuce
- Scallions
- Shallots
- Snap peas
- Sorrel
- Spinach
- Sprouts
- Squash: Officially a fruit.
- Stinging nettles
- Tomatoes: Officially a fruit. Both fresh and Sun dried.

- **Watercress**
- **Wild greens, edible:** From your region of the planet.
- **Yams:** Grate them over salads and raw soups. Use shredded yams in recipes for dehydrated crackers. Some people steam thin slices of them in a steamer basket.
- **Zucchini:** Officially a fruit. Shred with a spiralizer and use as pasta.

Fruits and berries of all sorts, especially those that are seasonal, organically grown, and not genetically engineered.

Don't mind if your fruits don't look picture perfect. Often if they are oddly shaped it may mean that they are of a variety that is closer to its natural state, less hybridized, and has not been waxed. Save the seeds and pits of fruits and plant them out in the wild.

If you grow fruit or berries in pots, buckets, or other containers, occasionally put a handful of rich soil from the ground into the container. This will help transfer fungus from the ground or compost pit into the container soil. The fungus will help transfer nutrients from the soil into the roots of the plant, resulting in a better tasting fruit.

- **Apples:** All varieties. Especially seek out or grow organic and Heirloom varieties. Malic acid in apples is a liver cleanser. The boron in apples is good for building strong bones.
- **Apricots**
- **Asian pears**
- **Avocados** of all varieties.
- **Bananas:** Freeze them and put them through a Champion juicer with the blank plate on. Mix with agave nectar syrup, vanilla, and fruit and/or berries. This is raw vegan ice cream. Make sure to purchase or grow only organic bananas. The farming chemicals, including dibromochloropropane, used on bananas have a history of causing great harm to farmers, wildlife, and the environment. There are many varieties of bananas coming on the market. Some are less hybridized than the typical yellow banana. If you live in a region that does not experience freezing temperatures, you can likely grow your own bananas.
- **Berries** of all varieties: blackberries, blueberries, cranberries, goji, Inca berries, mulberry, raspberries, strawberries, etc. Blueberries are often singled out as the best source for antioxidants, and for their ability to lower cholesterol because they contain pterostilbene, which also regulates blood sugar. But all edible berries contain beneficial nutrients. There are likely places near you that have wild berries growing. If not, plant some.
- **Cantaloupe**
- **Cherimoya**
- **Cherries**
- **Cranberries:** Cranberries are beneficial to the health of the bladder. The tannins in cranberries prevent bacteria from attaching to cells in the urinary tract. For a

drink that maintains bladder health and prevents urinary tract infections, blend a handful of fresh cranberries with water, several freshly crushed grapefruit seeds, and fresh squeezed lemon juice and/or fresh seeded (not "seedless") purple grapes. Drink this on an empty stomach. After a half hour or more, eat some fresh papaya, dried papaya spears, or papaya juice to calm the stomach.

- Cucumbers
- Cumin powder
- Currants
- Curry
- Dates
- Dragon fruit
- Durian
- Eggfruit
- Feijoa
- Figs: Many people have only eaten dried figs. But fresh figs are a wonderful treat. This is another fruit tree that grows very well in many locations. If you purchase dried figs, avoid those that have been treated with sulfur.
- Grapefruit: Save the seeds. See cranberries in list above.
- Grapes: With seeds, not seedless. Grapeseeds are a source of high-quality essential fatty acids. Grape leaves are edible and can be used as a wrap. It is likely that you can grow your own grapes.
- Guava: Rich in lycopene, a cancer-fighting plant chemical. Guava is ranked second to blueberries in antioxidant content.
- Honeydew melon
- Kiwi
- Kumquats
- Lemons
- Lime
- Litchis/lychis/lichis
- Longan
- Loquat
- Mamey
- Mandarin oranges
- Mango
- Mangostein
- Melon of all varieties.
- Nectarines
- Noni
- Olives: Make sure they are raw, not heated (see Sunfood.Com).

- Oranges of all varieties
- Papaya of all varieties
- Passion fruit
- Peaches
- Pears
- Peppers
- Persimmons
- Pineapple
- Plantain
- Plums and prunes
- Pomegranates
- Prickly pear
- Raisins: With seeds, not seedless.
- Rambutan
- Sapodilla
- Sapote
- Soursop
- Starfruit/Carambola
- Sugar apple
- Tangerines
- Watermelon: With seeds, not seedless.

Herbs, spices and natural flavorings:
- Allspice
- Anise
- Basil
- Cardamom pods
- Cayenne pepper
- Celery seed
- Chili powder
- Chipotle pepper: fresh or dried
- Chives
- Cilantro
- Cinnamon
- Cloves
- Coriander
- Cumin seeds
- Currants

- Curry leaves
- Dill
- Fennel seeds
- Garlic
- Ginger
- Lavender
- Lemongrass
- Licorice
- Mace
- Marjoram
- Mint
- Mustard seed
- Nutmeg
- Oregano
- Paprika
- Parsley
- Peppercorns
- Peppermint
- Rosemary
- Sage
- Spearmint
- Thyme
- Turmeric
- Vanilla beans

Nuts, seeds, and beans for sprinkling in salads, on cold soups, and as an ingredient in dehydrated foods. Also for soaking and sprouting (see Sprouting, and Rejuvelac).

- Aduki
- Almonds
- Brazil nuts
- Broccoli seeds
- Cabbage seeds
- Cashews
- Chia seeds
- Clover seeds
- Coconuts and coconut oil: The saturated fats in raw coconuts are medium chain triglycerides and are burned as energy. Triglycerides are a combination of three

fatty acids with glycerol, the natural form of plant fats. They aren't the damaging saturated fats found in animal products. Coconuts also contain lauric acid, which is anti-microbial and anti-viral.

- **Fenugreek seeds**
- **Filberts**
- **Flax seeds**: A good source of omega-3 fatty acids
- **Garbanzo beans**/chick peas: raw, dry seeds. Not canned.
- **Hazelnuts**
- **Hemp seeds**: The best source of a balanced ratio of essential fatty acids. (see Hemp)
- **Kamut**
- **Lentils**
- **Macadamia nuts**
- **Millet**
- **Mung beans**
- **Mustard seeds**: For making your own mustard, and for sprouting.
- **Oat groats**
- **Onion seeds**
- **Peas**
- **Pecans**
- **Pine nuts/Pignolis**
- **Pistachios**
- **Poppy seeds**
- **Pumpkin seeds**
- **Quinoa**
- **Radish seeds**
- **Red clover seeds**
- **Sesame seeds**: Make sure they are raw and unhulled. These are one type of seed that are often sold "toasted." They are also a very nutritious seed containing vitamin E as well as calcium, copper, iron, manganese, and zinc. Sesame seeds are a rich source of phytosterols, which are helpful in balancing the cholesterol.
- **Spelt**
- **Sunflower seeds**
- **Triticale**
- **Walnuts**
- **Wheat berries**: wheat seeds, for sprouting (See Wheatgrass Juice).
- **Wild rice**: rice can be softened by soaking in water for several hours, then keeping moist for a day or two instead of boiling.

Sweeteners: Get rid of all white sugar, corn syrup, and artificial sweeteners.
- **Agave nectar**: From the agave cactus, which is also used to make tequila. But Sunfoodists use agave as a sweetener. When purchasing this make sure the label says that it is raw — otherwise you will likely be buying something that has been heated to prevent fermentation.
- **Date sugar**: Dehydrated date powder.
- **Honey**: Raw, and preferably from your local region. While some Sunfoodists use honey, others choose to avoid it. There are valid ethical and environmental reasons to stay away from honey and other bee products. See: Honey.
- **Sweetwater**: Make this by soaking such dried fruits as raisins, dates, or currants in water. You can also use a high speed blender to blend these into the water, but you will likely have to use a sharp knife to cut the dried fruit into small bits before blending. Otherwise you may simply have large chunks sticking to the blender blade not getting blended.
- **Yacon root syrup**: Pressed/cold-processed. Not boiled.

Food items are typically found in a Sunfood kitchen include (make sure they are raw, unheated, and preferably organic):
- **Agar agar**
- **Almond butter**
- **Aloe vera gel**
- **Amaranth**
- **Apple cider vinegar**
- **Bee pollen:** this is a bee product, which some choose to avoid.
- **Blue-green algae powder**
- **Cacao butter**: Raw. This is true white chocolate. Melts at 90° Fahrenheit (see: Chocolate).
- **Cacao**: This is raw chocolate (see: Chocolate)
- **Carob powder**: Make sure it is raw, not toasted or heated
- **Coconut butter**
- **Coconut, shredded**
- **Coconut water**
- **Dulse** powder or flakes
- **Edible flowers**
- **Flax oil**
- **Garlic oil**: Oil with garlic soaking in it. Usually made with olive oil, but grape seed oil is also a good match for the flavor of garlic.
- **Ginger**: Raw root. It can also be soaked in oil, such as olive or hemp oils, to give flavor to the oil.
- **Ginseng**

- Goji berries
- Grapeseed oil
- Habanero pepper
- Hemp seed butter
- Hemp seed oil
- Himalayan pink salt
- Honey: Some choose to refrain from consuming honey. See Honey.
- Horseradish: Easily made by grating horseradish root (grow it in your garden) and mixing with salt and vinegar. For added color and sweetness, you can add grated beet.
- Jalapeno peppers: dried.
- Jungle peanuts
- Kamut grain
- Kelp powder
- Kombucha tea culture
- Maca powder: Make sure it is raw, not toasted.
- Mesquite powder
- Millet grain
- Miso: Fermented soybean curd. If you buy it at the natural foods store, purchase it unpasteurized. Some raw foodists avoid consuming miso because it is originally a cooked soybean product. After it has been fermented, which brings in enzymes, some people consider it to be a raw product. I usually choose to avoid it.
- MSM powder
- Mushrooms
- Nettles
- Nama shoyu: Similar to miso, the creation of nama shoyu involves some cooking. After a period of fermentation it is rich in enzymes. If you purchase it, make sure the label states that it is unpasteurized. It has a taste similar to soy sauce or tamari sauce. I usually choose to avoid this product.
- Nori sheets
- Nutritional yeast
- Oat groats
- Olive oil: If you purchase this, make sure the label states that it is organic and "cold-pressed" or "cold processed."
- Poppy seeds
- Pumpkin butter
- Quinoa grain
- Raisins
- Rose hips: Make sure they are from an organic source, and not from plants that

have been grown using chemical fertilizers or treated with other toxic chemicals, such as pesticides and fungicides.

- **Salt**: Himalayan pink salt, or other unheated, unbleached natural salt. Avoid table salts that have been processed.
- **Sea vegetables**: wakame, dulse, kelp, nori, hijiki, arame, etc.
- **Soaking raisins or date bits**: By soaking about a cup of raisins or chopped dates in about 1.5 cups of water for a few hours you can make sweet juice that can be used in various recipes. Keep container covered and in a cool place, or refrigerator.
- **Spelt grain**
- **Spirulina powder of flakes**
- **Tabasco sauce**: This can be made by drying and grinding chili peppers, then mixing the powder with vinegar and salt.
- **Tahini**: This is the paste of sesame seeds. You might call it "sesame seed butter." Make sure it is organic, raw/unheated. It is most commonly used to make hummus, but can also be used to make vanilla desert sauces, such as when it is blended with lemon, vanilla, soaked nuts, agave syrup, and a pinch of salt. It is also used in raw brownies, cookies, and pie crusts.
- **Teff grain**
- **Thai coconuts**
- **Vanilla**: Made from the beans of the pod of the tropical American climbing epiphytic orchid.
- **Vinegar**
- **VitaMineral Green** or other raw green nutritional powder

Kitchen Equipment

A bout juicers: There are juicing machines that are favored above others, but it seems to be a matter of taste and function.

Our oven sits as a relic of ancient times, and is used as a storage cabinet. Sometimes it is used to heat water for tea. We have no use for toasters, toaster ovens, or microwaves.

You may be able to buy new or slightly used kitchen equipment by checking the community board at your local natural foods store.

- **Asian or kimchi (also spelled *kim-chee*) crock**: For making kimchi and sauerkraut. Get one and learn how to use it. Asian markets often sell them. Another possibility is a Harsch crock made by a company in Germany. Raw fermented foods made from organic produce are nutrient rich.

- **Bamboo sushi roller**
- **Blender:** There are a variety of blenders on the market. However, a strong, restaurant-quality blender is great for making all sorts of things, from hummus to sauces, and smoothies. The VitaMix brand blender with manual speed control knobs is pretty common in raw vegan kitchens. This requires an investment (presently about $400), but I have seen them for sale on the community bulletin board at the local natural foods store. For those who don't have electricity in their living space, there is at least one company that makes a hand-crank blender. There is another that makes a solar blender.
- **Bowls:** You need a variety of bowls. Stick with those that are made of glass, ceramic, and wood. Stay away from aluminum, plastic, and bowls that can rust, degrade, or release chemicals as food is soaking or stored in them.
- **Champion juicer:** Often used a lot. Save the pulp from the vegetables you juice, mix them with oil of olives or flax seeds, hemp seeds, or grapeseeds; mix in some Himalayan sea salt, minced garlic, diced onion, chopped tomatoes, or scissor-cut pieces of dried tomatoes, chopped Italian herbs, soaked seeds of pumpkin, flax, sesame and sunflower; mix in some nutritional yeast, then spread on your dehydrator sheets, and dehydrate at about 108° for 24 hours (less or more depending on your desired level of crispness). Cut into squares and store in a cool place in a big glass jar. Use for dips, spreads, guacamole, and other recipes from raw vegan recipe books.
- **Citrus juicer:** A mechanical juicer is a basic. A small, hand-held juicer can be useful if you only need to squeeze the juice from one lemon or other citrus fruit.
- **Citrus zester**
- **Coffee grinder:** Used to grind cacao, flax seeds, pumpkin seeds, hemp seeds, herbs, etc.
- **Cuisinart food processor**
- **Cuisinart mini prep:** For making salad dressings and sauces.
- **Cutting boards** made of bamboo. Keep them dry and clean. Don't use soap on them.
- **Dehydrator,** or a solar food dryer. If you purchase an electric dehydrator, seek out one that has an adjustable heat control. I tend to stay away from dehydrated foods because they make me feel dehydrated. But a dehydrator is useful for making vegetable crackers out

of pulp left over from juicing vegetables. They are also handy for making seed and nut cheeses, pizza crust, granola, pie crusts, and raw vegan nut cheese cake crusts. They can always be used to dehydrate tomatoes and other soft fruits and vegetables for winter storage. Chefs I know are constantly making all sorts of experimental foods in their dehydrators. Some taste good. Some do not. Probably my favorite dehydrated food item is rawmasean that is made right, which involves several days to make rejuvelac, and blending this with soaked pignolis (pine nuts), mixing this with nutritional yeast (not brewers' yeast), and letting this ferment covered with a cloth for a day in a warm/dark place before adding Italian herbs and salt, then, spreading on dehydrator sheets and dehydrating for a day at low heat.

- **Funnel**
- **Garlic press.** I rarely use this item. I put the garlic on a cutting board, place the side of the chef's knife on top of it, and hit the knife. The garlic breaks open and the skin is easy to remove.
- **Ginger grater:** Made of porcelain.
- **Grater and shredder**
- **Green Star juicer:** Used much less often. I've heard others say that this is their favorite juicer.
- **Icing bag:** This can be used for decorating foods with creams and sauces.
- **Jars:** Big glass ones for making herbal Sun teas; making and refrigerating rejuvelac; storing seeds; sprouting; storing dehydrated foods; making wine (don't ask!), etc.
- **Knife sharpener**
- **Knives:** Professional chef quality. Chef's knife, paring knife, serrated knife, cleaver (for opening coconuts).
- **Mandolin:** For cutting vegetables in fancy ways.
- **Measuring cups and spoons.** I rarely use them. But a glass measuring cup often comes in handy.
- **Melon baller**
- **Misting bottle** containing hydrogen peroxide for misting produce before rinsing, and for sanitizing cutting boards and other surfaces (hydrogen peroxide breaks down into oxygen and water).
- **Mortar and pestle:** This is useful tool for making mustard, and for

grinding seeds and fresh herbs.

- **Norwalk juicer**: Some people swear these are the best juicers. I don't own one.
- **Peeler**
- **Pie plates**
- **Rolling Pin**
- **Salad spinner**: To spin rinsed greens free of water.
- **Scissors**: A sturdy pair of kitchen scissors often comes in handy, especially for cutting herbs in the garden just before use, and for cutting up the herbs over various dishes.
- **Screened shelf or box**: Used to store fruits and vegetables, and to keep bugs away. Easy to create using a stapler or tacks on a small hinged door.
- **Serving utensils**: Triangular spatula, salad spoon and fork, tongs, soup ladle.
- **Solar power panel** on the roof or in the yard for creating electricity.
- **Spice grater**
- **Spatulas**
- **Spiralizer/Saladacco**: For making zucchini "pasta."
- **Spoons**: Metal and wooden. A small wooden spoon, or a ceramic spoon, is good to use in honey and miso.
- **Sprouter**: Fresh Life Automatic Sprouter, or Biosta tiered sprouter, or other sprouter. You can also use a large jar, or glass casserole with clear glass cover. We like to use glass jars and glass casserole dishes rather than plastic sprouters because plastic can leach toxins into the food (see: Sprouting).
- **Strainers**: Both hand held mesh strainers and bowl-type strainers with legs are useful. Another way of straining water out of salad is a salad spinner, or by spreading salad on a towel, and gently rolling the towel into a roll to absorb water.
- **Steamer basket or double boiler**: For those wishing to steam vegetables at low heat.
- **Torte pans**: These are two-piece pie pans that come in a variety of depths and sizes for creating free-standing cakes, pies, tarts, tortes.
- **Towels**: There is always something that is in need of drying, wip-

ing, or cleaning. Cleanliness in food preparation is a very good thing. Organic cotton is good, but hemp towels will last longer because the fibers are sturdier. Don't worry about getting them stained, because they will. Once they are too old to use in the kitchen they can be used for household cleaning. They can easily be cleaned in a big bowl with some biodegradable dish soap, and hung out in Sun to dry. If they are 100 percent natural fiber (no polyester or other plastic fiber) they can eventually be cut up and tossed into the compost pile. Avoid using paper towels; we don't need to be cutting down our forests to throw them away.

- **Vegetable peeler**
- **Wheat grass sprouter and juicer** (See Wheatgrass)

Laundry and Dry Cleaning

Also see:
- Cleaning Soaps and Detergents

P lease choose to use cleaners that are nontoxic, biodegradable, and plant-based.

Laundry pollution has become an enormous problem that is often overlooked. It pollutes our ground water, rivers, streams, lakes and oceans, poisoning wildlife and killing off water plants that support wildlife and healthy ecosystems. It also causes algae blooms that kill many varieties of marine life. Most natural foods stores sell nontoxic, biodegradable, plant-based laundry detergents.

If you take your clothes to a dry cleaner, please choose a cleaner that uses nonperchloroethylene (perc) alternatives. Avoid purchasing clothes that need to be dry cleaned.

Did you know that most commonly used laundry detergents and other household cleaners are made from petroleum chemicals and contain toxic chemical dyes to make them appear more vibrant? In the soap industry these dyes are referred to as "optical brighteners." Most common laundry soaps also contain chemical fragrances to give them a scent that people consider to be the smell of soap.

Did you know that when you wear clothes and sleep in bedding that have been washed in these chemical soaps some of the chemicals get absorbed into your skin? If you removed the chemical dyes and scents these soaps and detergents contain they would look much like the natural products sold in natural foods stores. But they would still be highly polluting because they are made from petrochemicals and byproducts of various chemical industries, including phosphates, which are not good for the environment or wildlife.

Unlike soaps made from plant extracts, soaps made from petroleum are damaging to the environment in a number of ways. Petroleum is a non-renewable resource. The production of petrochemicals cause great harm to the environment: first, in the drilling and extraction from Earth; then in the transportation, refinement, and synthesis, which are all energy-intensive processes that create more pollution. All these pollutants accumulate in the air, water, and in plants, wildlife, and humans.

Many of the chemicals contained in the most commonly used house-hold cleaners are Persistent Organic Pollutants (POPs), which are not good.

"POPs include many pesticides, industrial chemicals like PCBs, organochlorines, and by-products of a variety of manufacturing and waste incineration processes like dioxins. Because it is a new kind of chemical category based on health and environmental effects, not chemistry, any compound can be labeled a POP as long as it has these characteristics:
- It resists biodegradation and therefore persists in the environment.
- It builds up in body fat and accumulates in ever higher levels as it migrates up the food chain.
- It travels efficiently throughout the atmosphere and global waters.
- Many POPs are linked to serious hormonal, reproductive, neurological, and/or immune disorders."
— From SeventhGeneration.Com, 2006

Get your family and friends to stop using soaps and household cleaners containing toxic chemicals that pollute the air, water, and land. Using plant-based soaps is also one more way we can disconnect from the petroleum industry.

Don't use chlorine bleach, which is highly toxic, persists in the environment, results in toxic organochlorines, such as chloroform and dioxin; and can cause cancers, birth defects, learning disabilities, mimic hormones in the body, and disrupt hormonal balances in wildlife. Instead, use hydrogen peroxide-based bleaching agents, because these simply break down into water and oxygen.

The following companies produce plant-based cleaners that are biodegradable, do not contain harmful chemical dyes or fragrances, and have not been tested on laboratory animals.

Bio-Pac.Com

Bio-Pac sells Oasis Biocompatible laundry detergent that breaks down into plant nutrients. They also sell other household cleaners, such as those made from natural plant oils and enzymes.

Bio-Pac donates a part of its profits to groups involved in wilderness preservation.

DrBronner.Com

Dr. Bronner's biodegradable soaps are made from hemp oil, and their bottles are made from recycled PET plastics.

Ecover.Com

Ecover produces a full line of biodegradable household cleaners. They began producing a phosphate-free cleaning powder before it was well known that phosphates are damaging to the environment. They are so environmentally concerned that they even built a factory that has a grass-covered roof.

Earth Friendly Products, Ecos.Com

GreenEarth.Com

HangersDryCleaners.Com

Seventh Generation, SeventhGeneration.Com

Seventh Generation not only produces nontoxic, petroleum-free, biodegradable household cleaners, they also provide a wealth of information about the typical toxins that nonenvironmentally sound soap companies use in their products, such as phosphates, petrochemicals, chlorine, and other persistent organic pollutants. Check out the "Chemical Glossary" on the site to find out about some of the most common toxins found in the typical American home.

Leather

Also see:
• Vegetarian Groups, Web Sites, Restaurants & Stores

When people think of leather they often think of cow skin, which is mostly a by-product of the meat industry. But there are many types of animal skins used to make wallets, purses, luggage, shoes, boots, belts, hats, watchbands, and other clothing, accessories, and furniture. These items may be made of the skins of deer, pigs, alligators, snakes, ostriches, and a wide assortment of other animals. In addition to millions of animals raised on farms specifically for their skin, a large variety of wild animals, including rare and endangered animals, are killed each year for their skin and fur.

One of the most ecologically disastrous forms of "leather farming" is that of crocodiles in Cambodia. The crocodile farmers of Cambodia are responsible for the depletion of fish in the country's waters. Because the populations of fish have been depleted, the crocodile farmers have turned to feeding their crocodiles with millions of snakes taken from the wild. This is depleting the snake populations so quickly that it is having an impact on other wild animals that feed off the snakes; in turn, other wildlife that depend on predator animals are also suffering. The snakes the farmers don't give to the crocodiles are sold off for their skins and meat.

Like most people, I was unaware of the impact that the leather industry is having on the environment. I have some old leather shoes purchased during my less enlightened years, but whenever I purchase new footwear I seek out those made from nonleather "pleather" or fabric. In the Vegetarian Groups section of this book I list stores that sell vegan shoes, belts, wallets, and other accessories.

Lighting and Pollution

Also see:
• Solar Energy

The use of electricity in homes and businesses contributes greatly to air pollution. It is estimated that electric utilities are responsible for over two-thirds of sulfur dioxide emissions, nearly a third of nitrogen oxide emissions, and more than a third of carbon emissions. These toxins are major factors in smog, haze, acid rain, mercury contamination, and global warming.

Compact fluorescent light bulbs use 75 percent less energy than conventional bulbs. Replace your standard light bulbs with compact fluorescent bulbs and you will save a lot of energy and money, and cause less pollution.

Turn off your lights when they aren't needed.

If you use lanterns, put hemp oil in them instead of kerosene or other petroleum oil. Hemp oil burns cleaner and brighter.

If you burn candles, avoid candles made from petroleum wax. Instead, seek candles that are made from such substances as hemp oil, soy, vegetable glycerin, and other nontoxic substances. When you burn candles, collect the wax, and then use it to make your own candles. As mentioned earlier, if you are vegan you likely want to avoid candles made from beeswax.

Ever wonder why so many companies, office towers, schools, malls, restaurants, car lots, and other commercial and government structures leave their lights on all night? According to OneEarth.Org, over 30 percent of the energy used in the U.S. goes for office buildings, and over 30 percent of offices leave their equipment on 24 hours a day. This is a tremendous waste of electricity and world resources, and results in a dependence on petroleum. It also contributes an exorbitant amount of pollution to the environment. The millions of tons of coal and tens of millions of barrels of oil used to create electricity for lighting spews tons of carbon dioxide (CO_2), a greenhouse gas; sulfur dioxide (SO_2), which is found in acid rain; and nitrogen oxides (NO_x), a common ingredient in smog.

If those businesses that are leaving their lights on at night are worried about safety, they should install motion detectors that turn on the lights only when there is motion within a certain area.

As outdoor advertising and commercial and government buildings have been built around the world, lighting pollution has become a global problem. Satellite photos of Earth show how intrusive outdoor lighting is. The glare from lights in cities and towns and along roads and highways can be seen from outer space.

The haze from outdoor lighting reduces our ability to see the stars; disrupts migratory bird populations; interferes with sea turtle nesting and disorients their hatchlings; intrudes on nocturnal wildlife feeding patterns; and affects some types of plants.

Many millions of birds every year die at night because of outdoor lighting. This is because many types of birds migrate at night. They become disoriented because of the lights of skyscrapers, airports, radio towers, cell phone towers, billboards, and often slam into the structures.

Sea turtle hatchlings will go the wrong direction, toward land, instead of toward the ocean, when they hatch at night and see electric lighting. They confuse the electric lights of cities, towns, and roads for the flickers of light reflecting off the ocean water in the night, and they head toward the lights instead of the ocean. This results in their death from dehydration within several hours. All varieties of sea turtles are endangered.

Darkness for humans during sleep is better for the brain and body tissues. Light regulates human physiology. Light affects everything from our body temperature to the chemistry of our urine to the production of hormones in the brain and our moods. The pineal gland of our brain produces melatonin in connection with our exposure to light, which affects our sleep patterns. Researchers at the University of Pennsylvania and the Children's Hospital of Pennsylvania found that young children who slept in a room with a night light were more likely to develop nearsightedness.

Turn off outside lighting when it doesn't need to be on. If you are concerned about security, connect a motion detector to exterior lighting. Put top shields on outside lights so the light does not go up into the sky, but goes down to what you want illuminated.

Get your local governments to pass laws restricting the use of commercial lighting at night, such as in car lots, restaurants, empty office buildings, and malls; to require star guards on outside lighting to prevent lighting from going skyward; and to turn off lights in buildings that aren't occupied.

Citizens for Responsible Lighting, CRLAction.Org

> "Animals and plants, moreso than mankind, have lived in an outdoor environment with natural diurnal and nocturnal circadian and circannual rhythms governed by photoperiods brought forth by the Sun and Moon and varying natural light duration imposed by the change of seasons since the dawn of time. Their DNA through the process of evolution and natural selection requires specific periods of darkness for them to survive in many if not most cases."

Dark-sky List Forum, Groups.Yahoo.Com/Group/DarkSky-List/

International Dark-Sky Association, DarkSky.Org

Lighting Research Center, LRC.RPI.Edu

NativeEnergy.Com

Virginia Outdoor Lighting Taskforce, Volt.Org

Locally Grown Food

Also see:
• Farmers' Markets

Local Harvest, 831-475-8150; LocalHarvest.Org
Site lists farmers' markets, family farms, and sources for food grown locally in your area.

Love

"Neither a lofty degree of intelligence nor imagination nor both together go to the making of genius. Love, love, love, that is the soul of genius."
— **Wolfgang Amadeus Mozart**

Love is in an essential nutrient. Love needs to be both synthesized within us and obtained from outside sources. This nutrient helps us to manifest Divinity.

Love permeates all, is the strongest power of all, and is the only superpower.

When love is present, people learn, heal, play, think, feel, and sleep better. Love is necessary for a life to be healthy. Love uplifts and brightens. It helps those who are sad to become happy. The nurturing energy of love brings people to prosper by uplifting them and getting them to use their intellect, talents, and abilities.

To bring love into your life, you must first love yourself. Love for self includes taking care of yourself, respecting your being, as well as other life forms, such as the animals of the land, sky, and water. It includes believing that your essence is worthy of love. Knowing that you are worthy of love will drive you to improve your life in every way.

Emotions that are in alignment with love include kindness, forgiveness, patience, encouragement, and respect for the talents, abilities, and intellect of others. Nothing good can happen without love. So if you want good in your life, you must align yourself with the energy of love, which is good.

Work to love everyone. Sometimes you may find it difficult, especially with the way certain people conduct themselves. But you will be better off doing it than not.

Just because others select words, actions, and expressions that are opposite of love does not mean that you have to participate in the same behavior.

Refuse violence. Refuse to participate in war. Dispose of weaponry.

Choose to take the higher road. Follow and be led by love. Evolve through love.

Magnetizing Your Life

Also see:
- Brain
- Love
- People
- Thinking
- Television
- Yoga

"It's not what you are that holds you back, it's what you think you are not."
— **Denis Waitley**

Stop looking away from those parts of your life that need attention. Instead, turn and face them.

"One of the great lessons I've learned in athletics is that you've got to discipline your life. No matter how good you may be, you've got to be willing to cut out of your life those things that keep you from going to the top."
— **Bob Richards, Olympic Pole Vaulting Champion**

You cannot continue to eat a degenerating diet and expect to generate health. In the same way, you cannot think negative thoughts and expect positive actions out of your body.

Work to dispose of that which is negative. Included in that should be the negative influence of other people. As Wolfe says, "Stop listening to people who are not getting the results in their life that you desire to have in your life."

Take every element of your life and place it where it works for you. Make it function. Form it into what is best for you.

Work yourself away from that which holds you back. Work toward that which brings you health, happiness, and success. Arrange your atmosphere into that which brings about health. Clean and organize your belongings and surroundings in a way that allows you to function at a higher level.

You have the power within you to heal yourself and to create the life you want. As long as you have the desire to do so, you can begin to work it. As a being that has abilities, you can formulate yourself into what you are capable of.

You are in charge of how happy and healthy you can become. If you do not like the health you are experiencing, you can change it. If you do not like the thoughts and visions in your mind, you can change them. If you do not like the atmosphere you are living in, you can change the scenery. If there is anything in your life that you do not like, work to change it.

The mind is an incredible tool that constantly seeks answers for what it needs to know. But it can only work if the person cooperates in voicing the words that make up the questions. Those who seek can find. Those who ask, receive. Those who ask receive an answer.

There is a law of Nature that works in all life forms. Some call it the "law of attraction." It can be seen in all living things, and even in the elements and energy. Similar to the way a nail is drawn to a magnet, certain things are attracted to other things

Things are naturally attracted to that which helps them to exist. One way the law of attraction is displayed is when you see how the leaves of a plant turn toward Sun. Another way this is displayed is in how the roots of a plant are drawn to damper soil, and deeper into the nutritious, mineralized soil. You can plant a seed in a cup that has one side packed with rich soil, and the other side packed with sand. The roots of the plant will naturally become more abundant in the soil-filled side of the cup.

The law of attraction also works with people. The difference is that people can play a part in where their roots, or attention and energy, travel. It is your choice to associate with energies, situations, people, and elements that will help you grow in a positive way, or with those that will lead to self-destruction. This element of your person is active whether you are aware of it or not.

"Your mind is a living magnet. You automatically draw people, things, and circumstances into your life in harmony with your dominant thoughts and desires."
— **David Wolfe**

You can feel better about yourself. You can experience better health. You can think better and respond better to that which is presented to you. All this is what you can do with the goal of improving and building things into the way you want them to be for your life.

Your thoughts and actions play a major role in what types of people, situations, and elements appear in your life. What you think about results in the awareness and the actions that draw you to act and react in a way that creates an atmosphere. The atmosphere is created by everything you do, what you wear, what you say, where you go, what you accumulate, what you seek, what you eat, what you listen to, and what you think.

If you want certain things in your life, then you should focus on those things. Visualize them in your life. Plan and work for them to happen and become present in your life. Magnetize yourself to them, and them to you. The more effort you put into attaining the images in your thoughts, the more likely they are to materialize.

If you want your life to be organized and experienced in a certain way, work to attract the things that will help you live your life in that way. Like plant roots that grow toward the most fertile areas of soil, your life will be guided into the energies and elements that you want to absorb — as long as you set the power of your mind to work in that direction. To attract a most radiant and abundant life filled with satisfied goals and people who love and respect you as you love and respect them, work to attract that situation.

Constantly develop and prepare yourself to receive the situation you want. Do it through healthful food choices of the highest quality; through physical preparation of exercise and a confident stance; through dress; through mental awareness, knowledge, focus, visualization, and rationalization; and through using your intellect, talents, and abilities to set the stage for magnetizing your life to draw in the life that you want.

When you begin to follow a Sunfood diet your life will change. This is especially true if you had been eating devitalized, unhealthful, deadened, processed commercial food. Opportunities will arise that you may never have considered. Things will happen that you didn't think were a possibility, or were not even in your concept of how things could happen. You will find yourself thinking differently than before. Your perceptions will change. Foods, music, and designs of things may seem different to you. Activities in which you may never have thought about participating may draw your attention. The way you eat, dress, think, play, and the general way you participate in life may all go through a radical change. The higher frequency that you tune into by eating more vibrant foods can ignite your passions in intense ways you never thought possible.

Do not give in to people who doubt that you are capable of succeeding. Do not allow yourself to think that you are not capable or that you are not worthy.

People may doubt your words, but they can't doubt your actions. The originating force in your actions is what you are thinking. Begin now to think yourself healthy and successful. Take continuous intentional actions toward creating your life into the life you want.

Contained within you are all the pieces of the puzzle you need to build the life you need. You have talents, use them. You have intellect, plug into it. You have abilities; work with them. You are capable. And you know it.

> "Wasted is every thought, feeling, or vibration which is out of harmony with your true pattern of life. Learn to live by the pattern of life that is contained within you. You already know what it is. Now it is time for you to remember."
> — David Wolfe

The power of your soul is what formulated your tissues and it is what is animating you. It is making you think. It is making your heart beat and your lungs breathe. It is making your cells function, and your body parts to move. It is what is making you desire and to seek what you want. It is pushing you to constantly work out your thoughts through actions. You can make it work for you. It is your power source. Honor it with rightful living, self-respect, and vibrant foods.

Purify your diet in a way that your body is getting what it needs to build a healthy, strong structure. Do not pollute your body with low-quality foods. Do not allow yourself to eat deadened or otherwise processed foods that would lower your frequency and that would leave residues of toxins in your tissues that clog your system. Eat high-quality foods that enliven your body, that bring about the beauty of health, and that improve your level of consciousness. Partake in the living power of Nature that is contained in raw fruits, vegetables, nuts, seeds, herbs, sea vegetables, and edible flowers. Let these ignite your passions, talents, confidence, and thought patterns.

Grab onto courage and confidence. Bravely take charge of your days and set out a plan to succeed. Be determined to rid yourself of that which clutters your path and holds you back. Do not look back toward your failures. Instead, look forward to that which you can attain through perseverance. Like an athlete who constantly works toward victory you too will break your own records in ways that you never thought you could.

As you go forward into a healthier life, and learn of the benefits of the good things you are doing for yourself, you will be able to surpass the limits under which you once lived. You will be able to see that you are capable of attaining good things for yourself that are truly improving your life.

Give energy to thoughts that work toward your success. Let the thoughts of success power you rather than the thoughts of fear. Allow yourself to be propelled toward a better life by visualizing your life the way you want it to be and making it happen through intentional living.

Keeping a journal of your progress, of your thoughts, and of your goals and dreams can help you along in your process of self-improvement. Write down what inspires you. Write down what you want to overcome and how you plan to overcome it. Write down the thoughts that motivate you.

Plan out your way to live and live out your plan to live.

Milk from Animals

"Scant evidence supports nutrition guidelines that focus specifically on increasing milk or other dairy product intake for promoting child or adolescent bone mineralization."
— *Pediatrics*, March 2005

"Dairy cows are truly sick, miserable, abused creatures that are fed a high-protein (often animal-based) diet counterproductive to their health. They are then often drugged with bovine growth hormones and antibiotics, and abused to provide more milk than they have been created by Nature to give – little or none of which goes to their own young."
— Former Montana cattle rancher Howard Lyman, in his book *No More Bull: The Mad Cowboy Targets America's Worst Enemy: Our Diet*; MadCowboy.Com

"Of the beasts from whom cheese is made... The milk will be taken from the tiny children."
— Leonardo da Vinci, writing about how he thought taking milk from a cow is stealing from the calf. da Vinci was a vegetarian and outspoken about his beliefs in protecting the animal kingdom.

"Interestingly, many long-term studies have now examined milk consumption in relation to risk of fractures. With remarkable consistency, these studies do not show reduction in fractures with high dairy product consumption. The hype about milk is basically an effective market-

ing campaign by the American Dairy industry."
— **Walter Willet, M.D., M.P.H., Dr.P.H., Harvard School of Public Health's Nutrition chairman,** *Scientific American,* **January 2003**

"There's no reason to drink cow's milk at any time in your life. It was designed for calves, not humans, and we should all stop drinking it today."
— **Dr. Frank A. Oski, former Director of Pediatrics, Johns Hopkins University**

Cow milk is for baby cows. If you think you are doing yourself a favor by drinking cow milk, or any milk from an animal, you may want to reconsider. The milk may not be doing the good you that you may believe it is doing for your body, your heart, your cellular structure, your joints, or your bones. Numerous studies have concluded that the more milk you drink and the more meat you eat, the more likely you are to suffer from osteoporosis, arthritis, kidney disease, diabetes, colon cancer, and glandular cancers.

Commercials often claim that milk is a good source of calcium. What is the best source of calcium for humans? Raw green-leafed vegetables and other raw fruits and vegetables.

Learn how to make nut and seed mylks (spelled "mylk" when made out of nuts). There are many recipes for them in the raw vegan recipe books.

However, if you do choose to drink animal milk, as mentioned earlier in the book, only consume milk that is from organic dairies that allow the cows or goats to graze in open fields, that don't treat the animals with milk stimulant drugs, and that don't pasteurize the milk. This raw, organic milk from animals consuming a natural diet contains beneficial nutrients, such as helpful lactic-acid-generating bacteria; enzymes, and higher levels of omega-3 and omega-6 essential fatty acids. Pasteurization of milk damages these nutrients. In this way, even though I do not consume milk, I am a proponent of raw, organic milk from open field-grazed cows.

People who once drank pasteurized milk and milk products from factory farms and who then switched to raw, organic milk that is from field-grazed cows have noticed a reduction in or disappearance of certain allergies and skin conditions.

Milk that is from cows that are grain fed, that don't graze in open fields, and that are treated with milk stimulants and antibiotics is unhealthful. This milk, which is from factory farms, should be pasteurized. Humans also shouldn't consume it.

The same standards apply to goat milk: organic, raw milk from field-grazed animals is the way to go.

Cheese, cream, kefir, and yogurt should also be from these quality sources, and never from factory farmed animals.

Because each state seems to have a different law regarding raw milk and raw cheeses, if you are going to consume dairy products, you may need to do some research to know where to get organic, raw dairy products. In some states you may have to join a farm co-op to get quality raw dairy products. A sort of "underground" activist movement has formed around this very topic.

Campaign for Real Milk, RealMilk.Com

Compassion for Farm Animals, TorturedCows.Com

Mindfully.Org/Plastic/Dairies-Glass-Bottle-Milk.htm
Provides a list of dairies that sell their milk in glass instead of plastic.

Not Milk, NotMilk.Com
A slew of information on why humans shouldn't drink cow milk.

Organic Pastures Dairy Company, Fresno, CA; OrganicPastures.Com

PETA's cow page, UnhappyCows.Com
"California's dairy cows are crammed into huge lots, where they live covered in mud and their own feces for most of their miserable lives. They are pumped full of drugs to keep them producing such unnatural amounts of milk that their udders often become swollen and infected – in fact, at any given time, roughly one-third of California's cows suffer from painful udder infections, and more than half suffer from other painful infections and illnesses. They are forcefully impregnated every year to keep them producing milk, and their male babies often end up chained by their necks in veal crates before being slaughtered at just 16 weeks old [their meat is sold as 'veal'].

More than a fourth of California's dairy cows are slaughtered each year, generally because they've become crippled from painful foot infections or calcium depletion. At this point, they are trucked to the slaughterhouse through all weather extremes, many collapsing and arriving crippled. Slaughter is gruesome and often terrifying and painful. Said one former USDA slaughter inspector, 'In the summertime, when it's 90, 95 degrees, they're transporting cattle from 1,200 to 1,500 miles away on a trailer, 40 to 45 head crammed in there, and some collapse from heat exhaustion. This past winter, we had minus-50-degree weather with the windchill. Can you imagine if you were in the back of a trailer that's open, and the windchill factor is minus 50 degrees, and that trailer is going 50 to 60 miles an hour? The animals are urinating and defecating right in the trailers, and after a while, it's going to freeze, and their hooves are right in it. If they go down – well, you can imagine lying in there for ten hours on a trip.'"

Minerals

Some people think that they have to eat meat and dairy to get good nutrition, and especially minerals. But the truth is that meat and dairy are not the best sources of minerals. Far from it. When you look at the natural diet of cows, giraffes, gorillas, elephants, deer, and other large animals, you can clearly see that they get their nutrition from eating green-leafed vegetation. These large animals are the substances of leaves transformed through the miracle of life into living body tissues. It is no coincidence that calcium is the primary mineral in leaves, and is also the chief mineral in the human body.

If you want to get high-quality minerals into your body, as well as an amazing assortment of other nutrients, be sure to regularly eat raw, green-leafed vegetables. The colloidal minerals that your body needs to construct and maintain your tissues are contained in raw plants. Leafy vegetables have a good balance of magnesium, manganese, and silicon, which are needed to assimilate calcium. Spinach is an ideal source of all these minerals. Water vegetables are especially rich in minerals.

Money and Investing

"I make myself rich by making my wants few."
— Henry David Thoreau

"Try not to become a man of success, but rather try to become a man of value."
— Albert Einstein

Some seem to think that if you are rich you must be destroying the planet. But if you participate in socially responsible investing (SRI), you can actually help to protect Earth, although it does have its limits.

While there were people always seeking to avoid investing in companies involved in questionable activities, such as the slave trade, SRI became more common in the 1960s when people didn't want to invest in companies that had military contracts. In the last couple decades people have avoided investing in companies associated with South Africa's apartheid government, and also in the seriously corrupt diamond trade and in much of the chocolate market. Presently investors are avoiding companies that invest in those that directly or indirectly are associated with slave farms in Africa; in companies that have anything to do with military contracts; in companies involved in genetic engineering of food plants; and in companies that have a large influence in factory farming, in major causes of global warming, and in destruction of the environment.

Because more and more people are becoming aware of global warming and war issues, there is a whole lot more money going into companies that are involved in less destructive activities. Many of the funds that focus on SRI are producing high financial returns. One reason for this is that companies focusing on socially responsible practices are less likely to get sued, and are more likely to pay and treat their workers in a responsible manner.

If you have money to invest, research the growing number of financial organizations that seek to invest in such things as solar energy, organic farming, nontoxic cosmetics, industrial hemp, and vegan food companies. Look to invest in companies that donate part of their profits to environmental and wildlife protection. Move your money into a "green bank" or credit union focused on environmentally responsible investing.

One of the most common ways to invest is through a mutual fund. These are funds that invest in a diversified group of companies. Listed below are mutual fund companies that focus on companies identified as socially responsible. Your initial investment in a mutual fund may be as little as a few hundred dollars, then you agree to put a certain amount of money into the account every month. The mutual fund managers maintain the account by deciding which stocks to invest in, and when to sell them. Investing in a mutual fund instantly diversifies your money and saves on trading commissions paid when you invest in individual stocks. Be sure to investigate if the mutual fund invests in companies that are in tune with your ideas of a green company.

If you have a 401(k) retirement plan, check to see if they offer socially responsible investing options. If they do not, kindly inquire if they would start providing this option. You might help this happen by providing a list of 401(k) plans that are involved in SRI. (Check the details of your 401(k) plan to see if it is secure from being pilfered by your company or embezzled by company management. Keep an eye on quarterly statements that may detail unexplained dips in balance, changes to investments you did not authorize, and changes in investment managers. The company president may be the sole manager of the account, and able to take "loans" from the account that may never be repaid. The fidelity bond insurance may cover 10 percent or less of the plan's assets. Annual independent audits don't have to be done on 401(k) plans of smaller companies, so problems may take years to be discovered. You may find that other types of savings plans are more secure, and more likely to qualify as SRI.)

Do you have a lot of money? Invest directly in companies that are considered to be environmentally green, and then donate any profits to an organization that works to protect and preserve wild plants, land, water, and animals. Write a Will that includes a gift to an environmental charity, such as organizations working to protect the forests of the planet.

Establishing a gift fund or a foundation can turn you into a philanthropist. Gift funds, which are offered through a limited number of mutual fund companies, are less expensive to start and maintain than foundations. Gift funds also have tax and other benefits that foundations do not.

Before you invest in anything, research where your money is going. Avoid investing in companies involved in weaponry, nuclear power; petroleum exploration; mining; genetic engineering of food plants; farming chemicals; factory farming; pharmaceutical drugs; the grain industry; chocolate farming that uses slaves; the fur trade; the diamond trade; vivisection, or lumber.

Avoid investing in U.S. government bonds, else you may be helping to fund war, nuclear bombs, and the military/industrial complex. Municipal bonds are likely a much safer investment because they are usually used to fund local citizen projects. But municipal bonds may also fund highways and power plants.

When you purchase stock in a company you are allowed to vote on corporate policy. In this way you can work to make a company more environmentally responsible. It's called "shareholder activism." It has worked in some cases, such as by getting office supply chains to start selling recycled paper.

There are investment funds that work to purchase into companies with histories of bad environmental policy. They do this with the goal of making the companies more environmentally friendly by changing its policies. But some funds don't always engage in this even when they say it is their goal. If you invest in funds that claim they are working to be shareholder activists, make sure the funds stick to their word.

Some of the following may be helpful when seeking to invest your money in socially and environmentally responsible ways. Also, publications such as *Mother Jones*, *Utne*, and *E Magazine* often carry advertisements from investment companies focused on investing in environmentally friendly ways – at least more environmentally friendly than most companies.

AsYouSow.Org
Promotes corporate social responsibility.

Business Ethics Magazine, Minneapolis, MN; Business-Ethics.Com

Calvert Financial Group, Bethesda, MD; 800-248-0337; CalvertGroup.Com
Mutual funds.

Chittenden Bank, Brattleboro, VT, 800-772-3863;
SociallyResponsible.Chittenden.Com

Citizens Funds, Portsmouth, NH; 800-223-7010; CitizensFunds.Com
Mutual funds.

Clean Yield, Greensboro, VT; 800-809-6439; CleanYield.Com
Asset management.

Coalition for Environmentally Responsible Economies, Ceres.Org

Domini Social Investments, Providence, RI; 800-225-3863; Domini.Com
Mutual funds.

Dreyfus Corporation, Dreyfus.Com
Mutual funds.

First Affirmative Financial Network, Colorado Springs, CO; 800-422-7284;
FirstAffirmative.Com
Asset management.

Green Century Funds, Boston, MA; 800-934-7336; GreenCentury.Com
Mutual funds.

GreenMBA.Com

Green Money Journal, Santa Fe, NM; GreenMoneyJournal.Com

HopeDance.Org

Published an issue about socially responsible investing.

Interfaith Center on Corporate Responsibility, New York, NY; ICCR.Org

Investor Responsibility Research Center, Washington, DC; IRRC.Org

KLD Research & Analytics, Inc., Boston, MA; KLD.Com
Compiles and maintains profiles on 3,000 U.S. companies. Keeps information on global industry practices. Maintains socially responsible investing indexes.

Latino Community Credit Union, 219 West Main St., POB 25360; Durham, NC 27702; CoOperativaLatina.Org

National Green Pages of Co-Op America, 1612 K St., NW, Ste. 600, Washington, DC 20006; CoOpAmerica.Org
Contains a financial section for those interested in socially responsible investing.

Natural Investment Services, NaturalInvesting.Com

Neuberger Berman Mutual Funds, New York, NY; 800-877-9700; NB.Com

New Alternatives Fund, Melville, NY; 800-423-8383; NewAlternativesFund.Com
Mutual funds.

Parnassus Investments, San Francisco, CA; 800-999-3505; Parnassus.Com
Mutual funds.

Pax World Funds, New York, NY; 800-229-1172; PaxFunds.Com
Mutual funds.

Pension Rights Center, 202-296-3776; PensionRights.Org

Permaculture Credit Union, 4250 Cerrillos Rd., Santa Fe, NM 87592; 866-954-3479; PCUOnline.Org
Offers savings accounts, various types of loans, and a Visa card.

Portfolio 21, Progressive Investment Management, Portland, OR; Portfolio21.Com
Mutual funds.

Principle Profits, Amherst, MA; 800-972-3289; PrincipleProfits.Com
Asset management.

Progressive Asset Management Network, Oakland, CA; 800-786-2998; ProgressiveAssetManagment.Com

Progressive Investor monthly newsletter, SustainableBusiness.Com

Real Money bimonthly newsletter on socially responsible investing, Co-Op

America; RealMoney.Com

Rocky Mountain Humane Investing, GreenInvestment.Com
   Customized portfolios.

Self-Help Credit Union, Durham, NC; 800-966-SELF; Self-Help.Org

ShoreBank Pacific, Ilwaco, WA; 888-326-2265; Eco-Bank.Com

Sierra Club Mutual Funds, San Francisco, CA; 415-863-6300;
SierraClubFunds.Com

Social Investment Forum, Washington, DC; SocialInvest.Org
   Trade organization for socially responsible investing.

SRI World Group, Brattleboro, VT, SRIWorld.Com; and SocialFunds.Com

Trillium Asset Management, Boston, Boise, Durham, San Francisco; 800-548-5684; TrilliumInvest.Com

Winslow Green Growth Fund, Portland, ME; 888-314-9049;
WinslowGreen.Com

MSG: Monosodium Glutamate

Book:
• *In Bad Taste: The MSG Syndrome*, by Dr. George Schwartz, M.D.

Avoid foods that contain MSG. This toxic food additive is created in a fermenting process that includes starch, sugar beets, sugar cane, or molasses. Consuming foods that contain it can lead to, contribute to, or aggravate health conditions, including headaches, asthma, depression, irritability, nausea, weakness, congestion, and allergy-type symptoms.

In popular use by many food companies as a "flavor enhancer," MSG can sometimes be found anonymously listed as "natural flavoring" and "natural seasoning" on ingredient labels. Under Food and Drug Administration regulations, MSG must be listed as "monosodium glutamate" on food ingredient labels. Lots of companies break that rule. It is most commonly found as an additive in processed foods, canned foods, frozen foods, junk foods, fast-foods, and especially in Chinese foods.

On its Web site, the FDA says, "Injections of glutamate in laboratory animals have resulted in damage to nerve cells in the brain." The report also states rather unconvincingly, "Consumption of glutamate in food, however, does not cause this effect." This is a rather confusing claim, especially when the same FDA document also goes on to say, "The Federation of American Societies for Experimental Biology (FASEB) report identifies two groups of people who may develop a condition the report refers to as 'MSG symptom complex.' One group is those who may be intolerant to MSG when eaten in a large quantity. The second is a group of people with severe, poorly controlled asthma. These people, in addition to being prone to MSG symptom complex, may suffer temporary worsening of asthmatic symptoms after consuming MSG." The following confusing sentence is also in the same report: "In 1986, FDA's Advisory Committee on Hypersensitivity to Food Constituents concluded that MSG poses no threat to the general public but that reactions of brief duration might occur in some people." So, it's a threat, but it isn't a threat? The report goes on to say, "Between 1980 and 1994, the Adverse Reaction Monitoring System in FDA's Center for Food Safety and Applied Nutrition received 622 reports of complaints about MSG. Headache was the most frequently reported symptom. No severe reactions were documented, but some reports indicated that people with asthma got worse after they consumed MSG. In some of those cases, the asthma didn't get worse until many hours later."

The same report defines "MSG symptom complex" as a condition characterized by one or more of the following symptoms:

• Burning sensation in the back of the neck, forearms, and chest

• Numbness in the back of the neck, radiating to the arms and back

• Tingling, warmth and weakness in the face, temples, upper back, neck, and arms

• Facial pressure or tightness

• Chest pain

• Headache

• Nausea

• Rapid heartbeat

• Bronchospasm (difficulty breathing) in MSG-intolerant people with asthma

• Drowsiness

• Weakness

It appears that the FDA can't make up its mind as it is saying that MSG is safe, but it is also not safe at all. (To read the full report, access VM.CFSan.FDA.Gov/~LRD/MSG.html.)

> "Behavioral and physical problems of children, such as incontinence and seizures, as well as attention deficit disorder (ADD), have been diagnosed and successfully treated as MSG disorders."
> — NaturoDoc.Com/Library/Nutrition/MSG.htm; September 2006

I don't believe MSG is safe. If you care about your health you won't be eating foods containing MSG.

Some professional athletes have it written into their contract that they are not allowed to consume any foods containing MSG.

Do yourself a favor and keep MSG out of your food, and out of your body. Stick to real foods created by Nature in the form of raw, organically grown fruits, vegetables, nuts, and seeds, and foods made of them.

Nuclear Energy

Books:
- *Insurmountable Risks: The Dangers in Using Nuclear Power to Combat Global Climate Change*, by Dr. Brice Smith
- *Killing Our Own: The Disaster of America's Experience with Atomic Radiation*, by Robert Alvarez

> "You can't fix a problem with a problem. Nuclear power just has too many downsides. It is not a renewable energy. There is mining of uranium involved. The radioactive waste has a horrifically long lifespan and cannot be disposed of safely. The reactors are dangerous and accidents can be disastrous, deadly, and have long-term health and environmental ramifications. The proposal of addressing our energy needs with nuclear power is symptomatic of the short-term thinking that politicians are known for. There are so many other options out there. We need to start employing those options and funding research on others immediately."
> — Daryl Hannah, *VegNews*, December 2006; VegNews.Com

Don't believe the propaganda put out by the nuclear power industry claiming that nuclear energy is clean and environmentally safe. The nuclear energy industry donates large amounts of money to political campaigns to support politicians most likely to vote in favor of what the nuclear energy industry wants.

Study up on the contamination issues and the environmental destruction caused by nuclear power plants, and look at the problem of nuclear waste, as well as nuclear power plant and nuclear waste safety concerns. You will understand where the nuclear energy industry has misinformed the public in favor of huge profits and at great harm to life.

Do you think nuclear power is safe? Consider what would happen if a nuclear power plant near you had a meltdown, or was somehow destroyed. The result would be radiation fallout over a vast area, many thousands dead, and millions exposed to enough radiation to cause long-term health problems. The wildlife in the region would experience the same.

What do we do with nuclear waste that will need to be stored for thousands of years? Who can determine what potential storage area is not going to experience an earthquake, flood, tsunami, volcanic eruption, or other natural disaster during those thousands of years? Will people in a thousand years want to, or know how to, deal with this radioactive trash? How about people in a hundred years? Or even the people who are alive now? Local governments are refusing nuclear waste. The U.S. government has plans to store more and more of the stuff on Indian reservations. The U.S. government also wants to build more nuclear energy plants. There are already over 100 nuclear power plants in the U.S.

Nuclear energy is not a good thing.

Close nuclear power plants. Work to prevent new ones from being built.

CitizenAlert.Org

Mindfully.Org/Nuclear

Natural Resources Defense Council, NRDC.Org/Nuclear/Default.asp

Nuclear Information and Resource Service, NIRS.Com
"Once-through cooling technology is used exclusively in 48 nuclear reactors with 11 additional reactors employing the technology in conjunction with cooling towers and canals. These reactors, situated on coastal waters, major rivers, and lakes can draw in as much as a billion gallons of water per reactor unit a day, nearly a million gallons a minute, in order to dissipate the extraordinary amounts of waste heat generated in the fission process.

The initial devastation of marine life and ecosystems stems from the powerful intake of water into the nuclear reactor. Marine life, ranging from endangered sea turtles and manatees down to delicate fish larvae and microscopic planktonic organisms vital to the ocean ecosystem, is sucked irresistibly into the reactor cooling system, a process known as entrainment. Some of these animals are killed, either through impingement (animals are caught and trapped against filters, grates, and other reactor structures), or, in the case of air-breathing animals like turtles, seals, and manatees, drown or suffocate."

Physicians for Social Responsibility, PSR.Org

Public Citizen's Critical Mass Energy Program, Citzen.Org/CMEP

RedwoodAlliance.Org

Shundahai Network, Shundahai.Org

SierraClub.Org/NuclearWaste

Union of Concerned Scientists, UCSUSA.Org

Off-Road Vehicles: The Plague of the Wildlands

"In the entire National Forest system – covering more than 190 million acres in 155 forests – only two forests, the Hoosier in Indiana and the Monongahela in West Virginia, do not allow off-road vehicle use... The [George W. Bush] administration and snowmobile industry agreed in 2001 to work together to overturn a decision by the National Park Service to protect Yellowstone and Grand Teton National Parks by phasing out snowmobiles. In January 2003, the [Bush] administration issued a rule that will make it easier for off-road vehicle interests and developers to use a Civil War-era law – passed to encourage settlement of the West – to build roads and expand off-road vehicle use in National Parks, Monuments, and Forests."
— **The Wilderness Society, Wilderness.Org; 2006**

Off-road vehicles in the shape of "dirt-bike" motorcycles, dune buggies, all terrain vehicles (ATVs), pickup trucks, Jeeps, snowmobiles, and even jet skis and swamp buggies are causing severe damage to wildlands at an alarming rate. There are well over 60,000 miles of dirt roads that have been created by renegade off-road vehicles throughout the wildlands of the U.S., and that number continues to grow every year.

Off-road vehicles ruin the soil base for plants; kill small plants, bushes and trees; degrade the soil leading to flash flooding and soil loss; disrupt feeding, nesting, breeding and sleep patterns of wild animals while reducing their habitat; kill small animals, especially their young; and reduce pristine areas to dirt trails void of plant life where invasive weeds take root and compete with native vegetation.

What is often left behind on much of the off-road trails deep in the wild are rutted trails; damaged stream banks; altered rock beds; areas strewn with beer and soda cans, broken bottles, wax-coated and foil and plastic food wrappers, cups and utensils, cigarette butts; spent cartridge shells; wads of toilet paper; broken Styrofoam containers; and motor oil spills. Off-road vehicles also leave behind polluted air, broken bushes and trees, reduced water quality, and terrified and injured wildlife.

Natural Trails and Waters Coalition, NaturalTrails.Org

The Wilderness Society,
Wilderness.Org/OurIssues/ORV/Index.cfm?TopLevel=Home

WildLandsCPR.Org
Specifically targets off-road vehicle abuse of public lands and actively promotes wildland restoration, road removal and the prevention of new road construction.

Organic Issues

Also see:
• Gardening and Farming

"Pesticides are a $35 billion a year industry. They are chemical concoctions created to kill living things, usually in gardens and human dwellings. But pesticides are known to cause various types of birth defects, cancers, mental disabilities, and also damage and kill wildlife, as well as poison the water, air, and land. They have been directly linked to the demise of certain animal and beneficial bug and insect populations, as well as to deformities in wildlife. The companies producing these chemicals work very hard to help governments form laws allowing for the use of the pesticides."
  — **Pesticide Action Network North America, PANNA.Org, 2006**

"Organic agriculture is an ecological production management system that promotes and enhances biodiversity, biological cycles and soil biological activity. It is based on minimal use of off-farm inputs and on

management practices that restore, maintain and enhance ecological harmony... Organic food handlers, processors and retailers adhere to standards that maintain the integrity of organic agricultural products. The primary goal of organic agriculture is to optimize the health and productivity of interdependent communities of soil life, plants, animals, and people."
— **The National Organic Standards Board, 2005**

According to Consumer Reports, the fruits and vegetables that have the highest concentration of toxic pesticides include:
- Apples
- Bell peppers
- Cucumbers
- Green beans
- Peaches
- Pears
- Spinach
- Strawberries
- Tomatoes
- Winter squash

Acres USA, POB 91299, Austin, TX 78709; AcresUSA.Com
   Monthly magazine.

AllOrganicLinks.Com

California Certified Organic Farmers, POB 8136, Santa Cruz, CA 95061; CCOF.Org

Rachel Carson Council, POB 10779, Silver Spring, MD 20914, Members.AOL.Com/RCCouncil/OurPage/
   In 1962 Rachel Carson wrote the book *Silent Spring*. It sounded the alarm about the hazards of chemical pesticides.

RachelCarson.Org

Community Alliance with Family Farmers, POB 363, Davis, CA 95617; 916-756-8518; CAFF.Org
   Publishes *The National Organic Directory*.

Environmental Working Group, 1718 Connecticut Ave., NW, Ste. 600,

Washington, DC 20000; 202-667-6982; EWG.Org

Farm Verified Organic Program, POB 2747, 274 Riverside Ave., Westport, CT 06880; ICS-Intl.Com/FVO.htm

Green People.Org
Contains a list of organic food companies and sellers.

HawaiiOrganicFarmers.Org

International Federation of Organic Agriculture Movements,
IFOAM General Secretariat, c/o Okozentrum, Imsbach, D - 6695 Tholey-Theley, Germany; IFOAM.Org

Mindfully.Org/Pesticide

National Coalition Against the Misuse of Pesticides, 701 E St., SE, Ste. 200, Washington, DC 20003; BeyondPesticides.Org

National Farmers' Retail & Markets Association (FARMA), FarmShopping.Com
Farmers' markets in England.

NewFarm.Org

Northeast Organic Farmers Association, POB 135, Stevenson, CT 06491; NOFA.Org

Northwest Coalition for Alternatives to Pesticides, POB 1393, Eugene, OR 97440; Pesticide.Org

Oregon Tilth, Salem, OR; Tilth.Org

OrganicAlliance.Org

Organic Consumers Association, 6101 Cliff Estate Rd., Little Marais, MN 55614; 218-226-4164; PureFood.Org; OrganicConsumers.Org

Organic Crop Improvement Association, Rt. 1, Box 163, Marquette, NE 68854; 402-854-3195; 308-382-2707; OCIA.Org

Organic Farming Research Foundation, POB 440, Santa Cruz, CA 95061; 831-426-6606; OFRF.Org

Organic.Org

TheOrganicPages.Com

Organic Trade Association, Greenfield, MA; OTA.Com

Organic Trade Services, OrganicTS.Com

OrganicTrading.Com

Pesticide Action Network, North America, 49 Powell St., St. 500, San Francisco, CA 94102; 415-981-1771; PANNA.Org

PureFood.Org

SeattleTilth.Org

SoilAssociation.Org
  England's organic food certification organization.

Paints and Finishes

Also see:
• Building Materials and Supplies

Consider the paint or finishes on your walls, ceilings, floors, and furniture. Are they made from petroleum products, or are they made from plant extracts? Most commonly used paints contain volatile organic compounds (VOCs) that release toxic gasses. When purchasing paints and finishes, look for those that are no-VOC. Also seek paints that do not contain preservatives called biocides, which are especially bad for women planning on becoming pregnant, for pregnant and nursing mothers, and for babies and children (basically they aren't good for anyone).

AFM Enterprises, 619-239-0565; AFMSafeCoat.Com

AglaiaPaint.Com

Antique Drapery Rod Company, 214-653-1733; AntiqueDraperyRod.Com

Auro, 888-302-9352; AuroUSA.Com

BestPaintCo.Com

BioShield, 505-438-3448; BioShieldPaint.Com

ChemSafe Paints, EcoWise.Net/Interiors/Paint/Chemsafe

EcoSafeProducts.Com

KeimMineralSystems.Com

Miller Paint Company, 503-255-0190; 206-784-7878; MillerPaint.Com

SafeCoat, AFMSafecoat.Com

SpectraPaint.Com

Palm Oil: Terrible for Wildlife and the Environment

Palm oil is the most widely produced food oil. It is an extract of the fruit of the oil palm tree. Palm kernel oil is extracted from the seeds of the fruit.

The sprawl of oil palm plantations is wiping out thousands of species in Malaysia and Indonesia where more than 25,000 square miles of hardwood rainforest have been cleared and are being used to grow palm oil. In 2006 Malaysia was the world's lead producer of palm oil with a palm oil industry that brings in about $6 billion, second only to their electronics industry.

One of the chief reasons why orangutans on Borneo and Sumatra are facing extinction is because vast expanses of the forests where they have lived have been cleared using fire to expand oil palm and tropical wood plantations. Included in the list of species that are facing extinction because of these plantations are the Sumatran rhinoceros, Asian elephant, and Sumatran tiger. Several hundred people have also died in recent years defending their land against the expansion of the palm oil industry.

Oil palm plantations and production of palm oil damages the environment by reducing the soil base, poisoning the rivers, and polluting the air. Because peat swamps of Southeast Asia are also being drained to grow oil palm plantations, this increases environmental damage as the carbon escaping from the dried peat contributes to global warming. Roads created to manage the plantations cut through waterways, destroy more wildlife habitat, and provide ways for hunters of exotic animals to gain easy access to endangered wildlife.

Palm oil, which is high in saturated fat and low in polyunsaturated fat, is often cited as unhealthful oil that promotes heart disease. It is especially harmful to health after it has been heated.

It is often cited that raw palm oil is beneficial to health because it contains carotenoids, co-enzyme Q-10, magnesium, vitamin K, omega fatty acids, and tocotrienols. Because of its betacarotene content, raw palm oil has an orange tint, but when it is heated the carotenoids and other nutrients are destroyed and the oil becomes white and very unhealthful.

There are many fruits and vegetables that are excellent sources of the nutrients found in palm oil, and that do not cause damage to the environment and wildlife.

Often palm oil is labeled as "vegetable oil" in everything from chocolate to bread, cookies, margarine, shortening, and microwave popcorn. It is also used in makeup, lotions, soaps, shampoos and conditioners, in toothpaste, and in detergents. It has been used as an industrial lubricant for machinery.

More recently palm oil is being used as an ingredient in biodiesel. As demand increases for biodiesel, the governments of Southeast Asia have been seeking to take advantage of this market and are promoting the export of palm oil. A much more environmentally safe and sustainable oil to use for combustible engines is hemp oil.

Please avoid purchasing products containing palm oil and palm kernel oil. Help to educate others about the environmental damage and species degradation caused by oil palm plantations.

Center for Science in the Public Interest,
CSPINet.Org/PalmOilReport/Index.html
This site contains downloadable information about the environmental destruction and animal extinction being caused by the palm oil industry.

Orangutans.Com/UA

Paper That Isn't from Trees

Ecosource Paper Inc., 111-1841 Oak Bay Ave., Victoria, British Columbia, Canada, V8R 1C4; 800-665-6944; 250-595-4367; IslandNet.Com/~Ecodette/EcoSource.htm

Evanescent Press, Mendocino County, California; Tree.Org
An amazing little company that publishes original books on their own handmade paper, printed letterpress from hand-set type, and hand-bound. They make paper from hemp, kenaf, abaca, cotton, linen, and other natural fibers, including local weeds

that grow wild in the surrounding mountains.

Living Tree Paper, 1430 Willamette St., Ste. 367, Eugene, OR 97401; 800-309-2974; 541-342-297; LivingTreePaper.Com

Old Growth Free, Markets Initiative, POB 489, Tofino, BC V0R 2Z0 Canada; 250-725-2950; OldGrowthFree.Com

Peace

"As a nation, this is the moment to start seriously investing our time, energy and resources into proven methods of reducing violence, both within our nation as well as internationally. The cost of violence to our culture and our children is simply not sustainable. I have learned that in the United States, youth homicide rates are more than ten times that of other leading industrialized nations. This is just one example of the challenges we face. Is this really a legacy we want to leave our children? There is a better way."
— **Joaquin Phoenix, ThePeaceAlliance.Org; 2006**

"There are no national boundaries. The whole globe is becoming one body. In these circumstances, I think war is outdated.
Destruction of your neighbor is actually destruction of yourself."
— **Dalai Lama speaking to teenagers from 31 countries at PeaceJam, Denver, Colorado; September 2006**

AntiWar.Com

AntiWarPosters.Com

Central Committee for Conscientious Objectors, Objector.Org

CodePink4Peace.Org

Common Dreams, POB 443, Portland, ME 04112-0443; CommonDreams.Org

Cursor.Org

EndSelectiveService.Org

Grandmothers for Peace, 9444 Medstead Wy., Elk Grove, CA 95758; 916-684-8744; GrandmothersForPeace.Org

Earth Charter Initiative, University for Peace Campus, POB 138-6100, San Jose,

Costa Rica; EarthCharter.Org

EatingForPeace.Org

NotInOurName.Net

OregonPeaceWorks.Org

PeaceSupplies.Org

The Peace Worker, Oregon PeaceWorks, 104 Commercial St. NE, Salem, OR 97301; OregonPeaceWorker.Org
    Published monthly, except January and August.

Rocky Mountain Peace and Justice Center, POB 1156, Boulder, CO 80306; 303-444-6981; RMPJC.Org

School of the Americas Watch, SOAW.Org

Science for Peace, ScienceForPeace.SA.UToronto.CA

Truth Out, POB 55871 Sherman Oaks, CA 91413; TruthOut.Org

YouthLeadersInAction.Org

Peak Oil

Also see:
- Biking
- Biodiesel
- Gardening and Farming
- Hemp Farming: Work to Legalize It

Book:
- *Powerdown: Options for a Post-Carbon World*, by Richard Heinberg

CultureChange.Org

EclipseNow.Org

EndOfSuburbia.Com

FromTheWilderness.Com

HubbertPeak.Com

LifeAfterTheOilCrash.Net

NewUrbanism.Org

Odac-Info.Com

OilAwareness.Meetup.Com

OilCrash.Com

PeakOilAction.Org

PeakOil.Net

Portland City Repair Project, CityRepair.Org

PostCarbon.Org

PowerFromSun.Com

SurvivingPeakOil.Com

People

Also see:
• Love
• Magnetizing Your Life
• Thinking

The people around you are power sources. The power they carry can be helpful or harmful, or pretty evenly divided.

Some people will leach off the energy of the people around them, using them, stealing their power, or at least taking whatever they can get, and drawing others into their problems and drama. It is unhealthful for you to be around these types of people. They are like parasites, and are dependent on others to continue their behavior.

People who live off the energy of others may be so used to doing this that they lead their lives through other people's energies. They may appear strong and in control, but they are likely weak, and unable to carry themselves on their own energy, flailing about when they have no one to leach from.

As you understand these concepts, you will be able to recognize those people who are takers of your time, energy, resources, and talents. You will be able to see it in the lives of those around you. You can see them placing dependence on others. This may be done to the extent that they may keep others under control by working on deconstructing the self-esteem of those off whom they leach. There may be negative comments where there should be compliments, insults where there should be kindness, cutting down where there should be building up. Once you have recognized these people in your life you will be able to put a stop to their vacuuming of your life energy. Not doing so is enabling them to continue their actions, cheating yourself out of your life force, and degrading your power.

Not making changes to improve your life and not disconnecting parasitical people from your energy will be contributing to your victimization, and an underutilization of your potential.

Many people are actually their own worst enemy. This may be so because they don't live up to their own power, and allow themselves to be influenced by the negative energy of others.

It is amazing how many people allow themselves to be treated as if they are inferior to others; how many people don't use their own power to get ahead in life; and how many people are stuck in the circular motion of self-deceit. Many people have been in these types of situations their entire lives. It has become their norm. Anything outside of what is normal to them may become uncomfortable – even if healthier. Recognize if you are one of these types of people who allow their lives to be overtaken by the lives of others. Take an assessment of the people in your life. Identify the relationships in your life that are wearing you down. Also, identify the relationships in your life that are healthy.

If you don't like what you find in the assessment of the people in your life, take action to change things.

Keep in mind that it is unproductive to blame others for your situation. It is also not productive to expect others to improve your life. It is up to you to make the changes in your life that you want.

You may know of people who have many talents, skills, and high levels of intellect, and who do nothing with these attributes. They likely are involved in self-destructive behavior, or mindless activities, such as staring at the television, or hanging out with other people whose lives are tragedies. Perhaps you see some of your traits in them. Maybe they are some of the people who are closest to you. If your life is highly unsatisfactory to you, it is likely that you are surrounding yourself with similar people. This has likely become your norm, but it is not your natural, and it never can be.

Some energy-zapping people will be able to deal with your actions to take control of your life. They may recognize what they were doing, correct their ways, and be able to conduct themselves with respect to your life in a way that benefits both of you in great ways. Others may get upset and respond like spoiled children as you stop allowing them to continue the unhealthful relationship. Still others may feel overwhelmed by the change they see in you and become a nuisance and a problem to you. The latter should be a sign to you that you need to disassociate yourself from them.

Stop allowing others to steal your life. Stop letting yourself to be influenced by that which brings you down.

Living a life conforming to the projections of others is one way to limit yourself to a small fraction of what you can be. You may be playing a part in supporting someone else's life by subjecting yourself to their visions and dreams, while living little of your own. If that is the way you want to live, that is your right. Maybe it works for you, but maybe you are cheating yourself, underestimating your abilities, and denying yourself the expression of your talents and intellect. By conforming to the lives of others, what you may be doing is truly setting yourself up for deep regret when you realize that you have not established and worked toward the expression of your own talents, abilities, and intellect.

No matter how you are living, it could be an interesting exercise to make a list of things you want, things you want to do, and things you need to do to bring about the life that you would like to have. Ideally you would be able to work on this with the person with whom you are in a relationship, and align your goals, priorities, needs, and wants. Then work together to attain those things.

> "People do not lack courage, they simply are overburdened by an abundance of conformity. Persistence requires courage, while quitting requires conformity."
> — David Wolfe

There is bravery, courage, and dignity in working to improve your life.

Look at your life as though it were a garden. Eliminate that which chokes the beauty and damages the harvest of good things that you should get out of life. Live your life as if your days are golden, and not stolen.

Changing your life from what it is to what it can be, especially if the change is radical, may require strengths you have never exercised, and perhaps strengths you never knew you had. If people have become lazy in their lives, spending years living an unhealthful lifestyle, eating the same unhealthful foods, requiring little of their faculties to get through their days, and doing the same things over and over, breaking away from their life may feel incredible in an uncomfortable way, but may also feel amazingly liberating.

As you change your life and become different from what you used to be, you may also find yourself getting attention that you are not used to – including criticism that you have not experienced. When people are accustomed to seeing you live and look a certain way, and then they see you differently, they also may feel uncomfortable. You will be breaking out of the role that you have been playing. People will have to recast you in their mind as not the person they thought you were, and maybe the person they thought you couldn't be.

When you become healthy, people notice. Your skin, shape, and movement change. Your confidence and energy improve. It is then that people may be interested in what it is that you are doing that changed you.

Improving your life may be as difficult or as easy as you make it, or that you allow it to be. But it is better to use your energy to achieve your goals and live your life rather than to allow others to take them from you.

Don't waste time in trying to tell others what you are capable of doing. It is always more empowering to plan and then accomplish your goals. Others may or may not acknowledge your accomplishments. Whether they do or do not recognize your achievements does not devalue your work. Don't expect praise. Keep moving along toward accomplishing your goals.

Nurture your life with good things. Recognize that you are worthy and capable of improving your life. Work with visualization techniques. Keep a journal to help you build and journey toward a better life. Work daily to achieve your list of goals. Raise your standards to that which will bring about good things in your life. Allow yourself to be inspired by good things. Build your life by using your intellect, talents, abilities, and energy to work for you. Surround yourself and associate yourself with the elements, sounds, literature, food, actions, and people that will work to uplift you and help propel you into a better life. Experience joy, respect, satisfaction, kindness, and love in your life. Let this be your norm.

Realize that there is no competition. You are only working to improve yourself, regardless of what others are doing. Comparing yourself to others is degrading to your spirit, to others, and weakens you. Set the pace for yourself to improve your own situation, and you may be surprised how it can help to inspire others to do the same.

When you relieve yourself of the feeling that you are not competing with others, you will begin to understand the concept that there is no competition. All you are doing is working to improve your life regardless of what others are doing.

Allow the good of others to affect you. Reject the negative. Accept the positive. Acknowledge the good.

Nurture the things you like about people. Recognize that your thoughts and words can seduce the best qualities from people, and from yourself. Complimenting, encouraging, and nurturing good in others is doing the same for yourself.

Treating others in a way that respects their intellect, talents, and abilities creates an atmosphere of respect within you that will bring about the respect of your own intellect, talents, and abilities. This is why you should work to acknowledge the positive aspects of those around you. It is in alignment with the theory that you should treat others as you would like to be treated.

Pesticides

Also see:
• Organic Issues

Pesticides are toxic chemicals designed to kill living things. They also lead to birth defects, learning disabilities and cancers in humans and animals.

Farmers who work on farms where pesticides are used are at the greatest risk, as are those who live in farm communities where the pesticides lurk in the air, land, and water. Children who live in farm communities where pesticides are used on nearby fields have higher than average rates of asthma and other ailments. People who work in the pesticide factories, and those who live near the factories are also at risk.

When you purchase food, cosmetics, and fabrics, seek out those that have been grown without the use of pesticides.

BeyondPesticides.Org

FoodNews.Org

Mindfully.Org/Pesticide

Pesticide Action Network International, PAN-International.Org

Pesticide Action Network of North America, PANNA.Org

Pet Care

Consider what you are feeding your pet. Many pet food companies include substances in their products that are not only bad for pet health, but for the environment as well. Refrain from purchasing pet food that contains artificial dyes and flavors, synthetic preservatives, pesticides, hormones, and other toxins. When in doubt, contact the pet food manufacturer and ask for a list of the ingredients in their products.

A raw food diet is healthier for your pet.

Consider that the chemicals you are applying to your pet for flea and tick control are also toxic to the pet, to you, and to the environment. Seek natural pet care products that won't harm us.

Consider that the cat litter you are using may be toxic for you as well as your pet. Use natural cat litter.

If you live in an area where you must clean up after your pet, use biodegradable poop bags, or a scooper.

PETA.Org

VeganCats.Com

VegetarianDogs.Com

Plastics, Packaging, and Pollution

At this point, how can we get plastics and packaging out of our lives?

While you may not be able to get rid of plastics and packaging from every area of your life, you can work to eliminate some of them.

Instead of fabric and clothing that contain synthetic materials, choose those that are made from natural, plant-derived fibers.

Instead of buying packaged foods, purchase from the bulk section at your local natural foods store.

Instead of keeping your food in plastic containers, keep them in glass, ceramic, wood, and/or bamboo containers.

Instead of a bed and blankets that contain synthetic fabrics, choose bedding that is made from natural fibers.

Look for plastics that are biodegradable, which is a plastic that degrades from the activities of naturally occurring microorganisms, including algae, bacteria, and fungus.

Biodegradable plastics are different from compostable plastics, which may not completely degrade or get assimilated by microorganisms.

How a plastic degrades depends on what it is exposed to in the environment: heat, cold, wet, dry, oxygen, surrounding organisms, etc.

All plastics will degrade in that they will eventually warp, shrink, fall apart, or turn into a powder or smaller fragmented pieces. But some plastics contain more harmful chemicals than others. Plastics that don't degrade into the soil are called recalcitrant plastics.

Some companies are making plastics that are made from corn or other vegetable matter, such as potato peels. These may degrade completely into harmless matter.

Other plastics that are labeled compostable are blended with petroleum-based polymers, and these are not the best for the environment.

Some companies that label their products as biodegradable are not telling the truth. Some disposable diaper companies label their products as biodegradable, but the plastics are a mix of starch-based plastic with petroleum plastic, which does not completely biodegrade, but only breaks into smaller parts.

"Soft plastics and phthalates: PVC plastic – those pliable, gummy-like plastics – are laden with phthalates, chemicals that have been linked to premature birth, reproductive defects, early onset of puberty in girls, and reduced sperm quality in adult males. PVC is used in everything from home building materials to food packaging to children's toys. Phthalates can leach out of these products, which is particularly concerning for children who explore the world by putting things in their mouths. While many manufacturers have removed phthalates from toys and other products intended for very young children, there is no law requiring this and very few products are labeled as such.

Hard plastics and bisphenol-A: Polycarbonate plastic, which is hard, shatter-resistant and often clear in color, contains bisphenol-A, a hormone-disrupting chemical linked to Down's syndrome, early onset of puberty, obesity, hyperactivity, and breast and prostate cancer. Almost all plastic baby bottles are made from polycarbonate plastic, as well as popular camping water bottles (like some Nalgene brand bottles) and large water cooler jugs. In addition, a resin made with bisphenol-A coats the inside of aluminum and tin food cans. Bisphenol-A leaches readily into food and liquids. There is no law prohibiting its use, and currently very few manufacturers have taken any action to stop using polycarbonate plastic in their products.

- Avoid: Food containers with polycarbonate or PVC plastic.
- Avoid: #7 recycling code or 'PC' (polycarbonate) and #3 (PVC) on the bottom/underside of the product.
- Avoid: Foods wrapped in 'cling' plastic.
- Choose: 'PVC Free' labels on toys.
- Choose: Plastic food containers labeled with #1, #2, #4, or #5 recycling code on the bottom.
- Do not: Heat foods in plastic containers.
- Choose: Glass for baby bottles and food containers. Look for glass options rather than plastics or cans.
- Do not: Allow children to put plastic toys in their mouths.
- Do not: Allow baby milk to stand in plastic bottles for long periods."
  — **EnvironmentCalifornia.Org; 2006**

Biodegradable Products Institute, BPI.World.Org

EnvironmentCalifornia.Org

Mindfully.Org/Plastic

US Composting Council, CompostingCouncil.Org

Politicians

Also see:
- Activist Directories

Don't wait around for politicians to change the world and make it into a better place. Start with yourself, working in your community to create good happenings and change things for the better, and spread it from there.

Get involved in supporting the environmental groups listed in this book.

Want to change the world? Be your own revolution. Start with what you eat and how you spend your time, energy, and resources.

Your actions and words are the blossoms of your thoughts. Want to improve your life? Improve your thoughts.

Consider running for office. Get involved in your community. Work for a more environmentally safe and sustainable culture that doesn't use fossil fuels.

Prisoner Rights

Also see:
• Hemp Farming: Work to Legalize It

America has the largest prison population on the planet. Home of the free.

Amnesty International, AIUSA.Org

Anarchists Prisoner Legal Aid Network, 818 SW 3rd Ave., PMB 354, Portland, OR 97204; APLAN@Tao.CA

Civil Liberties Defense Center, 259 East Fifth Ave., Ste. 300, Eugene, OR 97401; CLDC.Org

Critical Resistance, 1904 Franklin St., Ste. 504, Oakland, CA 94612; 510-444-0484; CriticalResistance.Org

Drug Policy Alliance, DrugPolicy.Org

Earth Liberation Prisoner's Support Network, SpiritOfFreedom.Org.Uk

Friends of MOVE, POB 19709, Philadelphia, PA 19143

Human Rights Watch, HRW.Org

The Moratorium Campaign, MoratoriumCampaign.Org

North American Earth Liberation Prisoners Support Network, POB 11331, Eugene, OR 97440; NAELPSN@Tao.CA

Prison Activist Resource Center, POB 339, Berkeley CA 94701; 510-893-4648; PrisonActivist.Org

Prison Dharma Network, POB 4623, Boulder CO 80306; 303-544-5923;

PrisonDharmaNetwork.Org

The Sentencing Project, SentencingProject.Org

Stop Prisoner Rape, SPR.Org

Protein

Books:
- *Diet for a New America*, by John Robbins
- *Diet for a Small Planet*, by Frances Moore Lappé
- *The Food Revolution*, by John Robbins

Some vegetarians and vegans get caught up in eating all sorts of soy bean products – soy milk, soy ice cream, soy yogurt, tofu everything, soy burgers, soy powders, soy cheese, and soy custards and puddings. This is done with the belief that soy protein is needed in the diet.

Proteins are made out of chains of amino acids. There is an abundance of amino acids in raw fruits and vegetables. The body makes the protein it needs out of the amino acids.

Again, I use an example: All the numerous types of animals that are natural vegans, such as cows, horses, gorillas, giraffes, deer, goats, elephants, etc., eat plants. Their bodies make protein out of the substances within the plants.

I don't depend on soy, or any one particular plant, for protein in my diet. I eat a variety of fruits, vegetables, herbs, nuts, and seeds, and my body gets more than enough protein-building properties in the form of amino acids.

"Perhaps the biggest misconception in the field of nutrition is the confusion between fat and protein. When someone says, 'I need protein,' what they really need and want is fat. Most people and nutritionists cannot distinguish between the desire for fat and the desire for protein. Many raw-food advocates have recommended nuts for protein, when in reality the value of nuts is in their fat. People can give up steak much easier than cheese, because steak is mostly protein, whereas cheese is mostly fat."
— **David Wolfe**

The fiber of our physical body is made up of protein. So people tend to think that we need to eat protein in the form of flesh to build our tissues. This is a huge misconception that drives people to focus on eating diets that are chiefly protein, and which are rough on the system. It also has helped to fuel the animal farming industry, slaughterhouses, the heart attack industry, deforestation, the colon cancer industry, the hospital industry, the pharmaceutical industry, and animal cruelty on a massive scale.

You do not need to eat animal flesh to get protein.

If you don't eat animal flesh, you do not need to eat soy to get protein.

Your body needs amino acids to build protein. A Sunfood diet provides an abundance of amino acids from a variety of raw plant sources.

Even when a person eats animal protein, the body does not simply transfer that protein into the tissues of the body. The body takes the amino acids from the protein to form the type of amino acid chain that it needs, forming its own protein.

As Wolfe points out, even in the time of life when the body is going through an amazing increase in size, the first year of life after birth, the breast milk one relies on at that time is only about 2 percent protein, and is mostly fat.

In addition to the protein-dominant foods of legumes, mushrooms are also protein-dominant. But they are not a plant, they are a fungus. They are okay to eat in moderation. They contain the mineral potassium as well as nutritional compounds that improve the immune system and may prevent cancer.

I have paranoia about picking my own mushrooms from the wild, as I know that certain types of mushrooms can make you very ill, and others can kill you. Of course there are also mushrooms that can open your mind. Mushrooms that fall under the poisonous category make up only a small fraction of the thousands of mushroom species. There are only a few hundred types of mushrooms that are considered to have a good taste. I prefer to buy my mushrooms at the market, or from people who are educated about mushrooms – such as the family who have a mushroom stand at the local farmers' market.

Protein-dominant seeds are legumes. These include chickpeas (also known as garbanzo beans), kidney beans, lentils, mung beans, and soybeans. Protein-dominant foods can be harsh on the system. To increase the presence of amino acids and enzymes in legumes, soak them for several hours in water, or sprout them over three to six days (being sure to rinse them at least once a day, and preferably twice). Soaking will make them less heavy and harsh on the digestive system, and provide more nutrients, such as enzymes.

> "Real strength and building material comes from green-leafed vegetables, seeds, and superfoods where the amino acids are found. These are our true 'protein foods.' They contain all the amino acids we require. We might look at the gorilla, zebra, giraffe, hippo, rhino, or elephant and find they build their enormous musculature on green-leafed vegetation and grass seeds exclusively."
> — David Wolfe

> "Carrot tops have several times more nutrition than the roots, but the opinion that greens are for rabbits, sheep, and cows, has been preventing us from eating carrot tops in our salads. We routinely throw away the most nutritious part of the carrot plant! The roots are much more palatable to human taste than the tops because the roots contain significantly more sugar and water. The tops are bitter from the abundant amount of nutrients in them."
> — Victoria Boutenko in her book *Green for Life*, RawFamily.Com

> "The Benefits of Green-Leafed Vegetables (Raw):
> - Insure good, daily elimination.
> - Chlorophyll, Nature's medicine.
> - Counteract acid-forming foods such as nuts, seeds, avocados, cooked foods, apple cider vinegar, proteins, animal products.
> - Counteract acid-forming air toxins such as carbon dioxide, carbon monoxide, sulfuric acid, nitrous oxide, chlorine, etc.
> - Greens are the lung cleansers.
> - Deactivate, combine with, and help wash out heavy metals.
> - Alkaline-forming foods. Greens make the body alkaline.
> - Best source of minerals (calcium, sodium, magnesium, trace minerals).
> - Balance the endocrine system (especially if wild greens are eaten).
> - Green-leaves naturally brush and clean the teeth.
> - Green-leaves naturally broom out the entire digestive tract as they pass through the body.
> - They ground the mind.
> - They calm the system.
> - They are karmically neutral."
> — David Wolfe, *The Sunfood Diet Success System*

Don't believe the nonsense put out by the meat and dairy industries that tell you to consume meat, milk, and eggs to get protein into your diet. Even the United States government programs that supposedly "establish" nutrition "requirements" – such as the food triangle – are flawed, and are strongly influenced by the financial interests of the meat, dairy, and egg industries.

In addition, much of the nutritional information presented to children in their classrooms is flawed, and much of it is provided free to school systems from organizations supported by the meat and dairy industries. Included in this biased and flawed information that they hand out is the advice that humans should eat a large amount of animal protein, according to the U.S. Recommended Daily Allowance (USRDA), and the government's food triangle, which are largely nonsense.

Those people who consume the largest amounts of animal protein also experience degenerative diseases, such as heart disease, diabetes, arthritis, cancers, etc., in conjunction with the amount of animal flesh, milk, and eggs they consume.

A diet that is abundant in animal oils and animal protein leads to a clogged body system. When a person eats the kind of animal protein-laden diet that is recommended in the U.S. Government "food triangle," the cells, blood system, and lymph system slow down as the body becomes saturated with heavy fats, cholesterol, and undigested and indigestible animal protein. This provides a bed for toxins to settle into; strangles the cells from necessary nutrients they need to function efficiently; and taxes the energy of the cells and system as they try to deal with all the unnecessary substances of a protein-dominant and cooked food diet. In the long term, a diet heavy in meat and dairy begins to break down and degenerate as a result of being too acidic and out-of-balance with Nature. The result is the types of diseases that are common among people who eat a lot of dairy, eggs, and meat: heart disease, arthritis, cancers, bone distortion, diabetes, etc.

To detox and balance a body that is out-of-balance, all one needs to do is start following a Sunfood diet, and run with it – raw vegetables; raw fruit; raw berries; raw herbs; raw seeds; and raw nuts; water vegetables; quality water; daily exercise; and a brain that is exercised through use of its intellect, talent, and skills, and that generates positive thought processes through intentionally goal-oriented living.

Publications

100Fires.Com
  Sells books, CDs, DVDs, videos, cassettes, periodicals, and other items relating to the environment, peace, ecology, and more.

Clamor Magazine, POB 1225, Bowling Green, OH 43402; ClamorMagazine.Org

Earth First! Journal, POB 3023, Tucson, AZ 85702; 520-620-6900; EarthFirstJournal.Org; EarthFirst.Org

Earth Island Journal, 300 Broadway, Ste. 28, San Francisco, CA 94133; 415-788-3666; EarthIsland.Org

Earth Light magazine, 111 Fairmount Ave., Oakland, CA 94611, USA; 510-451-4926; EarthLight.Org

Eco-LogicBooks.Com, England

E the Environmental Magazine, 28 Knight St., Norwalk, CT 06851; POB 5098, Westport, CT 06881; 203-854-5559; EMagazine.Com

Green Anarchy, POB 11331, Eugene, OR 97440; GreenAnarchy.Org

Green Teacher magazine, Canada: Green Teacher, 95 Robert St., Toronto, ON M5S 2K5; United States: Green Teacher, POB 452, Niagara Falls, NY 14304-0452; 416-960-1244; 888-804-1486; GreenTeacher.Com

Herbivore magazine, 5519 NE 30th Ave., Portland, OR 97211; HerbivoreMagazine.Com

Hope Dance, POB 15609, San Luis Obispo, CA 93406; HopeDance.Org

ImpactPress.Com

LanternBooks.Com

Living Nutrition magazine, POB 256, Sebastopol, CA 95473; 707-829-0362; LivingNutrition.Com

MotherEarthNews.Com

Mother Jones magazine, POB 334, Mt. Morris, IL 61054; 800-438-6656; 415-665-6637; MotherJones.Com

NaturalHomeMagazine.Com

Orion, The Orion Society and Myrin Institute, 187 Main St., Great Barrington, MA 01230; OrionSociety.Org

Permaculture Activist, POB 5516, Bloomington, IN 47407; PermacultureActivist.Net

Permaculture magazine: Solutions for Sustainable Living, PermaCulture.Co.UK

Satya, 539 1st St., Brooklyn, NY 11215; SatyaMag.Com

Revolution Books, 206-325-7415; SeattleRevolutionBooks.BlogSpot.Com

The Sun, POB 469061, Escondido, CA 92046; TheSunMagazine.Org

Terrain, Northern California's Environmental Quarterly, 2530 San Pablo Ave., Berkeley, CA 94702; EcologyCenter.Org

Threshold, Student Environmental Action Coalition, POB 31909, Philadelphia, PA 19104; SEAC.Org

The Trumpeter: Journal of Ecosophy, C/O Athabasca University, 1 University Dr., Athabasca, AB T9S 3A3, Canada; 800-780-9041; TheTrumpeter.AtHabascaU.CA

Utne reader, 1624 Harmon Pl., Minneapolis, MN 55403; 613-338-5040; Utne.Com

Vegan Voice magazine, POB 30 Mimbin, NSW, 2480, Australia; Veganic.Net

Wild Earth, POB 455, Richmond, VT 05477; 802-434-4077; Wild-Earth.Org

Z magazine, 18 Millfield St., Woods Hole, MA 02543; 508-548-9063; ZMag.Org
  Z Video has produced over 50 videos on politics, economics, foreign policy, etc. These are available for personal, classroom, and organizing use.

Raw Vegan Potlucks and Support Groups

Also see:
- Raw Vegan Web Sites
- Restaurants, Cafes and Delis Providing Raw Cuisine

RawFoodInfo.Com

RawFood.Meetup.Com

Sunfood.Com

Raw Vegan Web Sites

Also see:
- Raw Vegan Potlucks and Support Groups
- Restaurants, Cafes and Delis Providing Raw Cuisine

Matt Amsden, Santa Monica CA and New York, NY; RawVolution.Com

Michelle Audria, MAudria.Com

BarakaFoods.Com

Sergei Boutenko, HarmonyHikes.Com

CilantroLive.Com

AlissaCohen.Com

Creative Health Institute, CreativeHealthUSA.Com

Kerrie Cushing, DancingButterfly.Net

Dr. Richard DeAndrea, M.D., N.D., 21DayDetox.Com

Ekaya Institute of Living Food Education, TheGardenDiet.Com

TheEuphoriaCompany.Com

Foodology.Com
  Company produces some packaged raw vegan products.

FunkyRaw.Com

RoeGallo.Com

TheGardenDiet.Com

GardenOfHealth.Com

GoJuvo.Com

Dr. Douglas Graham, D.C., FoodNSport.Com

Healthful Living International, HealthfulLivingIntl.Org

Health Force Nutritionals, HealthForce.Com

Hippocrates Health Institute, HippocratesInst.Com

Roxanne Klein, RawRox.Com

Live-Food.Com

LivingFoodInstitute.Com

Living Light Culinary Arts Institute, RawFoodChef.Com

Living Nutrition magazine, LivingNutrition.Com

Living and Raw Foods, Living-Foods.Com

Living Tree Community Foods, LivingTreeCommunity.Com

North Bay Living Foods Community, BeRaw.Com

OneLuckyDuck.Com

PearMagazine.Com

Pure Joy Living Foods, PureJoyLivingFoods.Com

AmyRachelle.Com

RawAndJuicy.Com

RawBakery.Com

Rawcreation Ltd. / Shazzie, Shazzie.Com

RawCuisine.Co.UK

Raw Family & Victoria Boutenko, RawFamily.Com

RawFoodChat.Com

RawFoodChef.Com

Raw Food Equipment Store, RawFoodEquipment.Com

RawFoodLife.Com

RawFood.Meetup.Com

RawFoodSuperStore.Com

RawForLife.Com

RawLife.Com

TheRawGourmet.Com

RawLifeLine.Com Shipped Raw Meals, RawLifeline.Com

RawNewEnglandCommunity.Com

RawPower.Info

The Raw Raw Girls, Eugene, OR; RawRawGirls.Com
  Enewsletter available through TheRawRawGirls@Yahoo.Com

RawReform.Com

RawRob.Com

RawRox.Com

Rawsheed.com

RawSpiritFest.Com

Rawstock.US

RawTimes.Com

RawVeganNetwork.Com

Rawvolution.Com

Rejuvenative Foods, Rejuvenative.Com

Rhio's Raw Food, RawFoodInfo.Com

Chad Sarno/Vital Creations, RawChef.Org

SomeLikeItRaw.Net

SproutMan.Com

SunfoodLiving.Com

Sunfood Nutrition, Sunfood.Com

SuperSprouts.Com

Tree of Life Rejuvenation Center, TreeOfLife.Nu

TreeSong.Org

Renée Loux, EuphoricOrganics.Com

Vital Creations, RawChef.Org

Woody Harrelson and Laura Louie, VoiceYourself.Com

Ann Wigmore Institute, AnnWigmore.Org

David Wolfe, DavidWolfe.Com

Recipe Books for a Raw Vegan Kitchen

Recipe books (not "cook" books) that may be helpful in your raw vegan kitchen. For the latest list, access:
Sunfood Nutrition, 11653 Riverside Dr., Lakeside, CA 92040; 800-205-2350; 888-RAW-FOOD; International: +001-619-596-7979; Sunfood.Com

- *Angel Foods: Healthy Recipes for Heavenly Bodies*, by Cherie Soria
- *The Balanced Plate*, by Renée Loux
- *The Complete Book of Raw Food*, by Lori Baird, editor
- *A Cup Of Sunshine: Recipes Straight from the Garden*, by Dianne Onstad
- *Detox Delights*, by Shazzie
- *Detox Your World*, by Shazzie
- *Dining in the Raw*, by Rita Romano
- *Eating without Heating*, by Sergei and Valya Boutenko
- *Food for a Golden Age*, by Urs Hochstrasser-Maharaj
- *Garden of Eden Raw Fruit & Vegetable Recipes*, by Phyllis Avery
- *Green for Life*, by Victoria Boutenko
- *The Hippocrates Diet and Health Program*, by Ann Wigmore
- *Hooked on Raw*, by Rhio
- *The Joy of Living Live: A Raw Food Journey*, by Zakhah
- *Lifefood Recipe Book*, by Annie Padden Jubb and David Jubb
- *Living Cuisine: The Art and Spirit of Raw Foods*, by Renée Loux
- *Living Foods for Radiant Health*, by Elaine Bruce
- *Living in the Raw*, by Rose Lee Calabro
- *Living with Green Power*, by Elysa Markowitz

- *Love Your Body*, by Viktoras Kulvinskas
- *Naked Chocolate*, by David Wolfe and Shazzie
- *Rainbow Green Live Food Cuisine*, by Dr Gabriel Cousens M.D.
- *Raw Family*, by Victoria, Igor, Sergei and Valya Boutenko
- *Raw Foods for Busy People*, by Jordan Maerin
- *The Raw Gourmet*, by Nomi Shannon
- *Raw in Ten Minutes*, by Bryan Au
- *Rawsome!*, by Brigitte Mars
- *Raw Transformation*, by Wendy Rudell
- *The Raw Truth*, by Jeremy Safron
- *RawVolution Gourmet Living Cuisine*, by Matt Amsden
- *Recipes for Longer Life*, by Ann Wigmore
- *SmartMonkey Foods: The Art of Raw*, by Ani Phyo and Ede
- *Smoothies and Other Scrumptious Delights*, by Elysa Markowitz
- *The Sprouting Book*, by Ann Wigmore
- *Sproutman's Kitchen Garden Cookbook*, by Steve Meyerowitz
- *Sunfood Cuisine*, by Frederic Patenaude
- *Thank God for Raw: Recipes for Health*, by Julie Wandling
- *Uncooking with Jameth & Kim*, by Jameth Sheridan, N.D. and Kim Sheridan, N.D.
- *Vibrant Living*, by James Levin, M.D. and Natalie Cederquist
- *Vital Creations: An Organic Life Experience*, by Chad Sarno
- *Warming Up to Living Foods*, by Elysa Markowitz

Recycling

BioCycle: Journal of Composting & Organic Recycling,
JGPress.Com/BioCycle.htm

Earth911.Org
  Site contains abundant information about recycling and toxic and hazardous waste disposal. Enter your zip code to view your local environmental information.

EcoCycle.Org

FreeCycle.Org

  "The Freecycle Network was started in May 2003 to promote waste reduction in Tucson's downtown and help save desert landscape from being taken over by landfills. The Network provides individuals and non-profits an electronic forum to 'recycle' unwanted items. One person's trash can truly be another's treasure."

Global Recycling Network, GRN.Com

National Recycling Coalition, NRC-Recycle.Org

NWMaterialsMart.Org

Recycle.CC

ZeroWasteAmerica.Org

Rejuvelac

Rejuvelac is fermented water. It is rich in B vitamins, vitamins C and E, enzymes, probiotic bacteria, lactic acid, and amino acids. Drinking rejuvelac is healthful for the digestive tract. It can also be used as an ingredient to add nutrients to salad dressings, and raw vegan soups.

Rejuvelac was advocated most notably by the late Dr. Ann Wigmore. It is easily made, but standards of cleanliness should be followed to prevent contamination.

Common seeds used to make rejuvelac include barley, buckwheat, millet, oats, quinoa, rye, and wheat, with the most common being wheat. The seeds should be from an organic source, and raw/unheated. Most are available at natural foods stores.

Soak the seeds for several hours in clean water.

Discard the water, rinsing the seeds in a mesh strainer.

Place the seeds in a clean sprouting jar, cover with a screen top or a clean, sheer cloth with a string holding it onto the top of the jar. They can also be placed in a glass casserole dish with a glass top. The key is to keep the seeds moist as they sprout, and not immersed in water.

Tip the jar with the bottom down at about a 45° angle by placing it in a big bowl and allowing the jar to tip sideways.

Place it in an area that is out of direct Sun light, in a low-light area.

Rinse the seeds two to three times a day by putting clean water in the jar, lightly swirling it, replacing the top, and tilting the jar over the sink, or outside.

After three to five days you should have seeds with little root tails on them.

Rinse the sprouts one more time, then put them into a four-inch-deep casserole dish, fill with water about 3/4 of the way deep. Some people use a large sprouting jar with a screen top. We like using a casserole dish because it provides a wide area for the cultures in the air to settle in and mix with the microflora on the surface of the grain. Keep the casserole partially covered with its glass top.

Set this in a clean, dry place at room temperature out of direct Sun light, in a dimly lit area, for 12 to 72 hours.

The fermenting time varies according to the type of seed you are using, and the temperature. When it is warmer, the fermenting kicks in faster. In cooler temperatures it takes longer. Sometimes the fermenting won't take place if the room is below 65 degrees.

The natural cultures in the air will be attracted to the water, mixing with the microflora on the grain, triggering the fermentation.

The soaking water should start to smell pungent, like a smelly cheese. It will start to become cloudy with a very slight yellow tinge. It should smell clean, and not rotten. The longer you ferment the water, the stronger the smell and taste will become.

Don't breathe on it. Don't dip a tasting spoon in it after you have put the spoon in your mouth. This is a live culture and you don't want to contaminate it with germs from your hands or mouth.

Up to 72 hours is about the extent of it. If it hasn't fermented by then, maybe it won't happen. I once made rejuvelac that didn't seem to start fermenting until after three days. When it finally did, it turned out great. The more you make rejuvelac the more you will learn when it is working, or when you need to toss it and start over.

When it smells nicely fragrant with a kind of sour and tangy smell, it is time to strain the sprouts out of the water. You can scoop out the sprouts using a straining or slotted spoon, or carefully pour the container into a strainer atop a bowl or large jar. Some people use a screened coffee strainer for this step.

The water is the rejuvelac. Keep it in a glass jar. It can be refrigerated for up to five to seven days.

Rejuvelac should have a pleasant but sour and tangy smell with a tart taste that may seem slightly carbonated. A slight clear to white or slightly yellowish film may form on the top; this is a good sign that it is very nutritionally strong.

If for any reason you are uncomfortable with the smell of the rejuvelac, toss it. As with any food that may be spoiled, when in doubt, toss it out.

You can drink rejuvelac by itself, or you can add lemon or other fruit juice or blended berries to make it more palatable.

It can also be used to make seed and or nut cheeses. One simple cheese is made by soaking pine nuts/pignolis in water for several hours, then strain the nuts and blend with rejuvelac, sea salt, and nutritional yeast (not brewer's yeast). You can also add fresh Italian herbs. Let this mixture stand in a clean bowl covered with a clean cloth for 12 to 24 hours to ferment at room temperature between 65 and 85 degrees Fahrenheit. You can use it as a soft cheese, or spread it on dehydrator sheets and dehydrate at 105° F for about 12 to 24 hours. The final product should be a flaky Parmesan-type cheese you can use in salads. If the cheese is well dehydrated, it can keep for several weeks in a covered container in a cool, dry place.

One book that has recipes for seed cheeses and dressings using rejuvelac is Renée Loux's *Living Cuisine: The Art and Spirit of Raw Foods*. It may be at your local natural foods store or library.

AnnWigmore.Com

HisHealingWays.Com/Rejuvelac/MakeRejuvelac.html

Renée Loux, EuphoricOrganics.Com

SproutPeople.Com/Cookery/Rejuvelac.html

Religion-Associated Environmental Groups

"I only went out for a walk and finally concluded to stay out till sundown, for going out, I found, was really going in."
— **John Muir, The Wilderness World of John Muir**

I am probably not the best person to listen to if you want to hear favorable things about organized religions. I'm not associated with any organized religion. Nor do I care to be.

However, studies have shown that people who regularly participate in a social community, such as through a church, club, or organization, are found to experience better health than those who do not. This appears to be particularly true with older people.

Too often it appears religion focuses on shame, limits potential, and drives people to lose the beauty of their individuality – all while working money out of people's pockets to support self-serving ministers.

To me it seems you will have a better chance of becoming a world-renowned artist by going to truck driving school than you will of becoming closer to God by associating with most of the churches that are in business.

To paraphrase Gandhi: I like Jesus, but I don't like these Christians, they don't remind me of Jesus. Too often they seem to have overlooked Jesus' teachings on love.

It would be nice if churches, which are major land owners on every continent, would stop building parking lots and buildings, and discontinued investing their money in commercial sprawl and in stocks of companies that are destroying the planet. Instead, it would be good if they became more involved in protecting this wonderful planet.

It seems to me that the humble person described in the *New Testament* wouldn't relate very well to a large number of those who call themselves "Christian." Many are often pro-war, live selfishly in opulent homes, think it is okay to spend more money building prisons than to build schools, support officials that allocate more money for the military than on protecting the environment, and appear to live with the attitude expressed through their actions that Earth and animals are here for us to violate and destroy.

To everyone's benefit, there are many people in all religions who are becoming involved in environmental issues, protecting wildlife, and following a diet that is more respectful of the treasures of Nature.

There are also some churches that are doing a good job at accepting a broad variety of personalities, including those who have been rejected by other churches. These churches are encouraging and nurturing people to bring out their talents, intellect, and individual beauty. Some incorporate dance, art, music, song, poetry, literature, environmental responsibility, yoga, and veganism into their gatherings. One of these is Agape International Spiritual Center in Culver City, California.

If you are churchgoer, consider organizing an environmental group among your fellow worshipers.

Some people may find interest in the following groups.

Agape International Spiritual Center, 5700 Buckingham Pkwy., Culver City, CA 90230; AgapeLive.Com

Buddhist Peace Fellowship, BPF.Org

Catholic Conservation Center, Conservation.Catholic.Org

Christians for Environmental Stewardship, RestoringEden.Org

Coalition on the Environment and Jewish Life, COEJL.Org

Earth Sangha (Buddhist-related), EarthSangha.Org

Episcopal Network for Stewardship, TENS.Org

Evangelical Environmental Network, CreationCare.Org

The Coalition on the Environment and Jewish Life of Southern California, Faith2Green.Com; info@CoejlSC.Org

Interfaith Council for Environmental Stewardship, Stewards.Net

Islamic Foundation for Ecological and Environmental Sciences, IFEES.Org

Jewish Vegetarians of North America, JewishVeg.Com

> "Economics was the initial reason I turned to vegetarianism. I had been teaching agricultural economics and became increasingly aware that it took up to 16 pounds of grain or other plant foods to produce one pound of meat. In earlier eras and poorer times, animals were only fed coarse plants and other things that humans could not digest. Today, in industrial societies, animals are fed grains, soybeans and other foods that could well be enjoyed by people. This makes meat and other animal foods a luxury; and, in a world where there are many hungry people, an increasingly extravagant luxury... Not only does moving toward a vegetarian diet save grains and beans for human consumption, the reduction of meat production saves water, energy, soil, and other scarce resources."
> — Vegetarianism: The Economic Reasons, by Roslyn Kunin, PhD; Spring 1996 issue of the *Jewish Vegetarian Newsletter* of the Jewish Vegetarians of North America.

National Religious Partnerships for the Environment, NRPE.Org

North American Coalition for Christianity and Ecology, NACCE.Org

Religious Campaign for Forest Conservation (Jewish related), CreationEthics.Org

US Conference of Catholic Bishops Environmental Justice Program, USCCB.Org/sdwp/EJP/Index.htm

Restaurants, Cafes, and Delis Providing Raw Cuisine

Also see:
- Raw Vegan Potlucks and Support Groups
- Raw Vegan Web Sites

For an up-to-date list of restaurants that serve raw vegan cuisine, access the following site: **RawFoodInfo.Com**

Vegetarian Resource Group, POB 1463, Baltimore, MD 21203; 410-366-8343; VRG.Org
In addition to links to other vegetarian sites, this site contains a list of vegetarian restaurants, and guides for vegetarian travelers.

Vegetarian-Restaurants.Net
Lists vegetarian restaurants and food stores in the U.S., Canada, England, Europe, and other areas of the world.

If you eat at restaurants, seek out those that serve organically grown food. As explained throughout this book, organically grown food is better for you. This is because it is grown without toxic chemicals that cause cancers, birth defects, environmental damage, and depleted soil. The roots of organically grown plants grow deeper, mining a wider variety of nutrients, which results in plants that are more vitamin and mineral rich, and have a stronger vibrancy.
One restaurant that is making food for dozens of people a day saves energy and resources.
If you don't have a raw vegan cafe in your town, start one! Get your recipes from any of the raw vegan recipe books that are now available. Buy produce from organic farmers in your region. Use biodegradable soaps, utensils and take-out containers. Furnish the restaurant with recycled and recovered wood furniture. Make the restaurant into a resource center and meeting place for those who are concerned about the environment and wildlife. Include bookshelves for a loaning library for literature concerning ecology and the environment. Let people perform music and poetry. Have a massage therapist set up a table to give your customers massages. Hold raw vegan food preparation classes. Do like Au Lac restaurant in Fountain Valley, California and have a bicycling club begin and finish a ride at your restaurant twice a month. Make fresh, organic baby foods and hemp milks for local mommies. Make nutrition bars for local athletes. And let the author of this book

know your restaurant is open.

The following restaurants are either completely raw, or have raw vegan cuisine on their menus. Many use organic ingredients, but some do not. Some have only a few items that are truly raw, while others serve nothing but raw/unheated cuisine. Some are not all vegetarian, and may be preparing meat in the same kitchen as their raw cuisine, while others may have a separate kitchen for their raw cuisine. Ask if their vegetable juices are truly raw, or if they are pasteurized (even flash pasteurized is not raw).

Alaska:

Juice Kaboos, 1330 E. Huffman Rd., Anchorage, AK 99515

Organic Oasis Restaurant & Juice Bar, 2610 Spenard Rd., Anchorage, AK; 907-277-7882

Arizona:

Anjali-Botanica/Botanic Restaurant, 330 E. 7th St., Tucson, AZ 85705; 520-623-0913; Anjali.Com

The Tree of Life, 771 Harshaw Rd., Patagonia, AZ 85624; 520-394-2589; TreeOfLife.NU

Rawesome Café, Gentle Strength Co-Op, Tempe, AZ; 480-496-5959; RawForLife.Com

Sedona Raw Café, 1595 W. Hwy. 89A, Sedona, AZ 86336; 928-282-2997; RawCafe@ESedona.Net

California:

Alive!, 1972 Lombard St., San Francisco, CA 94123; 415-923-1052; AliveVeggie.Com

Au Lac Vegetarian Restaurant, 16563 Brookhurst St., Fountain Valley, CA 92708; 714-418-0658; Aulac.Com

Beverly Hills Juice Club, 8382 Beverly Blvd., L.A., CA 94122; 323-655-8300

Café Gratitude, 2400 Harrison St. (@20th), San Francisco, CA; 415-824-4652; WithTheCurrent.Com/Café.htm

Café Gratitude, 1336 9th Ave. (@Irving), San Francisco, CA; WithTheCurrent.Com

Café Gratitude, 1730 Shattuck Ave. (@Virginia), Berkeley, CA;
WithTheCurrent.Com

Café La Vie, 429 Front St., Santa Cruz, CA 95060; 831-429-ORGN; LaVie.US

Café Muse, UC Berkeley Art Museum, 2625 Durant Ave., Berkeley, CA; 510-548-4266

Café Sangha, 31 Bolinas Rd., Fairfax, CA 94930; 415-546-5300

Castle Rock Inn, 5827 Sacramento Ave., Dunsmuir, CA 96025; 530-235-0782

Champions, 7523 Fay Ave., La Jolla, CA; 858-456-0536

Cilantro Live!, 315 1/2 3rd Ave., Chula Vista, CA 91910; 619-827-7401;
CilantroLive.Com

Cilantro Live!, 300 Carlsbad Village Dr., Carlsbad, CA 92008; 760-585-0136;
CilantroLive.Com

Couleur Alive Café, 7820 Broadway, Lemon Grove, CA 91945;
CouleurAliveCafe.Net

Elixir Teas and Tonics, 8612 Melrose Ave., West Hollywood, CA 90069; 310-657-9310

Erewhon Healthfood Store, Deli, and Cafe, 7660-A Beverly Blvd., LA, CA
90036; 323-937-0777; ErewhonMarket.Com

Euphoria Loves Rawvolution, 2301 Main Street, Santa Monica, CA 90405; 310-721-4222; 310-392-9501; 800-997-6729; EuphoriaCompany.Com;
Rawvolution.Com
    Recipe book author Matt Amsden's restaurant. Also has New York location.

Good Mood Food Deli Café, 5930 Warner Ave., Huntington Beach, CA; 714-377-2028; GoodMoodFood.Com

Green Life Evolution Center, 410 Railroad Ave., Blue Lake, CA 95525; 707-668-1781; GreenLifeFamily.Com

The Inn of the Seventh Ray (limited raw menu), 128 Old Topanga Canyon Rd.,
Topanga, CA 90290; 310-455-1311

Jenny's 118 Degrees (Inside The Camp natural stores mall), 2981 Bristol B5,
Costa Mesa, CA 92626; 949-295-4231; JennysRawEats.Com

Kung Food, 2949 5th Ave., San Diego, CA 92103; 619-298-7302; Kung-Food.Com
  Some raw items on menu.

Leaf Cuisine, 11938 West Washington Blvd., Culver City, CA 90066; 310-390-5720; LeafCuisine.Com

Leaf Cuisine, 14318 Ventura Blvd., Sherman Oaks, CA; LeafCuisine.Com

Leaf Cuisine, 8365 Santa Monica, Blvd. (at Kings Rd.), West Hollywood, CA; LeafCuisine.Com

Life Restaurant, Hillcrest, San Diego, CA; 800 384-6076; LifeRestaurant.Com

Living Light House, 1427 12th St., Santa Monica, CA 90401; 310-395-6337
  Not a restaurant, cafe, or deli, the Living Light House is a meeting place that holds raw vegan pot luck dinners.

Lydia's Organics, Lydia's Lovin' Foods, 31 Bolinas Ave., Fairfax, CA, 94930; 415-456-5300; 415-258-9678; LydiasOrganics.Com

Madeleine Bistro, 18621 Ventura Blvd., Tarzana, CA 91356; 818-758-6971; MadeleineBistro.Com
  Vegan. But limited raw menu.

Meshama at Mazy, 698 N. Coast Hwy, # 101, Encinitas, CA; 760-965-9018

Millenium Restaurant, Savoy Hotel, 580 Geary Street, San Francisco, CA 94102; 415-345-3900

Mother's Market & Kitchen, 19770 Beach Blvd., Huntington Beach, CA; 714-963-6667

Mother's Market & Kitchen, 225 E. 17th St., Costa Mesa, CA 92627; 949-631-4741

Mother's Market & Kitchen, 2963 Michelson Dr., Irvine, CA 92612; 949-752-6667

Mother's Market & Kitchen, 24165 Paseo De Valencia, Laguna Woods, CA 92653; 949-768-6667

Native Foods, 2938 Bristol St., The Camp, Costa Mesa, CA; 714-751-2151
  Vegan. Limited raw menu.

Native Foods, Smoke Tree Village, 1775 E. Palm, Palm Springs, CA; NativeFoods.Com

Native Foods, El Paso, Palm Desert, CA; NativeFoods.Com

Native Foods, Gayley Ave, Westwood Village, Los Angeles, CA; NativeFoods.Com

Oxygen Bar, 795 Valencia St., (Bet. 18th & 19th Sts.), San Francisco, CA

PaRawDise, 587 Post St., Union Square, San Francisco, CA; RawInten.Com

Rancho's Natural Foods Market, 3918 30th St., San Diego, CA 92104; 619-298-3339

Raw Energy Organic Juice Café, 2050 Addison, Berkeley, CA; 510-665-9464; RawEnergy.Net

The Santa Monica Co-Opportunity Natural Foods Store and Deli, 1525 Broadway, Santa Monica, CA 90404; 310-451-8902; CoOpportunity.Com

The Stand, 238 Thalia St., Laguna Beach, CA

Sunfood Nutrition Raw Superstore, 11653 Riverside Dr., Lakeside, CA 92040; 619-596-7979; Sunfood.Com

Taco Loco, 640 South Coast Hwy., Laguna Beach; 714-497-1635

Taste of the Goddess, 7373 Beverly Blvd., Los Angeles, CA 90036; 323-933-1400; 323-874-7700; TasteOfTheGoddess.Com

Wild Mango Café, 4120 Napier St., San Diego, CA; 619-335-1268; WildMangoCafe.Com

Voila! Juice Bar and Café, 510 Derby Ave., Oakland, CA 94601; 510-261-1138

Colorado:

Cafe Prasad, Boulder CoOp, 1904 Pearl St., Boulder, CO 80306; 303-447-COOP (2667); BoulderCoOp.Com

Karma Cuisine, 1911 Broadway Ave., Boulder, CO 80302; 303-440-9292
Not all raw.

Turtle Lake Refuge, 848 East 3rd Ave., Durango, CO 81301; 970-247-8395; TurtleLakeRefuge.Org

Connecticut:

The Alchemy Juice Bar Café, 203 New Britain Ave., Hartford, CT; 860-246-

5700; AlchemyJuiceBar.Com

Blue Green Organic Juice Café, Equinox Gym, 72 Heights Rd., Darien, CT 06820; 203-655-2300; BlueGreenJuice.Com

Florida:

5th Avenue Café and Market, 116 E. Fifth Ave., Mount Dora, FL 32757; 352-383-0090; 5thAvenueCafe.Com

Glaser Farms Organic Market, Coconut Grove in Miami, FL; 305-238-7747; GlaserOrganicFarms.Com

Grassroot Organic Restaurant, 2702 North Florida Ave., Tampa, FL 33602; 813 221-ROOT (7668); TheGrassRootLife.Com
Not all raw.

Health Station, 2500 N. Hwy. A1A, Indialiantic, FL 32903; 321 773-5678
Not all raw.

Living Greens, 205 McLeod St., Merritt Island, FL 32953; 321-454-2268; Living-Greens.Com

Rhythm and Roots Juice Bar, 111 N. M St., Lake Worth FL 33460; 561-588-2507; RhythmNRootsRawFoodCafe.Com

S & L Fruit Stand, 7805 W Irlo Bronson Memorial Hwy., Kissimmee, FL 34747; 407-396-1026

Georgia:

Café Life, 1453 Roswell Rd., Marietta, GA 30062; 770-977-9583; LifeGrocery.Com

Loving It Live, 2796 East Point St., Atlanta, GA 30344; 404-765-9220

Lush Life Café, 1405 Ralph D. Abernathy Blvd., Atlanta, GA 30310; 404-758-8737; FYLComMinc.Com/LushLifeCafe

Everlasting Life, 87 Ralph D. Abernathy Blvd., SW, Atlanta, GA 30310; 404-758-1110

Mutana Health Cafe and Marketplace, 1392 Ralph David Abernathy Blvd., SW, Atlanta, GA 30310; 404-753-5252

RAW, 878 Ralph D. Abernathy Blvd., Atlanta, GA; 404-758-1110

Hawaii:

Baraka Foods Café; 15-2945 Pahoa Village Rd., Pahoa, Big Island, HI 96778; 808-965-0305; DLawell@Yahoo.Com

Blossoming Lotus Café, 1384 Kuhio Hwy., Kaapa, Kauai, HI 96764; 808-822-7678; BlossomingLotusCafe.Com

Joy's Place, 1993 South Kihei Rd., Kihei, Maui, HI; 808-879-9258

Mandala Garden Juice Bar and Deli, 29 Baldwin Ave., Paia, HI 96779; 808-579-9500

Raisin' Cane, Makuu Market, Pahoa Village, Big Island, HI; 808-965-5486

Westside Natural Foods, 193 Lahainaluna, Lahaina, Maui, HI; 808-667-2855

Idaho:

Akasha Organics, 160 Main St., Ketchum, ID; 208-726-4777; Akasha@SVIdaho.Net

Boise Co-Opportunity, 888 W. Fort St., Boise, ID 83702; 208-472-4500; BoiseCoOp.Com

Illinois:

Chicago Diner, 3411 N. Halsted, Chicago, IL 60657; 773-935-6696; VeggieDiner.Com

Cousins Incredible Vitality, 3038 W. Irving Park Rd., Chicago, IL 60618; 773-478-6868; CousinsIV.Com

Karyn's, 1901 N. Halsted Ave., Chicago, IL 60614; 312-255-1590; KarynRaw.Com

Maryland:

Everlasting Life Healthfood Store, 9185 Central Ave., Capitol Hts., MD 20743; 301-324-6900; EverlastingLife.Net

The Yabba Pot, 2433 St. Paul St., Baltimore, MD 21218; 410-662-8638

The Yabba Pot, 771 Washington Blvd., Pigtown, Baltimore, MD; 410-962-8638

Massachusetts:

Organic Garden Restaurant and Juice Bar, 294 Cabot St., Beverly, MA 01915; 978-922-0004; VegDining.Com; OrganicGardenCafe.Com

Minnesota:

Ecopolitan, 2409 Lyndale Ave. S., Minneapolis, MN 55405; 612-87-Green (612-874-7336); Ecopolitan.Net

Nevada:

Go Raw Café, 2910 Lake East Dr., Las Vegas, NV 89117; 707-254-5382; GoRawCafe.Com

Go Raw Café, 2381 East Windmill Way, Las Vegas, NV 89123; GoRawCafe.Com

New Jersey:

Down to Earth, 7 Broad St., Redbank, NJ 07701; 732-747-4542

East Coast Vegan Restaurant, 313-A W. Water St., Toms River, NJ 08753; 732-473-9555; EastCoastVegan.Net

The Energy Bar Vegetarian Café, 307C Orange Rd., Montclair, NJ 07042; 973-746-7003; KHeperFoods.Com/EnergyBar.html

New Mexico:

Whole Body Café, The Body Center, 333 Cordova Rd., Santa Fe, NM 87505; 505-986-0362; BodyOfSanraFe.Com/Body_Cafe.Htm
  Not all raw.

New York:

Blue Green Organic Juice Café, 26 Jay St., First Fl., Brooklyn, NY 11201; 718-722-7541; BlueGreenJuice.Com

Blue Green Organic Juice Café, 248 Mott St., New York, NY 10012; 212-744-0920; 212-334-0805; BlueGreenJuice.Com

Blue Green Organic Juice Café; 203 E. 74th St., New York, NY 10021; BlueGreenJuice.Com

Bonobos Vegetarian, 18 E. 23rd St., New York, NY 10010; 212-505-1200; BonobosRestaurant.Com

Cafe Fresh, 431 West 121st St., New York, NY

Candle 79, 154 E. 79th St., New York, NY 10021; 212-573-7179; CandleCafe.Com

Caravan Of Dreams, 405 E. 6th St., New York, NY 10009; 212-254-1613; CaravanOfDreams.Net

Counter Vegetarian Restaurant, 105 First Ave., New York, NY 10003; 212-982-5870; CounterRestaurant.Com

Heirloom, 191 Orchard St., New York, NY; 212-228-9888
  Not all raw.

In the Raw, 65 Tinker St, Woodstock, NY 12498; 854-679-9494; WoodstockInTheRaw.Com

Jandi's Natural Market & Organic Cafe & Deli, 3000 Long Beach Rd., Oceanside, NY 11572; 516-536-5535; Jandis.Com

Jubbs Longevity Life Food Store, Organic Juice Bar & Patisserie, 508 E. 12th St. at Ave. A, New York, NY 10009; 888-420-8270; 212-358-8068; 212-353-5000; JubbsLongevity.Com; LifeFood.Com

Juice and Roots Bar, Safmink Holistic Center, 446B Dean Street, Brooklyn, NY 11217; 718-638-8250

Liquiteria, 170 Second Ave., New York, NY 10003; 212-358-0300

Organic Soul Café, Sixth Street Center, 638 East 6th St., New York, NY 10009; 212-677-1863; SixthStreetCenter.Org/Café_Index.html
  Not all raw.

Pure Food and Wine, 54 Irving Pl., New York, NY; 212-477-1010; PureFoodAndWine@Yahoo.Com

Pure Juice and Takeaway, 125 1/2 East 17th St., New York, NY; 212-477-7151

Quintessence, 263 East 10th St., New York, NY 10009; 646-654-1823

Raw Daily, Daily Soup, 241 West 54th St., New York, NY; 212-765-7687

Raw Soul Take-Out and Delivery, 745 St. Nicholas Ave., New York, NY 10031; 212-491-5859; RawSoul.Com

Rawvolution, 800-997-6729; EuphoriaCompany.com; Rawvolution.com
  Recipe book author Matt Amsden's restaurant. Also has Santa Monica, CA (Los

Angeles County) location and delivery service in both cities.

Sacred Chow, 227 Sullivan St., New York, NY 10012; 212-337-0863

North Carolina:

Natural Lifestyle Market, 16 Lookout Dr., Ashville, NC 28804; 800-752-2775; Natural-Lifestyle.Com

Smokey Mountain Natural Foods, 15 Aspen Ct., Ashville, NC 28806; 800-926-0974

Ohio:

Healthy Harvest, 8785 Mentor Ave., Mentor, OH 44060; 440-255-3468

Mustard Seed Market and Café, Montrose, West Market Plaza, 3885 W. Market St., Akron, OH 44333; 330-666-SEED (7333); MustardSeedMarket.Com

Mustard Seed Market and Café, Uptown Solon Shopping Center, 6025 Kruse Dr., Solon, OH 44139; 440-519-FOOD (3663); Café: 440-519-3600; MustardSeedMarket.Com

Nature's Bin Natural Food Store, 18120 Sloane Ave. Lakewood, OH 44107; 216-521-4600; Cornucopia-Inc.Org

Oregon:

The Blossoming Lotus, Yoga in the Pearl, 925 NW Davis, Portland, OR 97209; 503-525-YOGA; BlossomingLotus.Com

Mana: Life Friendly Foods, 85 Winburn Way (across from Lithia Park), Ashland, OR 97520; 541-482-2003; OurManna.Com
John, Humsa, and Crea.

Red Barn Natural Foods Store, 4th and Blair, Eugene, OR; 541-342-7503
  Sells some raw foods, also sells organic produce.

Ripe and Raw Roving Restaurant (catering), Portland, OR 97206; 503-771-5605; RawDiva@Earthlink.Net

Sundance Natural Foods, 24th and Hilyard, Eugene, OR; 541-343-9142
  Sells some raw foods, also sells organic produce.

Pennsylvania:

Arnold's Way, 319 West Main St., Store #4 Rear, Lansdale, PA 19446; 215-361-

0116; ArnoldsWay.Com

Kind Café, 724 N. 3rd St., Philadelphia, PA; 215-922-KIND; KindCafe.Com

Maggie's Mercantile, 320 Atwood St., Pittsburgh, PA 15213-4026; 724-593-5056

Maggie's Mercantile #2, 1262 Rte. 711, Stahlstown, PA 15687; 724-593-5056

Raw Life Line, Huntingdon Valley, PA; 800-RAW-9197; 215-947-1510; RawLifeLine.Com

Oasis Living Cuisine, Great Valley Shopping Center, 81 Lancaster Ave., Malvern, PA 19355; 610-647-9797; OasisLivingCuisine.Com

Texas:

Blueberry Market, Organic and Raw Foods Co-Op, 2819 Sandage Ave., Fort Worth TX; 817-703-3438

Daily Juice, Austin, TX; Kwahrer@Hotmail.Com

Oxygen Life Spa, The Rudra Center, 609 N. Locust St., Denton, TX 76201; 940-384-7946; OxygenLifeSpa.Com

Pure: A Living Foods Café, 2720 Greenville Ave., Dallas, TX 75206; 214-824-7776; PureRawCafe.Com

Sunfired Foods, 4915 MLK Blvd., Houston, TX 77021; 713-643-2884; SunfiredFoodsHouston.Com

Utah:

Living Cuisine, Herbs for Health, 1100 East Highland Drive/2144 S. Highland Dr., Salt Lake City, UT 84106; 801-467-4082

Sage's Café, 473 East 300 S., Salt Lake City, UT; 801-322-3790; SagesCafe.Com

Washington State:

Chaco Cayon Café, 4761 Brooklyn Ave. NE, 206-5 Canyon, Seattle, WA 98105; 206-522-6966; ChacoCanyonCafe.Com

Washington DC:

Everlasting Life Health Food Store, 2928 Georgia Ave. NW, Washington DC 20001; 202-232-1700; EverlastingLife.Net

Canada:

Live Health Café, 258 Dupont St., Toronto, Ontario, Canada; 416-515-2002

The Living Source Café, The Melting Pot Gallery, 1111 Commercial Dr., Vancouver, BC, Canada; 604-254-3335; LivingSourceCafe.CA

Papaya Island, 513 Yonge St., Toronto, Ontario, Canada; 416-960-0821; Papaya_Island@Hotmail.Com

Raw Health Café, 1849 W. 1st Ave., Vancouver, BC; 604-737-0420

Toronto Sprouts, 720 Bathurst St., Toronto, Ontario, M5S 2R4, Canada; 416-977-8929; TorontoSprouts.Com

Tout Cru Dans L'bec, 129, 7e rue, Rouyn-Noranda, Québec, Canada J9X 1Z8; ToutCruDansLbec@TLB.Sympatico.CA

WOW Wild Organic Café & Juice Bar, 22 Carden St., Guelph, Ontario, N1H 3A2, Canada; 519-766-1707

Raw, 1849 W. 1st Ave., Vancouver, British Columbia, V6J 5B8, Canada; 604-737-0420; RawHealthCafe.Com

Czech Republic:

Albiostyl; Albiostyle.CZ

England:

VitaOrganic (extensive raw and juice menu), Wholistic Restaurant, Alternative Café and Juice Bar, 279C Finchley Rd, London, NW3 6ND, England; 020-7435-2188; VitaOrganic.CO.UK

Jamaica:

Ashanti Foods Monthly Brunch, Yvonne Hope; 876-944-3316

Earl's Juice Garden, 16 Derrymore Rd., Kingston 10, Jamaica; 876-906-4287; 876 920-7009

Earl's Juice Garden #2, Shop #6, 6 Red Hills Rd., Kingston 10, Jamaica, 876-754-2425

Spain:

Organic, C. de la Junta de Comera 11, Barcelona, Spain 08001; 001 34 93 301

0902; Organic.ES

Thailand:

Rasayana Raw Food Café, 57 Soi Sukhumvit 39 (Prom-mitr), Sukhumvit Rd., Klongton-Nua Wattana 10110; Bangkok, Thailand, 66-2662-4803-5

Rodent Proofing and Humane Trapping

HelpingWildLife.Com/HouseMice.asp

Rodeo Animal Liberation

BuckStarbucks.Com and also SharkOnLine.Org
   Working to protest and stop Starbucks from sponsoring rodeos where many animals are terrorized, injured, and killed.

BuckTheRodeo.Com

European Anti-Rodeo Coalition, Anti-Rodeo.Org

RodeoCruelty.Com

SharkOnline.Org

Salt

The average American consumes about ten grams of salt per day, mostly through processed foods. The body needs only about a half gram per day, and more if the person is exercising or performing heavy labor. But the amount of salt that people eat isn't the only thing that is unhealthful; the most commonly used type of salt is also not good.

The most common kitchen salts have been processed at high heat, which damages the minerals, and they contain added substances like yellow prussiate of soda and alumino-silicate of sodium to prevent caking and moisture absorption. Processed salt contributes to such health maladies as high blood pressure, vision problems, skin issues, asthma, diabetes, osteoporosis, and diseases of the stomach and kidneys.

Get rid of your processed table salt. Instead of processed salt, use Celtic sea salt, or Himalayan pink salt. When purchasing sea salt, make sure that it was not processed in a drying kiln at high heat. Look on the label to see if it says "Sun-dried."

Your daily intake of salt is best obtained through uncooked organically grown vegetables, and especially by eating greens such as celery. The roots of these vegetables naturally mine minerals from the ground, and through Nature's magic of photosynthesis we get vegetables that provide us with perfect nutrients.

Sea vegetables are excellent sources of quality minerals, including salt. Powdered kelp or dulse can be used in place of salt in some recipes.

Sea Vegetables and Water Vegetation

Sea vegetables are sea plant leaves containing bountiful nutrients and spectrums of light drawn in from the ocean and Sun. They grow at or near the surface of water.

Although they all contain the green pigment of chlorophyll, the color of the seaweed can be anywhere from brown to green to red. The color depends on the variety of seaweed, and on what level of the spectrum of light they were exposed to while growing.

You may find water vegetables under the following names: agar agar, arame, chlorella, dulse, focus tip (also named bladderwrack), grapestone, hijiki, kombu, Nori (also known as mei bil, sea leaf, and porphyra), ocean ribbons, sea lettuce, sea palm, silky sea palm, sea whip, wakame, spirulina, and wild blue-green algae (Aphanizomenon flos aqua).

Not surprisingly, sea vegetables consist mostly of water. When dried they can have shrunk to less than 1/20 of their original size.

Sea vegetables are a source of the element iodine, which is fundamental to brain function and reduces stress. Other nutrients in water vegetables besides chlorophyll include amino acids, essential fatty acids, peptides, enzymes, vitamins A, C, D, E, and K; a variety of minerals; beta-carotene, folic acid and other B vitamins.

The nutrients in sea vegetables not only decrease the chances of a variety of cancers, but can also help to regenerate the cells, build the immune system, detoxify the body tissues, and aid in the absorption and utilization of nutrients. They also assist in the removal of heavy metals from the body; aid in the regulation of cholesterol; reduce cramps and anemia; alkalize the digestive tract and body; regulate the thyroid; restore endocrine deficiencies; improve antibody production; balance the hormones and insulin; improve kidney and adrenal function; and provide for better neural function. Sea vegetables contain more bio-available minerals than any other class of food.

The colloidal carbohydrate, alginic acid (sodium alginates), found in brown algae, binds with the heavy metals cadmium, lead, and mercury, as well as low-level radioactive material, and removes them from the body.

The calcium and iron in sea vegetables is of a better quality for the human body than the same nutrients found in animal meat or milk.

Raw and low-temperature dried sea vegetables contain healthy doses of enzymes. Out of the variety of sea vegetables, dulse contains the highest amount of the mineral manganese, which triggers the body to release more enzymes, improving digestion.

Maine Seaweed Company, POB 57, Steuben, ME 04680; 707-546-2875; AlcaSoft.Com/Seaweed/

Mendocino Sea Vegetable Company, POB 372, 255 Welding St., Navarro, CA 95463; 707-895-3741; Seaweed.Net

Ocean Harvest Sea Vegetables, POB 1719, Mendocino, CA 95460; 707-936-1923; OHSV.Net

Rising Tide Sea Vegetables, POB 1914, Mendocino, CA 95460; 707-964-5663; LoveSeaweed.Com

Sunfood Nutrition, 11653 Riverside Dr., Lakeside, CA 92040; 800-205-2350; 888-RAW-FOOD; International: +001-619-596-7979; Sunfood.Com

Seeds

Also see:
• Gardening and Farming

Book:
• *Breed Your Own Vegetable Varietiesz: The Gardener's and Farmer's Guide to Plant Breeding and Seed Saving*, by Carole Deppe

"Though I do not believe that a plant will spring up where no seed has been, I have great faith in a seed. Convince me that you have a

seed there and I am prepared to expect wonders."
— **Henry David Thoreau**

It has only been in the past hundred years that people have begun to depend on large companies, stores, and restaurants to supply food. Before that, most people grew or wild-harvested most or all their own food, and knew how to make dinner out of it.

Recently the number of food plants has been diminishing. Some have become extinct. This is because people are limiting themselves to certain food plants, are not involved so much in growing food, and have become dependent on multinational corporations and stores to provide food. Much of this began in the 1920s when the U.S. government funded programs that brought "hybrid" seeds into popularity. Farmers and gardeners then began buying more seeds while depending less on harvesting and saving their "heirloom" seeds.

Today most of the companies that sell food seeds either depend on larger companies for a large amount of their stock, or they are the companies that sell most of the seeds that are sold on the planet. Unfortunately, corporate greed is working to control the seeds stocks of the planet. Some of these companies are involved in genetically engineering food plants, and in putting international patent protection on the types of seeds they genetically engineer. This is often done with the help of the U.S. Department of Agriculture. Some of these companies are also involved in creating seeds that grow into self-sterilizing plants so that the farmers, or others, cannot keep a seed stock and have to purchase new seeds every year. Because of laws created by the seed industry, farmers have been sued or prosecuted for saving seeds, or for sharing seeds with other farmers. These are some of the activities that the World Trade Organization is involved in, enforcing seed patent laws.

Farmers are being sued for having plants growing on their property that contain the genes of patented plants. Monsanto, a company that owns a patent on genetically engineered canola has sued farmers who never planted the genetically engineered seeds. The crops have been contaminated with the pollen from neighboring farms where the genetically engineered seeds were planted.

If there is a law being created to protect patented crops and the seeds of them, it is likely that a company that will make money from the law is behind getting it passed.

In the recent wars on Iraq and Afghanistan the farmers in countries being attacked have seen their seeds stocks destroyed. These are cultures that have saved seeds for thousands of years. Now they are under the control of companies that are genetically engineering seeds.

The people of the world should work against the genetic engineering of plants and patent laws that prevent seed saving.

Formerly, people were connected to the seasons, to the plants, to their local environment, and to the ways of Nature that resulted in foods. They knew about how plants were pollinated by bees, butterflies, and bugs, as well as by birds and bats, by the wind, and by storms. Openly pollinated foods were the norm, and hybrid plants and genetically engineered foods were unheard of.

Now people expect their fruits and vegetables to look a certain way, and much of the produce sold in supermarkets is limited to what looks good on the shelf, and what ships easily. Even when most people plant food gardens they rely on store-bought seeds that must be purchased year after year because the hybridized plants often do not provide seeds that will produce the same quality of plant.

People need to get reacquainted with how Nature provides foods through open pollination; in collecting open pollinated seeds; in understanding soil organisms and helpful insects; and with growing foods that are genetically diverse and grown without the use of toxic chemicals.

Bay Area Seed Interchange Library, EcologyCenter.Org/BASIL
Working to preserve the world's seed stock.

National Farmers Union Seed Saver Campaign, 2717 Wentz Ave., Saskatoon, SK S7K 4B6, Canada; NFU.CA/SeedSaver.html

National Plant Germplasm Service, ARS-Grin.Gov/NPGS

Native Seeds/SEARCH, Tucson, AZ, 866-622-5561; NativeSeeds.Org

Oregon Tilth, Inc., Tilth.Org/Resources/OrganicSeeds.html
Site contains a list of seed companies that sell organic, heirloom, non-genetically modified seeds.

Organic Seed Alliance, POB 772, Port Townsend, WA 98368; SeedAlliance.Org

Osborn International Seed Co., OsbornSeed.Com

Peoples' Global Action, AGP.Org

Planting Seeds Project, New City Institute, Vancouver, CA; NewCity.CA/Pages/Planting_Seeds.html

Primal Seeds, PrimalSeeds.Org

Restoring Our Seed, POB 520, Waterville, ME 04903; GrowSeed.Org

Saving Our Seed, 286 Dixie Hollow, Louisa, VA, 23093; SavingOurSeed.Org

Scatterseed Project, POB 1167, Farmington, ME 04938; GardeningPlaces.Com/ScatterSeed.htm

SeedAlliance.Org

Seed and Plant Sanctuary for Canada, Salt Spring Island, BC SeedSanctuary.Org

SeedSave.Org

Seed Savers Exchange, Decorah, IA; SeedSavers.Org

Seed Savers Network, SeedSavers.Net

Seeds of Change, 3209 Richards Lane, Santa Fe, NM 87507; SeedsOfChange.Com
    This company is now owned by the multinational corporation M&M/Mars – a business that makes and sells a lot of unhealthful foods. Seeds of Change sells organic and heirloom seeds.

Seeds of Diversity, POB 36, Stn. Q, Toronto, ON M4T 2L7, Canada; Seeds.CA

Snow Seed Organic, 831-758-9869; SnowSeedCo.Com

Sow Organic Seed Co., POB 527, Williams, OR 97544; OrganicSeed.Com

Theodore Payne Foundation, TheodorePayne.Org
Promotes the preservation and use of native plants.

Underwood Gardens, Maryann Underwood, 1414 Ximmerman Rd., Woodstock, IL 60098; UnderwoodGardens.Com
    Maryann Underwood's company sells endangered and heirloom seeds; works to preserve genetic diversity of food plants; teaches people the ancient practice of saving seeds; and publishes books and videos on how to save seeds. The Web site features a forum where gardeners can share gardening tips, ask questions, and receive feedback.

United Plant Savers, POB 400, East Barre, VT, 05649; UnitedPlantSavers.Org

Solar Energy

American Solar Energy Society, ASES.Org

Green Energy News, NRGLink.Com

GreenHomeBuilding.Com

HatCreekPublishing.Com

Home Power Magazine, HomePower.Com

International Solar Energy Society, ISES.Org

Red Solar, CubaSolar.Cu
Site is in Spanish. The Cuban government has been very active in converting schools to solar energy.

Solar Energy Society of Canada, SolarEnergySociety.Ca

Solar Living Institute, POB 836, 13771 S. Hwy. 101, Hopland, CA 95449; 707-744-2017; SolarLiving.Org

SolWest.Org

Sprouting

Also see:
• Wheatgrass and Barleygrass juice

Books:
• *How to Grow and Use Sprouts to Maximize Your Health and Vitality*, by Ann Wigmore
• *Living Cuisine: The Art and Spirit of Raw Foods*, by Renée Loux

"Scientists have studied sprouts for centuries to better understand their high levels of disease-preventing phytochemicals, and how they contribute to better health, from prevention to treatment of life-threatening diseases. Major organizations including the National Institutes of Health, American Cancer Society and Johns Hopkins University have reinforced the benefits of sprouts with ongoing studies that explore various sprout varieties for their nutritional properties and to validate health claims.

According to Paul Talalay, M.D., in the American Cancer Society

NEWS, 'broccoli sprouts are better for you than full-grown broccoli, and contain more of the enzyme sulforaphane which helps protect cells and prevents their genes from turning into cancer.' His findings are consistent with several epidemiologic studies that have shown that sprouts contain significant amounts of vitamins A, C and D. Sprouts are widely recognized by nutrition-conscious consumers and health care professionals as a 'wonder food.'"

    – *Good Sprout News* of the International Sprout Growers' Association; ISGA-Sprouts.Org

Eating fresh sprouts is an excellent way to get phytonutrients (plant nutrients), such as enzymes (vital to all life), amino acids (for building protein), and chlorophyll (abundant in greens, especially baby greens). Sprouting is also one of the least expensive ways, besides growing your own garden, to get raw greens into your diet, which is important for anyone wanting to experience vibrant health.

The magic of a seed is that it is a plant-making kit. Seeds are amazing in that they can be eaten by an animal, pass through the digestive tract, and start to grow only after they have been excreted. Magically, what seeds need to grow is provided in the nutrient-rich feces. That is how many plants are spread through Nature, by being eaten by animals, who then unknowingly provide themselves as a vehicle to transfer the seed to a new location, where it grows.

Exposing seeds to moisture takes the seed out of its dormant state, shutting off the enzyme inhibitors, which mostly exist in the skin or shell, and igniting the nutrient factories that build the structure from a seed into a plant. The first few days of a plant's life is a time of exuberant energy and a microscopic storm of nutrient-making activity. By consuming the sprouts, you are transferring the concentrated vibrant nutrients of the young plant into your body.

As long as you have an area that is between about 50 to 100 degrees, and that has indirect Sun light, you can grow sprouts anywhere on the planet. You don't need anything special to grow sprouts. All it takes is something like a big glass jar and a screen to cover the top. You can also use a bowl covered with a screen, or a sheer cloth that allows light to get in. Of course, you also need clean water.

Probably the most common method of growing sprouts is to use a big jar covered by a screen, keeping the jar tilting at an approximate 45° angle in a big bowl to drain excess water.

There are a variety of sprouting trays and machines on the market that can make it easier to sprout seeds. Some sprouters automatically spray and rinse the sprouts so that you don't have to.

There are a variety of seeds that are good for sprouting. Seek those that are from organic sources.

Make sure your soaking and sprouting bowls, jars, and screens are clean, or else you will also be growing bacteria.

During the soaking time remember that seeds can die if they remain in water too long. The soak times listed below vary according to the temperature of the room and water. If it is cold, you may want to soak for the longer period; if it is warm you want to sprout for the shorter period. In warmer weather the seeds will also need to be rinsed more often. As you get more familiar with sprouting, you will learn what works best for the types of seeds you are using, and the environment of the room.

Unless you have an automatic sprouting machine that regularly mists the sprouting seeds, you will need to rinse them one to three times per day with clean water to keep them clean, fresh, and hydrated (moist). It is good to have a screened strainer for rinsing the smaller seeds, and a colander with smallish holes for rinsing the larger seeds/beans.

Sprouting takes place faster in warm weather, and also in a brighter location.

Most types of grain sprouts are sweetest when the tail on the seed has just started to grow. The longer the tail grows, the less sweet it will become.

Sprouts benefit from exposure to light, such as indirect Sun light, as this will trigger the development of chlorophyll in the sprouts.

Within a plant, chlorophyll transforms Sun light and CO_2 into sugar and oxygen. Chlorophyll is molecularly very similar to human blood plasma. There are strong nutritional qualities in chlorophyll as it helps strengthen the immune system in fighting off infections, and helps rid the body of toxins, especially those that gather in the liver. Because chlorophyll helps generate new cell growth, it also is important in the healing from wounds and illnesses.

Some sprouts are more chlorophyll-rich than others. With a content of about 70 percent chlorophyll, wheatgrass is the richest sprout of all.

If you are not going to use the sprouts right away, after the seeds have sprouted, you can slow down their growth by putting them in the refrigerator, or in a cold room (not freezing). Rinse and drain once a day with clean water and you should be able to keep them in a cold, slowed growing state for two to four days.

You can also slow soaked seeds from sprouting fully by keeping them in the refrigerator. Then, when you are ready to sprout them, remove them from the refrigerator, rinse, and let them grow at room temperature.

Sprouts are living, breathing plants. They need air. Don't put them into a sealed container. A screened jar or a casserole dish with a glass top work well because they both allow for air to enter the container. A jar with a screen fastened around the top and turned upside down at an angle in a jar works best for many seeds because it prevents them from sitting in water while letting in air. Just remember to rinse them two or three times a day to keep them from rotting.

One way of keeping sprouts fresh in the refrigerator is to store them in a bamboo bowl covered by a second bamboo bowl that has a dozen or more small holes drilled into it. This also provides an easy way to rinse them once a day by pouring water into the bowl, covering with the top bowl, and tilting upside down over the sink or outside to eliminate excess water before putting them back into the refrigerator.

The amount of time listed below for soaking can often be reduced to just a few hours. Some seeds can be soaked a lot longer, up to a day, but you risk killing the seeds.

Some people will drink the soak water as it contains enzymes that are released by the seeds.

Just as long as the soaked seeds are kept moist and you don't let them dry out, you break down the enzyme inhibitors, and nurture the seed to turn into a plant.

Again: Sprouts must be rinsed, and most are best if they are rinsed three times per day, although some may only require rinsing twice per day.

When the sprouts have reached the size you want them, put them in direct Sun for an hour or more. By doing this you will ignite the chlorophyll and nutrient-making factory within the sprouts, greatly increasing their nutritional value. Make sure not to allow Sun to bake them or let them dry out. Keep them covered with a screen or sheer cloth to keep little buggy friends away.

Popular seeds used in sprouting:

Seed:	Soak for:	Sprout for:
• Adzuki	6 to 7 hours	3 days
• Alfalfa	5 to 6 hours	2 to 4 days

- **Almond**   2 to 3 hours   Freshly soaked to 2 days
Toss into salads. Use as ingredient in smoothies, and desserts.

- **Blackeye peas**   7 to 9 hours   2 to 4 days

- **Broccoli**   5 to 6 hours   3 to 4 days
Strong taste. Use sparingly in salads, sandwiches, dressings.

- **Buckwheat**   5 to 6 hours   2 to 3 days
If you are to use the grain in only its soaked form, without sprouting them, you may want to put them through a process to activate the phytase enzyme. This breaks down the phytic acid, which is phosphoric, exists in the outer layer/bran of grains, and binds with minerals, preventing them from being absorbed into the digestive tract. After draining the water, soak the seeds in vinegar or lemon juice for about 30 minutes. Raw sauerkraut juice or kimchee juice also work in activating the phytase.

- **Cabbage**   5 to 6 hours   2 to 4 days

- **Cashew**   2 to 3 hours   Freshly soaked to 2 days
Toss into salads. Use as ingredient in smoothies, and desserts.

- **Chia**   5 to 6 hours   2 to 4 days

- **Clover**   5 to 6 hours   2 to 4 days

- **Corn**   7 to 9 hours   2 to 4 days

- **Dill**   5 to 6 hours   2 to 3 days

- **Fenugreek**   6 to 7 hours   2 to 4 days

- **Flax**   4 to 5 hours   Freshly soaked to 3 days
Not the easiest to sprout. It is good to use a large, wide-mouthed jar with a screen cover. This way the seeds can be rinsed by pouring water through the screen, and the upside-down jar kept at an angle to drain.
Time to use them depends on what you are using them for. If you are going to use them in raw dehydrated crackers, you may want to soak them only for several hours to ignite the enzymes. But for soft dehydrated breads and crusts you may want to sprout them a while longer. Also good for adding crunch to guacamole, salsa, and gazpacho.

- **Garbanzo**   8 to 10 hours   2 to 4 days
Make a sprouted garbanzo bean salad with olive oil, salt, lemon juice, chopped red bell pepper, chopped red onion, and pepper powder.

Blend into hummus after sprouting for two to four days (lemon juice, salt, raw tahini, garlic, olive oil. You can also add fresh Italian herbs, raw olives, chopped red bell pepper, and/or dried tomatoes).

• **Kamut**	5 to 6 hours	Freshly soaked to 3 days
• **Lentil**	6 to 8 hours	2 to 4 days
• **Macadamia**	2 to 3 hours	Freshly soaked to 3 days

Use as ingredient in smoothies, deserts, crusts, and fruit salads.

• **Millet**	7 to 9 hours	2 to 4 days

You can also make rejuvelac fermented water using sprouted millet soaked in water for 12 to 24 hours in a clean, warm place out of direct Sun light. (See Rejuvelac)

It is best to soak a small amount of millet in a big, screened jar to make them easier to rinse.

• **Mung beans**	6 to 8 hours	2 to 4 days

Mung bean sprouts will remain white if they are kept in the dark. If you expose them to light, they become green, but they also become bitter.

• **Mustard**	5 to 7 hours	2 to 4 days

Strong taste. Use sparingly in salads, sandwiches, and dressings.

• **Oat groats**	5 to 6 hours	Freshly soaked to 2 days

Use in crusts, or in breakfast bowl with berries and/or cut fruit, a bit of lemon juice, vanilla, shredded coconut, and soaked macadamia.

If you are to use the grain in only its soaked form, without sprouting them, you may want to put them through a process to activate the phytase enzyme. This breaks down the phytic acid, which is phosphoric, exists in the outer layer/bran of grains, and binds with minerals, preventing them from being absorbed into the digestive tract. After draining the water, soak the seeds in vinegar or lemon juice for about 30 minutes. Raw sauerkraut juice or kimchee juice also work in activating the phytase.

• **Onion**	5 to 7 hours	2 to 4 days
• **Peas**	6 to 9 hours	2 to 4 days
• **Pine nuts**	2 to 3 hours	freshly soaked
• **Pumpkin**	3 to 5 hours	Freshly soaked to 4 days

Toss onto salads. Blend into smoothies. Use soaked pumpkin seeds as an ingredient in raw dehydrated crackers.

- **Quinoa**   6 to 8 hours   2 to 3 days

Use in fresh or dehydrated crusts. You can also make rejuvelac fermented water using sprouted quinoa soaked in water for 12 to 24 hours in a clean, warm place out of direct Sun light. (See Rejuvelac)

- **Radish**   5 to 7 hours   1 to 5 days

- **Red clover**   5 to 7 hours   3 to 5 days

- **Rye**   7 to 9 hours   2 to 4 days

Use in fresh or dehydrated crusts.

- **Sesame**   4 to 6 hours   Freshly soaked to 3 days

- **Spelt**   5 to 6 hours   Freshly soaked to 3 days

- **Sunflower**   5 to 7 hours   Freshly soaked to 3 days

Toss into salads. Use soaked seeds in dehydrated raw crackers. You can also grow sunflower sprouts in a flat of organic soil, then after a few days, harvest them, including the roots, rinsing off the soil (or cutting off the roots), and using them in salads and as garnish for raw burgers (see raw vegan recipe books).

- **Triticale**   5 to 7 hours   2 to 3 days

- **Wheat berries**   5 to 7 hours   2 to 3 days, or for grass

Use in mixed sprouted grain salad.

Make rejuvelac (See Rejuvelac).

Use to grow wheat grass for juicing (See Wheat Grass).

If you are to use the grain in only its soaked form, without sprouting them, you may want to put them through a process to activate the phytase enzyme. This breaks down the phytic acid, which is phosphoric, exists in the outer layer/bran of grains, and binds with minerals, preventing them from being absorbed into the digestive tract. After draining the water, soak the seeds in vinegar or lemon juice for about 30 minutes. Raw sauerkraut juice or kimchee juice also work in activating the phytase.

- **Wild rice**   6 to 8 hours   3 to 5 days

Use in sprouted grain salad mixed with chopped soaked almonds or walnuts, raw oil, a little lemon juice, and Himalayan salt.

EatSprouts.Com

International Sprout Grower's Association, ISGA-Sprouts.Org

Mumm's Sprouting Seeds, Sprouting.Com

SproutMan.Com

SproutPeople.Com

Tim Tyler's Sprout Farm, Sprouting.Org

Talent

Also see:
- Brain
- Infinite Intelligence
- Love
- Magnetizing Your Life
- People
- Television

> "I cannot control the wind. But I can adjust my sails."
> — **An optimistic sailor**

The good and bad in things may be a matter of perception, and the way you perceive things has to do with the way you allow yourself to think.

> "A successful man is one who can lay a firm foundation with the bricks that others throw at him."
> — **David Brinkley**

As you are presented with situations throughout your day that may be less than ideal, look toward ways of remaining calm and dealing with them in a way that will bring about benefits. Through the power of thought you can transform your experiences from those that may damage into those that can benefit. This concept has to do with the frame of mind that you decide to carry.

Imagine if there were a Black child from a poor family who had a most unfortunate thing happen to him, such as losing his sight at an early age. Imagine that instead of working through that problem, and putting it in its place, he instead spent his life in the depths of self-pity. Imagine if he never discovered his talents and never developed his potential skills. Imagine that if instead of trying to make his life work, he stayed in his parents' home and never went anywhere, and did nothing with his time because he was too sad and too busy dwelling in self-pity. Imagine if his parents then died while he was still a young boy and he ended up living on the streets doing nothing with his time, and only took the smallest bit of effort to get by in his blind and self-pitiful state, allowing himself to be beaten down by the prejudices held by others who didn't like dark-skinned people and who didn't feel comfortable around blind people. Imagine if this boy grew into a man and never discovered what he could have become if he had discovered and used his talents.

> "Things turn out best for the people who make the best of the way things turn out."
> — Art Linkletter

Imagine a different set of life situations for that blind Black boy from the poor home. In this situation he had still lost both his sight and his parents at a young age. He also lived in a time when laws and people worked strongly against Black Americans. But this time the boy did not dwell in self-pity. Imagine that he went on to develop his talents, and despite some other life difficulties – including some of his own making – he broke through the obstacles that seemed to be chasing after him. Imagine that he used his intellect, talents, and abilities to become a very talented, world-famous musician who happened to be named Ray Charles.

> "If you have made mistakes, even serious ones, there is always another chance for you. What we call failure is not the falling down, but the staying down."
> — Mary Pickford

Understand that the life of Ray Charles turned out to be so incredible because he used the power of his mind to make it that way. When he fell down, he got back up.

> "I try to tell the young kids there are two cardinal rules: You should approach creativity with humility and have your success with grace. It's a gift from God. You don't deserve it. You are a vehicle of a higher power. Don't abuse it."
> — Quincy Jones

Throughout history, and in the lives of present-day people who have made great successes out of their lives, you can see a pattern of persistence in action, and a sustained focus on goals. They had faith that they could accomplish their goals, and then they demonstrated this faith through action. They didn't simply sit around talking and thinking about what they wanted to do, they went out and did it. Their concentration may have been broken on occasion, but they "kept on keeping on" and accomplished what they set out to do.

Living close to Nature through the Sunfood diet is connecting into the power of Nature, which is an astounding energy that is available to all because it is in and through all. By respecting yourself through taking care of your health on a natural diet, you are tuning into your strength, which has to do with being who you are as defined by your talents, intellect, and skills. It is in alignment with your spirit and essence. This is the power that triggers your cells to grow, and is connected to the power in the cells of all other living things. The most successful and happy people use this power in their life. It can work for you, if you choose to use it.

Know that you can attain the rightful things in life that you want to attain. Go about your days knowing that you are a unique individual capable of using your talents, intellect, knowledge, power, faith, and energy to create a life that is right for you.

Know that you do not have to compete with anyone; know that this is so because there is no competition, as you are a unique person capable of not comparing yourself to anyone but yourself, of attaining that which is right for you and nobody else.

"Having talent is like having blue eyes. You don't admire a man for the color of his eyes. I admire a man for what he does with his talent."
— Anthony Quinn

Telephone Services for Environmental Change

If you have a telephone, please try to get your service from a company that donates part of its profits to the environment.

If you use a cell phone, please do not throw unusable cell phones into the trash. Take them to a recycle center, or give them to an organization that recycles cell phones. Cell phones contain heavy metals and other toxins that are not good for the environment, and can turn a typical dump into a toxic waste dump. ·

BetterWorldTelecom.Com

ComeFromTheHeart.Com

EarthTones.Com

GreenLinePhone.Com

RedJellyFish.Com

WorkingAssets.Com

Television

If you have a TV, turn it off. TV is designed to keep you watching so that you watch as many commercials as possible with the goal of getting you to shop. On average, people who watch TV are heavier and less healthy than those who don't. Children who watch TV are more likely to have short attention spans and to eat unhealthful foods. Adults who watch a lot of TV are more likely to have more financial debt than those who watch little or no TV.

TV is king of the media-saturated and commercial-driven society. By avoiding TV, you are excluding the sensationalism and commercialism of television from your days and nights.

Television focuses on that which is energetically dark, such as greed, crime, and punishment. By focusing your attention on this form of "entertainment" you are absorbing this unhealthful energy into your life.

By watching TV you are removed from relating to people. There are people who think quality time with their family is spending their evenings watching TV shows together. They may become more emotionally connected to the characters on the TV shows than they are with the real people in their lives. Then, as a family activity they spend their weekend shopping for stuff they saw on TV. When they do finally spend time with the special person in their life they may do so only after they have gotten to some level of intoxication before feeling comfortable.

Watching TV is watching other people lead their lives. Watching TV is a waste of time and a waste of life. If you own a TV, put it in a place that is out of the way, or place a cloth over it and store away the remote to discourage yourself from watching it.

Instead of watching TV, spend time on working on your talents and intellect.

Make your life real, and make it based on your talents, abilities and intellect, and not on a commercially and celebrity-obsessed culture.

Thinking

Also see:
- Brain
- Infinite Intelligence
- Love
- Magnetizing Your Life
- People
- Talent
- Television
- Yoga

Books:
- *As You Think*, by Marc Allen, a revised and updated version of his father's book, *As a Man Thinketh*, by James Allen
- *Igniting Your Life*, by John McCabe

"Though we travel the world over to find the beautiful, we must carry it with us or find it not."
– **Ralph Waldo Emerson**

"I know of no more encouraging fact than the unquestioned ability of man to elevate his life by conscious endeavor."
– **Henry David Thoreau**

"All meaningful and lasting change starts first in your imagination and then works its way out. Imagination is more important than knowledge."
– **Albert Einstein**

You can resist damaging thought patterns. You can will away destructive emotions. You can consciously strengthen your abilities to think in a way that is more helpful to manifesting happiness in your life. You can eliminate damaging tendencies and retool your thoughts and actions in ways that can build a foundation for good things to manifest in your life.

The animation of your body is the emotion of your thought energy. Thoughts fuel actions. Actions that improve your life are the results of thoughts. If you want to improve your life, improve your thoughts.

> "Some folks are wise, and some otherwise."
> — Josh Billings

> "Opportunity is missed by most people because it comes dressed in overalls and looks like work."
> — Thomas Alva Edison

If you are waiting around for your life to begin, for things around you to change, for your days to be better to your liking, and to be in company that you would better enjoy, then you will be waiting a very long time. What you see around you is your life. If you don't like it, stop waiting for it to change, and start making it change.

> "We must all suffer one of two things: the pain of discipline or the pain of regret or disappointment."
> — E. James Rohn

Understand that the way you think helps to form your mind in a way that can greatly change your life. Work to change your life. Believe that you can do it. Conceptualize and know that your mindpower, talents, and what you can teach yourself through study and learning can bring about changes in your life. Bring all the right tools into your life to make the changes that need to happen. Improve your learning. Improve your way of thinking. Improve your diet. Improve your physical structure through daily exercise. Improve the way you spend your time. Improve the way you think of yourself as well as the way you think of others. Believe in yourself. Believe in your power and that you can shape your future.

> "What we are today comes from our thoughts of yesterday, and our present thoughts build our life of tomorrow: Our life is the creation of our mind."
> — Buddha

There is no better time to begin improving your life than the present. Now is the time to reach inside yourself to take control of your existence so that you can begin leading the best life you possibly can, through healthful eating, thinking, spirituality, and goal-oriented actions.

Many in life trip and stumble over the constant concern and worry about finances. But finances are the end result of actions. What drive your actions are your thoughts, and those are driven by your soul. The real power is the power of thought. The power of your thought is guided by your belief in what you are capable of doing mixed with the level at which you have tapped into the power of your essence and spirit, which is where your intellect, talents, and abilities dwell.

The essence of truth in enlightened teachings is that it inspires people to conduct themselves wisely, to respect themselves, and to respect wildlife. It instills a belief in power – the power to overcome, and the power to push forward and improve. It is the power to believe in yourself that can work miracles in your life.

> "When you undertake a Sunfood diet you will become more attached to the great workings of Nature and your true place and purpose will become more obvious to you. You will be compelled to let it unfold. Eating a raw, plant-based diet compels you to get into your true pattern of life."
> — David Wolfe

Move the obstacles out of your way. Do not dwell on the bad, unfortunate, and unfair things that happen to you. Don't let them shade your world or halt your progress. Refuse to be held bound by things and people that work against you. Do not make any time for self-pity in your days. Do not let your talents be caged in by the bars of regret.

> "Never regret. If it's good, it's wonderful. If it's bad, it's experience."
> — Victoria Holt

Look for the good in things, and build upon the good.

Start with what you have. Use it to bring yourself closer to the person you want to be. Work at this every day from the moment of awakening. Do so in a calm and determined manner that will propel you toward the person you want to become.

> "Realize that if you have time to whine and complain about something, you have time to do something about it."
> — Anonymous

Refuse to be overthrown by any problem that faces you.

What you think of as your greatest failure may actually turn out to be your greatest success, or a doorway to it. Keep using your intellect, talent, abilities, energy, resources, spirit, and the power of your thoughts to work toward creating the life you want to have.

Begin to think in a way that adjusts your energy to the frequency that you want to enjoy. Align yourself with good. Work to awaken the divinity that rests within.

Literature is food for the mind. People who read are found to have healthier brains with a wider variety of neural activity. Awaken your brain with reading. Read about things that have to do with what you want to do. Read about people who have succeeded in what you want to succeed in. Read things that will inspire you to become the person you want to be. Read what will nurture your thoughts to stay focused on your goals. Use literature to gain knowledge to better utilize your power.

Uplift yourself through inspirational thoughts. Let the common theme of your thoughts be that which empowers you. If it is a poem, think it. If it is a song, let it sing inside you. If it is an image, visualize it.

The ancient peoples of the world, the cave dwellers on every continent, the originators of religious teachings and philosophies, the creators of mythological stories that have been handed down for generations, everyone from the Aztecs and Buddhists to the Egyptians, Eskimos, Hebrews, Hindus, Hopi, Iroquois, Mayans, Polynesians, Upanishads, and every other group of people have shared the message that a person's happiness in life greatly relies on the choices of the individual to use his or her power.

"There is a you, lying dormant. A potential within you to be realized. It does not matter whether you have an intelligence quotient of 60 or 160, there is more of you than what you are presently aware of. Perhaps the only peace and joy in life lies in the pursuit of and development of this potential."
— Leo Buscaglia, Love: What life is all about

"We carry within us the wonders we seek without us."
— Sir Thomas Browne

"I shut my eyes in order to see."
— Paul Gauguin

"If you are seeking creative ideas, go out walking. Angels whisper to a man when he goes for a walk."
— **Raymond Inmon**

Don't think of creating your life as a way of finding it. It's not about finding it; it's about opening it. What you become is nurtured from within you. What moves you is your spirit. It is there. It is real. And you can use it any way you wish.

"You are not a human being in search of a spiritual experience. You are a spiritual being immersed in a human experience."
— **Pierre Teilhard de Chardin**

"A single gentle rain makes the grass many shades greener. So our prospects brighten on the influx of better thoughts."
— **Henry David Thoreau**

"Finally, brethren, whatever is true, whatever is honorable, whatever is right, whatever is pure, whatever is lovely, whatever is of good repute, if there is any excellence and if anything is worthy of praise, let your mind dwell on these things."
— **Philippians 4:8**

"You must be lamps unto yourselves."
— **Buddha**

"What gets us into trouble is not what we don't know. It's what we know for sure that just ain't so."
— **Mark Twain**

Stories originating from all parts of Earth carry a theme of people finding that the answers to their questions are right in front of them. For a time they may have been blind to the messages that surrounded them. Their stubbornness in their refusal to become enlightened made them unable to read the messages. They may have had resources of enlightenment surrounding them, but they did not recognize those. The tools may have existed, but they didn't do what it took to recognize them and know how to use them. Their possibilities and options were always there, but they did not notice them. But then a change of focus brought them to realize that they had the answers, the means, and the resources they needed to get what they needed.

"Often people attempt to live their lives backwards: they try to have more things, or more money, in order to do more of what they want so they will be happier. The way it actually works is the reverse. You must first be who you really are, then do what you need to do, in order to have what you want."
— **Margaret Young, as quoted in** *The Artist's Way*

Throughout world history as it is recorded on cave walls, in ancient scripts, in novels and plays, and in modern films there are similar representations of humans overcoming challenges. A common thread within these stories describe the change a person goes through within his or her mind that enables the person to overcome obstacles and achieve success in any situation. The message to be found is that it is up to the individual, using their intellect, to conquer and prosper starting from where they are by using their intuition, skills, talents, and intellect.

"If you don't set a baseline standard for what you'll accept in life, you'll find it's easy to slip into behaviors and attitudes or a quality of life that's far below what you deserve.
— **Anthony Robbins**

Just as your grandest successes may be self-created, so too may your greatest failures. It is up to you to decide which one of these options and possibilities may be realized. The message that transcends generations is that you are to decide which of your dreams becomes reality.

Your life does not have to be guided by the formula of the myth in which your strongest life-altering revelation arrives at your darkest moment. You do not have to depend on others for inspiration. Your personal revelations and inspirations can arrive at any time when you open yourself to the possibility of them. You may find this easier if you try to stay tuned to your self and use your attributes to propel your self into a better path.

"The mind is not a vessel to be filled, but a fire to be kindled."
— **William Butler Yeats**

How you visualize your life becoming is what your life is likely to become. If you want your life to be a certain way, start thinking about it being that way, and work your thoughts into actions that will create the life that you want. Pay attention to the things that will inspire your mind to bring this about.

When you begin to practice a task that requires a certain type of focus and movement, such as drawing, dancing, bike riding, or swimming, and you practice this task over and over during a period of weeks, months, and years, your brain actually rewires itself in coordination with the parts of the brain that control the movements you are making. That is a fascinating fact. This shows that what you think about, and what you do with your physical body, actually alters not only your muscles, but also the nerves inside your brain, and throughout your body tissues.

Understand that learning and doing keeps your brain growing and active. Do things that correspond with what you ideally see yourself doing. Teach yourself about the things you need to learn to live the life you want to have.

Whatever it is that you want to do, learn about it, and do it. Read books about it. Think about doing it. Plan on doing it. And do it mentally and physically.

Know that your thoughts are the sources driven by your spiritual force that will make you do what you want to do with your life.

> "The man without a purpose is like a ship without a rudder – a waif, a nothing, a no man. Have a purpose in life, and having it, throw such strength of mind and muscle into your work as God has given you."
> — Thomas Carlyle

There are patterns in things. Patterns in leaves, in seeds, in cells, and other living structures. There are patterns in your body, in your fingers, eyes, and through all the structures of your being. These structures erupt and are formulated by an inner power that directs the formation of the structures. Just as the notes of music put in a certain pattern can be either chaotic or pleasant, so too are the patterns of your thoughts and actions.

> "When you examine the lives of the most influential people who have ever walked among us, you discover one thread that winds through them all. They have been aligned first with their spiritual nature and only then with their physical selves."
> — Albert Einstein

There too are patterns in your essence. And there is power there. These powers are your talents, abilities, and intellect. And you can, with your power, use these to formulate your life and build it into what it should be. You have the strength within you to make this happen. You know it is there; it drives you to be attracted to, and to be pleased by, particular sounds, colors, shades, textures, smells, shapes, and feelings. Left to randomness they can be like all the pieces of a puzzle in a pile. Organized and managed, they can create the picture that is what your life is capable of becoming.

Make your life become what you want it to be. Understand that nobody can do it for you. You have to do it for yourself. Visualize it. Plan it. Nurture it. Do it. Become it. Live it.

Take care of your self, honoring your body with pure food from Nature that is Sunfood. This will help your life prosper.

Develop your talents and intellect, and trust in your heart.

Guide yourself more by love than by fear.

Be your own hero.

> "Go confidently in the direction of your dreams. Live the life you've always imagined."
> — **Henry David Thoreau**

Tissue Paper

Millions of trees are cut down every year to make tissue. When you buy tissue, buy the kind made from recycled paper.

Trauma Healing

Also see:
- Brain
- Infinite Intelligence
- Love
- Magnetizing Your Life
- People
- Talent
- Thinking
- Yoga

If you are in an abusive situation, leave it. Don't play the game in which you will always lose, and where there are no winners.

Many people get caught at the scene of the accident, and linger there for the rest of their lives, thus allowing their experience with negative events to define them.

Stop being upset with yourself. Move on toward better things through planning, goal setting, life reorientation, and connecting with your talents and intellect.

Take the remnants of your past and weave a better life. Compost the rest into a nurturing soil to grow the life you want.

> "Be not the slave of your own past – plunge into the sublime seas, dive deep, and swim far, so you shall come back with self-respect, with new power, with an advanced experience, that shall explain and over-look the old."
> — Ralph Waldo Emerson

While many of us have been subjected to negative, damaging situations, we do not have to dwell on those situations, or in the energy that surrounds those memories. We can break free of the things that have stopped us from succeeding in life. This includes releasing the energy surrounding negative personal relationships, cruel comments and actions, laziness, and bad food choices.

> "Great spirits have always encountered violent opposition from mediocre minds."
> — Albert Einstein

You can stop thinking bad thoughts about those in your life, and instead acknowledge the positive. You can stop rummaging around in the damage that was done to you and that you may have done with cruel words and unwise actions. You can begin to eat that which is most nutritional, and avoid foods that are damaging and unhealthful. Doing these things is liberating and empowering.

When the tissues of the body heal, they need nutrients. The better quality of the nutrients that are supplied to the tissues through high-quality foods, the better the tissues can heal. In a similar manner, if you are healing your life from one that has injured your spirit, mind, and body, you need to start feeding your life with those things that will help it to heal.

It all starts with the way you think.

Once you understand the source of what has damaged your life, you can begin to put those things out of your life. In your mind you can start to dispose of the clutter of damage that is creating a wall that blocks you from experiencing the life you should have.

Begin to replace thoughts of bad memories with thoughts of planning for a better future. Substitute thoughts that create good feelings for those thoughts that make you feel drained. Choose to think of the life you want to have instead of thinking of the life you had. This is the law of substitution: substituting positive thoughts in place of what were once negative thoughts.

"Go confidently in the direction of your dreams! Live the life you've imagined. As you simplify your life, the laws of the universe will be simpler; solitude will not be solitude, poverty will not be poverty, nor weakness weakness."
— Henry David Thoreau

This law of substitution is a concept spoken of by Brian Tracy in his book, *Maximum Achievement*. Tracy considers this to be one of the most important of all mental laws. It works to exercise your mind so that it holds positive instead of negative thoughts in ways that crowd out the negative. Because your mind is always working, make it work in the best way to suit your needs for a good life.

As negative thoughts lead to negative emotions, so too do positive thoughts lead to positive actions. Now think about that and consider what you most desire to have in your life. Do you want positive emotions? Then start to think positive. Doing so will enliven your body tissues. This is because thoughts release chemicals and energy into your body tissues. By working the power of your mind this way, you can bring positive thoughts to fuel your actions. Positive thoughts cannot fuel negative actions. Start thinking positively and you will naturally work your life in a more positive manner using the power of your positive thoughts.

"The key to life-long happiness is to systematically purge negative emotions from your life – to eliminate anything which triggers negativity or stress in your psyche. A garden-mind encumbered by negative thoughts repels health and prosperity. Purging negative emotions is not optional; it is necessary to achieve a vibrant state of health. This means you have to get away from negative friends, associates, or relatives as soon as possible. You cannot let their negativity dissuade you from your greatness."
— David Wolfe

As you start thinking positively you automatically start to become healthier. Make yourself constantly focus on thoughts that will uplift you. This will illuminate your life because thinking positive actually changes the electric charges throughout your body cells. By continuously thinking positive you are literally bathing the cells of your body in positive energy, positive emotions, and positive thought chemicals.

This is the start of the power that can take over your life. The power will drive you to think, act, plan, and communicate more positively. To build upon this you will need to provide your body with what it needs to grow more healthfully. This involves providing your body with the best nutrients; exercising your intellect by learning and practicing new things; and by getting daily exercise to make your body what it is capable of being. All these actions will work in symphony to drive your life forward into health.

The mind and body cannot perform at their peak without the necessary nutrients. The better nutrients your body receives, the better it can perform. The cleaner your diet, the less clogged will be the energy flow within your body. To change your life in the best ways you must provide your body with the best nutrients.

To guide you on your journey, create a strategy.

Write down your thoughts. Work them out like a puzzle to organize them into a workable pattern that you can work into your life. When you see what you want written on paper, it helps you visualize. Going through the list every morning helps you keep the life changes you want at the forefront of your mind. Thinking about the positive changes you want is the process that helps construct them and manifest them into your reality.

> "Character is formed in the stormy billows of the world."
> — Johann Wolfgang von Goethe

What you become from now on is up to you. There is no more blaming others, there is no more self-loathing and droning on and on about the past. Positive change happens at the present, and can be made in the future. Not in the past. It comes through motivational and inspired thoughts that elicit actions, not in depressing thoughts that create mental decay. It comes through providing the nutrients the body needs to function at a high level. These are the nutrients that are available in vibrant, alive plant substances containing the power of Nature. Not through a diet of dead foods. It comes through working toward established goals, and from organized priorities set to guide a person toward betterment. Not in disorganized randomness. It comes through daily exercise to enliven and strengthen the body. Not in sedentary slothfulness. It comes by choice, which happens in your mind. The mind that you need to change if you are going to change your life.

Reinterpret your past as something that can help you rather than something that harmed you. If it did harm you, then that is what happened. But that doesn't mean that you have to keep dwelling on it in a negative way. Rise above it.

Refuse to get caught in past regrets and the reverberating energy of unfortunate incidents. When you begin to feel the waves of bad memories flow through your being, choose to focus on thoughts that are more helpful and that will move you into more confident and uplifting thoughts.

Maybe the reason your life has not turned out the way you want is that you have allowed others to take it over, or have thought others would create a good life for you. You have given up your power.

Take charge of your life.

Consider others who have succeeded and gotten past horrible situations in their lives. Know that you too can bring yourself out of whatever rut you have been in. Understand that it is up to you to make the changes that will improve your life. Look toward the future and grow from where you are.

Work to eliminate those things from your life that are not part of the life that you want. This includes eliminating patterns of thinking, patterns of eating, patterns of acting, and patterns of activities that are not in alignment with the life that you want. By constantly focusing your life away from what you don't want, and onto what you do want, you will naturally be drawn to such things that you want. Freeing your life of those things that you don't want frees up your life to accept that which you do want.

By harboring the thoughts that are in alignment with the life that you want, you are planting the seeds that will grow into the life that you want.

Focus on your goals, not your obstacles.

For those of us who came from violent or otherwise abusive households, or who have experienced abusive relationships, some of the following may be of help.

Eye Movement Desensitization and Reprocessing Institute, EMDR.Com

Foundation for Human Enrichment, TraumaHealing.Com

Healing Sex: The Complete Guide to Sexual Wholeness, HealingSexTheMovie.Com

International Trauma-Healing Institute, TraumaInstitute.Org

National Coalition Against Domestic Violence, NCADV.Org

Travel

It is increasingly common to find organically grown produce in many towns and cities. There are Internet sights where you can locate farmers' markets as well as vegan restaurants that can satisfy your taste. Nearly every city has some sort of natural foods store where you can find organic produce as well as local magazines listing vegetarian restaurants and goings-on in town. (See the Restaurants and Vegetarian Web Site sections of this book to find what you may be seeking in the town you are visiting.)

Vegan dating sites also are a good source of information, and you may end up having a better time at your destination than you thought possible. (See the Dating section in this book.)

The travel industry creates enormous amounts of pollution. From airlines to hotels and from taxis to rental cars, the travel industry is very slowly starting to work on ways to clean up its act.

One way the travel industry pollutes is through its food. Tons of plastics and throwaway eating utensils are used every day by the airline industry. The hotel industry also causes massive amounts of pollution by not using recycled paper tissue, they don't recycle, they use enormous amounts of environmentally unfriendly cleaning materials, use chlorine products in their pools, dispose of hundreds of thousands of mattresses every year, construct and decorate their facilities using environmentally unsafe and nonsustainable materials, and use toxic pesticides, insecticides, weed killer and fertilizers in their landscaping.

If you travel, seek ways to reduce your impact on the planet. If you choose to travel by car remember that sharing car rides is always less polluting than traveling singularly. Check out the Internet rideshare boards that I've listed below.

Some of the following Web sites provide information on hotels that are working to become less toxic to the environment.

Adventure-Center.Com

Better World Club, 20 NW 5th Ave., #100, Portland, OR 97210;
BetterWorldClub.Com
 Provides everything from an "auto club" membership for roadside assistance for
bikes and cars; auto insurance for the environmentally minded traveler; maps and
travel services aimed at eco-travel; car rental discounts; and discounts for owners of
hybrid vehicles.

EcoClub.Com

EcoTourism.Org

EcoTravel.Com

EcoTravelSpecialists.Com

Gaiam.Com

GlobalExchange.Com

GreenHotels.Com

GreenSeal.Org/FindaProduct/Index.cfm

KindRideShare.Net

KindRideShare.Org/KindRideShare/

ResponsibleTravel.Com

StarsRainbowRideBoard.Org

Vegetarian Resource Group, POB 1463, Baltimore, MD 21203; 410-366-8343;
VRG.Org
 In addition to a links to other vegetarian sites, this Web site contains a list of veg-
etarian restaurants, and guides for vegetarian travelers.

Vegetarian-Restaurants.Net
 Lists vegetarian restaurants and food stores in the US, Canada, England, Europe,
and other areas of the world.

The White Pig Bed & Breakfast at Briar Creek Farm, Virginia;
TheWhitePig.Com

Trees and Plants

Also see:
* Environmental Protection

"Every year an amount of land the size of Greece is logged – some 32 million acres... Deforestation both reduces biodiversity and increases the presence of greenhouse gasses in the atmosphere."
— **Reuters, November 15, 2005**

"Most of the world's most valuable forests, especially in the tropics, are vanishing as fast as ever."
— **Simon Counsell, Rainforest Foundation, 2006**

Help plant trees, protect native flora, and reclaim land for the wild that has been damaged by human activities. Help support at least one of the following groups.

Action for Community and Ecology in the Rainforests of Central America; POB 57, Burlington, VT 05402; 802-863-0571; ACERCA.Org

Allegheny Defense Project, POB 245, Clarion, PA 16214; 814-223-4996; AlleghenyDefense.Org/

American Chestnut Foundation, ACF.Org
There were once billions of chestnut trees in North America. Now there are relatively few. Help bring them back; plant chestnut trees!

American Forests, AmFor.Org

Ancient Trees, Citizen's Campaign for Old Growth Preservation, POB 714, Ukiah, CA 95482; 707-923-1194; AncientTrees.Org

Bay Area Coalition for Headwaters Forest, 2530 San Pablo Ave., Berkeley, CA 94702; 510-548-2220; HeadwatersPreserve.Org/

Blue Mountains Biodiversity Project; HCR 82, Fossil, OR 97830; 541-468-2028

Botanic Gardens Conservation International, Japan, BGCI.Org

Budongo Forest Project, Budongo.Org

California Community Forests Foundation, CalTrees.Org

California Native Plant Society, CNPS.Org

Cascadia Rising EcoDefense, POB 12583, Portland, OR 97212; CascadiaRising.Org

Cascadia Wild, 1417 SE 34th Ave., Portland, OR 97214; 503-235-9533; CascadiaWild.Org

Cascadia Wildlands Project, POB 10455, Eugene, OR 97440; 541-434-1460

Center for Native Ecosystems, NativeEcosystems.Org

Center for Watershed Protection, Pipeline.Com/~mrRunOff/

ChicagoWilderness.Org

Children's Eternal Rainforest, Monteverde Conservation League, POB 124 - 5655 Monte Verde Puntarenas, Costa Rica; ACMCR.Org/Rain_Forest.htm

Circle of Life Foundation, POB 3764, Oakland, CA 94609; 510-601-9790; CircleOfLifeFoundation.Org
   This was founded by Julia Butterfly Hill who lived near the top of a California redwood tree for two years and brought international attention to the horrors of the lumber industry and the state of the environment. Hill authored a book titled *The Legacy of Luna*. Shortly after she left the ancient tree, someone with a chainsaw cut into the base of it.

Desert Harvesters, Tucson, AZ; DesertHarvester.Org
   Strives to promote, celebrate, and enhance, local food security and production by encouraging the planting of indigenous, food-bearing shade trees (such as the Velvet mesquite) in water -harvesting earthworks, and then educating the public on how to harvest and process the bounty.

Earth First!, Direct Action Fund, POB 210, Canyon, CA 91516; EarthFirstJournal.Org

Earth First!, POB 1415; Eugene, OR 97440; 541-741-9191; EarthFirstJournal.Org

Earth First! Journal, POB 3023, Tucson, AZ 85702-3023; 520-620-6900, EarthFirstJournal.Org

Earth Watch Institute, EarthWatch.Org

Eastern North American Native Forest Network, POB 57 Burlington VT 05402; Forests.Org

Forest Guardians, FGuardians.Org

Forests Forever, 973 Market St., Ste. 450, San Francisco, CA 94103; 415-974-3636; ForestsForever.Org

Forest Ethics, POB 3418, Berkeley, CA 94703; 510-533-8725; ForestEthics.Org
   Dedicated to protecting the ancient rainforests of British Columbia and endangered forests of North America by redirecting U.S. markets toward ecologically sound alternatives.

Forest Voice, ForestCouncil.Org
Published by Native Forest Council (listed below).

Fruit Tree Planting Foundation, FTPF.Org

FutureForests.Com

Gifford Pinchot Task Force, POB 11427, Olympia, WA 98508; 360-753-4185; GPTaskForce.Org

Granby Wilderness Society, POB 2532, Grand Forks, B.C. V0H 1H0 Canada; 250-442-2125; GrandbyWilderness.Org

Green Anarchy, POB 11331, Eugene, OR 97440; GreenAnarchy.Org

Green Korea United, GreenKorea.Org

Greenpeace.Org

Heartwood Forest Council, Heartwood.Org/ForestCouncil.htm

   "Heartwood's Forest Council is an annual event that seeks to bring together forest activists from throughout the eastern United States to share skills, learn about forest issues, and to support local forest protection efforts."

Heritage Forests Campaign, 1200 Eighteenth St., N.W., Washington, DC 20036; 202-887-8800; OurForests.Org

Illegal Logging at Suaq Balimbing, Duke.Edu/~MYM1/Suaq.htm

MangroveRestoration.Com

Mattole Forest Defenders, POB 117, Petrolia, CA 95558; 707-441-3828; MattoleDefense.Org

Mountain Justice Summer, MountainJusticeSummer.Org
   Focused on the tremendous ecological disaster being caused by mountain top removal mining in the Appalachian mountains of Tennessee, Virginia, West Virginia, and Kentucky.

The National Council for the Conservation of Plants and Gardens, England, NCCPG.Com

National Forest Protection Alliance, POB 8264, Missoula, MT 59807; ForestAdvocate.Org

National Tree Society, POB 10808; Bakersfield, CA 93389; 805-589-6912; Natural-Connection.Com/Institutes/National_Tree.html

National Tropical Botanical Garden, NTBG.Org

Native Forest Council, POB 2190, Eugene, OR 97402; ForestCouncil.Org

Native Forest Network, Northern Hemisphere: POB 8251, Missoula, MT 59807; 406-542-7343; Northern Hemisphere: Eastern North America, POB 57, Burlington, VT 05402; 802-863-0571; Southern Hemisphere: POB 301, Deloraine, Tasmania 7304 Australia; International +61 3 6369 5102; (Australia) 03 6369 5102; NativeForest.Org

North Coast Earth First!, POB 219, Bayside, CA 95524
  Working to protect the ancient forests of the Northern California. The Federal Fish and Wildlife Service allows lumber companies to cut down these ancient forests, killing many forms of wildlife. Please help stop this!

Northern Nut Growers Association, NorthernNutGrowers.Org, or NutGrowing.Org

Pawpaw Foundation, 147 Atwood Research Facility, Kentucky State University, Frankfort KY 40601-2355; PawPaw.KYSU.Edu

Theodore Payne Foundation, TheodorePayne.Org

Plantlife International: The Wild Plant Conservation Charity, England; Plantlife.Org.UK

Rainforest Action Network, 221 Pine St., Ste. 500, San Francisco, CA 94104; 415-398-4404; 415-398-2732; RAN.Org

Rainforest Foundation, 270 Lafayette St., Ste. 1107, New York, NY 10012; 212-431-908; SaveTheRest.Org

Rainforest Alliance, 665 Broadway, Ste. 500, New York, NY 10012; 212-677-1900; 888-My-Earth; RA.Org; Rainforest-Alliance.Org

RainForestPortal.Org

Redwood Action Team, POB 34, Garberville, Ecotopia 95542;

Stanford.Edu/Group/RATS

Save America Forest, POB 1023, Bowie, MO 20715

Save America's Forests, 4 Library Crt., SE, Washington, DC 20003; 202-544-9219; SaveAmericasForests.Org

Save the Redwoods League, 114 Sansome St., Rm. 605, San Francisco, CA 94104; SaveTheRedwoods.Org

Swamp Watch Action Team, SwampWatch.Org

Tasmanian Wilderness Society, EN.Wikipedia.Org/wiki/Tasmanian_Wilderness_Society

Tree Musketeers, TreeMusketeers.Org
   A kid-centered urban forestry-planting organization empowering young people to work to rescue Earth.

Tree People, 12601 Mulholland Dr., Beverly Hills, CA 90210; TreePeople.Org

Trees for Life, 1103 Jefferson, Wichita, KS 167203; TreesForLife.Org

Trees for the Future, TreesFTF.Org

Trees Foundation, POB 2202; Redway, CA 95542; TreesFoundation.Org

United Plant Savers, POB 400, East Barre, VT 05649; UnitedPlantSavers.Org

U.S. Forests Service Urban Forest Ecosystem Research Unit, FS.Fed.US/NE/Syracuse

TheWatershedProject.Org

World Rainforest Information Portal, RainforestWeb.Org

Veal: End This Cruel Industry

"Endless multitudes will have their little children taken from them, ripped open and flayed and most cruelly cut in pieces."
   — **Leonardo da Vinci, a vegetarian who was outspoken against the killing and consumption of animals**

"A newborn baby is taken from his mother and placed in a 'crate' so narrow he can't turn around or even lie down comfortably. Instead of nourishing mother's milk, he is fed a substitute liquid that is purposely deficient in iron and fiber – the better to keep his flesh pale. And since he can hardly move in his confined space, his muscles won't develop and he will stay soft and tender. He will endure this for four months... and then he'll be slaughtered and eaten.

Male calves are an unwanted 'by-product' of the dairy industry, as they cannot produce milk. They are trucked to livestock auctions within hours or days of being born and sold for just a few dollars to veal producers. If the calves are too weak or ill to sell after the grueling truck ride, they may be left to die in pens or back alleyways at the auction yards.

At the veal factories, each calf is chained at the neck in a crate only 22 inches wide, so he can't walk or turn around. Because the iron-deficient diet makes him anemic and sickly, his formula routinely contains drugs... that can get passed on to the unsuspecting consumer. The calf suffers from chronic diarrhea, and he is not even allowed to have water to drink – just the liquid diet that produces what is misleadingly labeled 'milk-fed' – and also 'fancy' or 'white' – veal.

Because this is considered a 'common agribusiness practice' it is typically exempt from animal-cruelty laws. As a matter of fact, the production of veal is specifically excluded from anticruelty laws in the majority of U.S. states. In Europe, several nations have banned the inhumane, severe confinement producer for calves that is standard operating procedure in the U.S. But, the meat and dairy industries are a wealthy, powerful lobbying and advertising force... and they have been defeating farm animal protection efforts for decades."

– **Farm Sanctuary No Veal Campaign; FarmSanctuary.Org**

Compassion Action Institute, PleaseBeKind.Com

Farm Sanctuary East, POB 150, Watkins Glen, NY 14891; 607-583-2225; FarmSanctuary.Org; FactoryFarming.Com; NoVeal.Org

Farm Sanctuary West, POB 1065, Orland, CA 95963; 530-865-4617; FarmSanctuary.Org; FactoryFarming.Com; NoVeal.Org

Humane Society of the United States, HSUS.Org

Vegetarian and Vegan Groups, Web Sites, Restaurants & Stores

"I have no doubt that it is a part of the destiny of the human race, in

its gradual improvement, to leave off eating animals."
   — **Henry David Thoreau**

"In the past half-century, most U.S. livestock production has moved
from small family farms to factory farms – huge warehouses where animals are confined in crowded cages or pens or in restrictive stalls. The
competition to lower costs has led agri-business to treat animals as
mere objects, rather than individuals who can suffer.
   Hidden from public view, the cruelty that occurs on factory farms is
easy to ignore. But more and more people are taking a look at how
farmed animals are treated and deciding that it's too cruel to support."
   — **Vegan Outreach, VeganOutreach.Org**

"Vegetarian diets offer a number of nutritional benefits, including
lower levels of saturated fat, cholesterol, and animal protein as well as
higher levels of carbohydrates, fiber, magnesium, potassium, folate, and
antioxidants such as vitamins C and E and phytochemicals. Vegetarians
have been reported to have lower body mass indexes than nonvegetarians, as well as lower rates of death from ischemic heart disease; vegetarians also show lower blood cholesterol levels; lower blood pressure;
and lower rates of hypertension, Type 2 diabetes, and prostate and
colon cancer."
   — *Journal of the American Dietetic Association*; **Vol. 103, No. 6; June 2003**

"If a man aspires towards a righteous life, his first act of abstinence is
from injury to animals."
   — **Albert Einstein**

"Contrary to what one may hear from the industry, chickens are not
mindless, simple automata but are complex behaviorally, do quite well
in learning, show a rich social organization, and have a diverse reper-
toire of calls. Anyone who has kept barnyard chickens also recognizes
their significant differences in personality.
   [It is] more economically efficient to put a greater number of birds
into each cage, accepting lower productivity per bird but greater productivity per cage... Individual animals may 'produce,' for example gain
weight, in part because they are immobile, yet suffer because of the
inability to move... Chickens are cheap, cages are expensive."
   — **Bernard E. Rollin, Ph.D.,** *Farm Animal Welfare,* **Iowa State University Press,
      1995**

"When I saw what life is really like for pigs on today's farms, I was
left feeling sick for days. I knew they lived on concrete, indoors in facto-

ry farms. However, I was not prepared for the awful reality of their boredom. In the gestation shed, sows continuously hit their heads against their cage doors as if trying to escape. After a while, some would give up and lie down, while others again took up the futile action.

I saw pens where pigs are fattened up for slaughter – essentially concrete cells, each holding about a dozen pigs. In one pen, there was a pig missing an ear. Another had a rupture the size of a grapefruit protruding from his stomach. A dead pig was constantly nudged and licked by the others. The stench in these places is overwhelming.

At the larger farms I visited in North Carolina, there were thousands of pigs housed in sheds. Dead pigs had been left in the pens with the living; other pigs had been tossed in the aisles – barely alive, unable to reach food or water."
— **Lauren Ornelas, VivaUSA.Org**

"They are not brethren; they are not underlings; they are other nations, caught with ourselves in the net of life and time, fellow prisoners of the splendour and travail of the earth."
— **Henry Beston**

"When we kill the animals to eat them, they end up killing us because their flesh, which contains cholesterol and saturated fat, was never intended for human beings."
— **William C. Roberts, M.D., editor of *The American Journal of Cardiology***

"Starvation, world hunger, cruelty, waste, wars – we must make a statement against these things. Vegetarianism is my statement. And I think it's a strong one."
— **Isaac Bashevis Singer**

"Vegetarianism preserves life, health, peace, the ecology, creates a more equitable distribution of resources, helps to feed the hungry, encourages nonviolence, and is a powerful aid for spiritual growth."
— **Gabriel Cousens, M.D.**

"Children who grow up getting their nutrition from plant foods rather than meats have a tremendous health advantage. They are less likely to develop weight problems, diabetes, high blood pressure, and some forms of cancer."
— **Benjamin Spock, M.D.**

"If the anticruelty laws that protect pets were applied to farmed ani-

mals, many of the most routine U.S. farming practices would be illegal in all 50 states. Are dogs and cats really so different from chickens, turkeys, pigs, and cows that one group deserves legal protection from cruelty, while the other deserves no protection at all?"
   – **OpposeCruelty.Org**

"There's a schizoid quality to our relationship with animals, in which sentiment and brutality exist side by side. Half the dogs in America will receive Christmas presents this year, yet few of us pause to consider the miserable life of the pig – an animal easily as intelligent as a dog – that becomes the Christmas ham."
   – **Michael Pollan, An Animal's Place,** *New York Times,* **November 10, 2002**

"For modern animal agriculture, the less the consumer knows about what's happening before the meat hits the plate, the better. If true, is this an ethical situation? Should we be reluctant to let people know what really goes on, because we're not really proud of it and concerned that it might turn them to vegetarianism?"
   – **Peter Cheeke, Ph.D., Oregon State University Professor of Animal Agriculture,** *Contemporary Issues in Animal Agriculture,* **2004 textbook**

"You put a baby in a crib with an apple and a rabbit. If it eats the rabbit and plays with the apple, I'll buy you a new car."
   – **Harvey Diamond, author of** *Fit for Life*

"Eating meat leaves behind an environmental toll that generations to come will be forced to pay.
   Land: Of all agricultural land in the U.S., 87 percent is used to raise animals. One acre of land can yield 20,000 pounds of potatoes or 165 pounds of beef.
   Water: Raising animals for food consumes more than half of all the water used in the U.S. It takes 2,500 gallons of water to produce a pound of beef, but only 25 gallons to produce a pound of wheat.
   Pollution: The meat industry causes more water pollution than any other industry. Animals raised for food produce about 43 tons of excrement every second. A typical pig factory farm generates raw waste equal to a city of 12,000 people.
   There are ten times more pesticides used for animal feed than for food production that is used directly for human consumption. The pesticides, which don't readily degrade, enter our waterways and poison us, and our food.
   Deforestation: Rainforests are being destroyed at a rate of 125,000 square miles per year to create space to raise animals for food. Fifty-five

square feet of land are consumed for every quarter-pound fast-food burger made of rainforest beef."
　— **MeatStinks.Org**

"It appears from Corsali's letter that Leonardo ate no meat, but lived entirely on vegetables, thus forestalling modern vegetarians by several centuries."
　— **Eugene Muntz in** *Leonardo da Vinci Artist, Thinker, and Man of Science,* **1898**

"Most of us think of vegetarians as nuts and I'm not a vegetarian but I wouldn't be surprised if we came to a time in 50 or 100 years when civilized people everywhere refused to eat animals. I could be one of them.
Of course, I'd be pretty old by then."
　— **Andy Rooney,** *60 Minutes,* **October 1, 2006**

"Certain infidels called Guzzarati [Hindus] do not feed upon anything that contains blood, nor do they permit among them any injury be done to any living thing, like our Leonardo da Vinci."
　— **Andrea Corsali, in a letter to Giuliano de' Medici, the brother of Pope Leo X, and patron of da Vinci; as quoted in Jean Paul Richter in** *The Literary Works of Leonardo da Vinci;* **1883**

"If you don't want to be beaten, imprisoned, mutilated, killed or tortured, then you shouldn't condone such behavior towards anyone, be they human or not."
　— **Moby**

Alaska Vegetarian Society, Wasilla, AK; RaysOfHope.Info

Albany Vegetarians, VegAlbany.Com

All Vegan, AllVeganShopping.Com
　A store in San Diego that sells everything from clothing to books and household items that are "cruelty free."

AmericanVegan.Org

Animal Rights Canada, AnimalRightsCanada.Com
　Web site contains a list of vegetarian groups.

Asian Vegetarians
　There are vegetarian groups in Hong Kong, Indonesia, Japan, Malaysia, Pakistan, Thailand, Mumbai, and Singapore. See VegDining.Com for links to vegetarian groups in Asia. Also, access the International Vegetarian Union Web site: IVU.Org

Bay Area Vegetarians, Montara, CA; BayAreaVeg.Org

Boston Vegetarian Society, BostonVeg.Com

Calgary Vegetarian Society, CalgaryVeg.Com

Canada Vegetarians
To locate a more complete list of vegetarian groups in Canada, see Vegdining.Com.
Also, access the Web site of the International Vegetarian Union: IVU.Org.

Chicago Vegetarians, VegChicago.Com

CosmosVeganShoppe.Com

DropSoul.Com

EarthSave International, 1509 Seabright Ave., Ste. B1, Santa Cruz, CA 95062;
831-423-0293; 800-362-3648; EarthSave.Org
Started by John Robbins, author of the books, *Diet for a New America, May All be Fed*, and *The Food Revolution*. EarthSave works to promote the many advantages – health, environmental, and otherwise – of following a plant-based diet. There are local chapters of EarthSave in many areas of the world.

EarthVegans.US

EcoVegEvents.Com
Information on ecology, animal rights, and vegan and vegetarian events.

Environ Gentle, 543 S. Coast Hwy. 101, Encinitas, CA 92024;
EnvironGentle.Com
Sells all sorts of items of interest to vegans, such as organic cotton and hemp products, including hemp-based foods. Also sells unusual things, such as recycled tire rubber belts, recycled inner tube rubber wallets, and nonpetroleum, biodegradable, compostable corn-based eating utensils.

Eugene Veg Education Network, EugVegeDuNet@Comcast.Net

European Vegetarians
There are vegetarian organizations in most European countries. Access
VegDining.Com for a list of them. Also access: European-Vegetarian.Org

FactoryFarming.Com

Food Fight Vegan Grocery, 4179 SE Division, Portland, OR; 503-233-3910;
FoodFightGrocery.Com
Food Fight sells vegan junk food. Their irreverent Web site contains current event

news regarding animal protection, political stupidity, world craziness, and wacky weird strangeness.

GarlicBoy.Com

Go Veggie, Chicago, IL; Go-Veggie.Org

Green People, GreenPeople.Org
Directory of eco-friendly products.

Daryl Hannah, DHLoveLife.Com

Happy Cow, HappyCow.Net
Guide to vegetarian restaurants and health food stores.

Hawaiian Vegetarians, VegHawaii.Com

Hong Kong Vegan Society, IVU.Org/HKVegan/

International Vegetarian Union, POB 9710, Washington, DC 20016; 202-362-VEGY; IVU.Org

Institute for Plant Based Nutrition, PlantBased.Org

Joruba.Com

LivingNutrition.Com

LondonVegans.Org.UK

Howard Lyman, MadCowboy.Com

Madison Vegetarians, VegMadison.Com

The Meat Free Zone, All-Creatures.Org/MFZ/

MeatStinks.Org

McLibelTheMovie.Com

McSpotlight.Org

New Zealand Vegetarian Society, VegSoc.Wellington.Net.NZ

North American Vegetarian Society, POB 72, Dolgeville, NY 13329; 518-568-7970; NAVS-Online.Org

North Connecticut Vegetarian Society, NorthCTVeg.Org

Ohio Vegetarians, Mercy for Animals, VegOhio.Com

OrganicAthlete.Org

PETA's GoVeg Campaign, 501 Front St., Norfolk, VA 23510; 757-622-PETA; GoVeg.Com

Philadelphia Vegetarians, VegPhilly.Com

RaveDiet.Com

Revolucion Vegana, RevolucionVegana.Org
Working to spread vegan principles to young people in Mexico.

San Diego Vegetarians, VegSanDiego.Com

Santa Cruz Vegetarians, VegSantaCruz.Com

Seattle Vegetarians, VegSeattle.Com

Sidecar for Pigs Peace, Seattle, WA; 206-523-9060; SideCarForPigsPeace.Com
Vegan supply store.

Southern California Vegetarians, Los Angeles, CA; SoCalVeg.Org

SoyStache.Com

Sunfood Nutrition, 11653 Riverside Dr., Lakeside, CA 92040; 800-205-2350; 888-RAW-FOOD; International: +001-619-596-7979; Sunfood.Com
    Sells books about raw veganism, and distributes kitchen equipment and food products. Runs seminars about Sunfood nutrition, and holds retreats in places like Hawaii, Costa Rica, Jamaica, and at Eden Hot Springs in Arizona.

SuperVegan.Com

SustainLane.Com

Toronto Vegetarian Association, Veg.Ca

TryVeg.Com, Compassion over Killing, POB 9773, Washington, DC 20016; 301-891-2458; TryVeg.Com; COK.Net

Vegan Action, POB 4288, Richmond, VA 23220; 804-502-8736; Vegan.Org
    Their Web site includes a list of suggested reading, as well as a list of companies that sell animal-safe, cruelty-free products, such as nonleather shoes.

VeganEssentials.Com

VeganForum.Com

Vegan Freak Radio, Podcast.VeganFreak.Com

VeganFreaks.Org

VeganHealthStudy.Com

Veganica.Com

Vegan Outreach, POB 38492, Pittsburgh, PA 15238-8492; 211 Indian Dr., Pittsburgh, PA 15238; VeganOutreach.Org

Vegans of Tijuana, VegTijuana.Com

VeganStore.Com

VegAnswers.Com

VeganUnlimited.Com

VegBay.Com

VegDining.Com
Online guide to vegetarian restaurants around the world.

Vegetarian.Meetup.Com

Vegetarian Network Victoria, Australia; VNV.Org.au

Vegetarian Resource Group, POB 1463, Baltimore, MD 21203; 410-366-8343; VRG.Org
In addition to a links to other vegetarian sites, this Web site contains a list of vegetarian restaurants, and guides for vegetarian travelers.

Vegetarian Resource Group of Tucson, AZ; VRGT.Org

Vegetarian-Restaurants.Net
Lists vegetarian restaurants and food stores in the U.S., Canada, England, Europe, and other areas of the world.

Vegetarians in Paradise, VegParadise.Com

VegetarianShoesAndBags.Com

Vegetarian Society of Colorado, VSC.Org

Vegetarian Society of Georgia, Norcross; VegSocietyOfGA.Org

Vegetarian Society of Hawaii, Honolulu; VSH.Org

Vegetarian Society of the District of Columbia, Washington, DC; VSDC.Org

VegetarianTeen.Com

Vegetarian USA, VegetarianUSA.Com

Vegetarian-Vacations.Com

Vegetarian/Vegan Society of Queensland, Australia, VegSoc.Org.AU

VeggieBite.Net

VeggieLA.Com

VeggieLiving.Net

VeggieRoomMate.Com

Veggies.Org.Uk

VeginOut.Com

VegKansasCity.Com

VegOhio.Com

VegSource.Com

Washington DC Vegetarians, VegDC.Com

The White Pig Bed & Breakfast at Briar Creek Farm, Virginia; TheWhitePig.Com

WildernessFamilyNaturals.Com

WorldFestEvents.Org

Vivisection: Extreme Animal Torture

Also see:
• Circus Animals

"Each year an estimated 28 million animals in the U.S. are used in research, testing, and education, including:
• 70,000 dogs
• 23,00 cats
• 54,000 nonhuman primates
• 266,000 guinea pigs
• 201,000 hamsters
• 280,000 rabbits
• 155,000 farm animals, including cattle, sheep, and pigs
• 165,000 others, such as gerbils, ferrets, and minks
• Approximately 20–25 million rats and mice."
   — A Voice for Animals, VoiceForAnimals.Net; 2006

"They laugh, like us. They are devoted to their families, like us. They show compassion, like us. They have unique personalities, like us. When they are confined, hurt, or experimented on, they get depressed, they get angry, they cry, and they grieve. Like us.
   — ReleaseChimps.Org

Animals kept in "science labs" are often purposefully injured, such as by burning them with a blow torch, breaking their bones, cutting off their limbs or facial parts, and having drills and surgical tools put into their brains and other parts of their body. Some have their eyes sewn shut. Others have harsh chemicals put into their eyes, on their skin, or into their mouths. Some have electrodes implanted into their skin, muscles, and brain. Some are exposed to extreme noise, nonstop wind, heat, cold, and other experiments. When they are of no more use to the lab workers these horribly abused animals are left to die, or are killed.

Who funds these laboratory experiments? Much of it is paid for by grants from the National Institutes of Health, which is funded by tax dollars. Another tax-supported agency involved with animal experimentation is the U.S. Department of Agriculture. Other labs are supported by businesses, such as those that manufacture various products. Some animal farming businesses use animals to experiment on to develop new ways of slaughtering farm animals.

"But aren't these experiments necessary to save human lives?
No, absolutely not. There are better ways to study human physiology, disease, and injury than inducing disease and injury in a different species.
Clinical human studies, autopsies, epidemiology, human tissue studies, and imaging technologies are only some of the better ways to study human health and disease."
— **New England Anti-Vivisection Society, NEAVS.Org**

Many cosmetics companies have been involved in animal experimentation. Federally funded agencies that have been involved in vivisection include the National Institute of Neurological Disorders and Stroke; the National Center for Research Resources; the National Institute of Diabetes & Digestive & Kidney Diseases; and the National Heart, Lung and Blood Institute. Many universities also run labs where animals are tortured. These include Boston University, Harvard University, the University of Massachusetts Medical School, and UCLA. But that is a very short list. For more information on companies, government agencies, schools and others conducting animal experimentation, contact the organizations listed in this section.

"In the past three years, approximately $15 million taxpayer dollars went into federally-funded cat experiments in the state of Massachusetts alone."
— **New England Anti-Vivisection Society, NEAVS.Org; 2002**

"If you agree with vivisection, go and be vivisected upon yourself."
— **Morrissey, during a concert in London, May 2006. He was commenting about a new £20 million animal testing lab at Oxford University. The week before, Oxford University won a legal appeal to keep demonstrators away from the "biomedical" animal torture facility.**

"What do they know – all these scholars, all these philosophers, all the leaders of the world? They have convinced themselves that man, the worst transgressor of all the species, is the crown of creation. All other creatures were created merely to provide him with food, pelts, to be tormented, exterminated. In relation to them, all people are Nazis; for the animals it is an eternal Treblinka."
— **Isaac Bashevis Singer, 1978 Nobel Prize winner**

"That vivisectors can look them in the eyes while perpetrating one atrocity after another on them is testament to the amorality that science permits itself. The poor, orphans, criminals, the mentally ill, Jews,

and African-Americans were all at some time within the vivisector's reach. Equally disturbing is that chimpanzees still are."
— **Theodora Capaldo, EdD, President of the New England Anti-Vivisection Society, NEAVS.Org**

"It is easy for me to see the connection between the entertainment industry and biomedical research for chimpanzees because I face it every day. I see their faces, and I think about what their lives were like before [arriving at The Fauna Foundation]. Half of my chimpanzee family began their lives in entertainment only to end up being used for biomedical research. I am ashamed by the lack of respect they were shown by humans. They deserve so much more."
— **Gloria Grow, Co-founder The Fauna Foundation; FaunaFoundation.Org**

"There are many reasons why the rat is an unsound model for toxicity testing and other experiments. Rat anatomy and physiology differ enormously from that of humans, and the dissimilarities render research invalid and harmful when extrapolated to humans. For example, rats rarely vomit; do not have a gall bladder; do not have sweat glands; cannot pant; are poor regulators of body temperature; have twice the concentrating ability for urine; and, have a heart rate four times that of a human.

Many drug studies on rats were inaccurate and dangerous when extrapolated to humans, including Flosint, an arthritis medication, which proved fatal to humans; Zelmid, an antidepressant, which caused neurological damage in humans; and Clioquinal, an antidiarrheal, which caused blindness and paralysis in humans – all despite animal testing."
— **New England Anti-Vivisection Society, NEAVS.Org; 2002**

American Anti-Vivisection Society, AAVS.Org

AnimalAid.Org.UK

Animal Protection Institute, API4Animals.Org

AnimalsNeedRights.Net

AnimalSuffering.Com

British Anti-Vivisection Society, BAVA.PWP.BlueYonder.CO.UK

British Union for the Abolition of Vivisection, BUAV.Org

CloseHLS.org

Coalition to Abolish Animal Testing, OHSUKillsPrimates.Com
Web site devoted to exposing the scientific and medical fraud committed at the Oregon Health Sciences University (OHSU) operated by the Oregon National Primate Research Center (ONPRC).

CovanceSucks.Com

Dawn Watch, DawnWatch.Com/Animal_Testing.htm

EmoryLies.Com

FreeAnimals.Org

FreeTheAnimals.Homestead.Com

The Humane Society of the United States, HSUS.Org

HuntingdonSucks.Com

In Defense of Animals, IDAUSA.Org; VivisectionInfo.Org

Irish Anti-Vivisection Society, IrishAntiVivisection.Org

Italian Anti-Vivisection Scientific Committee,
AntiVivisezione.IT/Engl.%20Sharpe.html

Last Chance for Animals, LCAnimal.Org

Liberation **magazine**, Liberation-Mag.Org.UK

National Anti-Vivisection Society, NAVS.Org

New England Anti-Vivisection Society, NEAVS.Org
"There are currently some 1,300 chimpanzees held in U.S. laboratories. Some in barren cages no larger than six feet, as allowed by law. Some are 'warehoused' for future use. Others are subjected to terrifying research procedures, like being shot with tranquilizer guns for even simple blood tests. They are infected with deadly viruses in tests that have proven to be of little or no value at all to help cure human disease. We must rescue each and every one of them so that they have the chance to live the remainder of their lives in safety and peace.

This is not a dream that is out of our reach. We have come so far already. Many other countries have already decided chimpanzees share too much in common with humans to justify their use and abuse by scientific researchers, especially since even the small amount of DNA that separates us from them makes tests done on chimpanzees irrelevant or misleading to humans. Many prominent researchers have acknowledged this failure and have stopped using chimpanzees in human disease research."

New Zealand Anti-Vivisection Society, NZAVS.Org.NZ

Northern Animal Rights Network, NARN-Online.Com

People for the Ethical Treatment of Animals, PETA.Org; StopAnimalTests.Com

Physicians Committee for Responsible Medicine, PCRM.Org

Stop Animal Exploitation Now, All-Creatures.Org/SAEN/

Uncaged.CO.UK

Vivisection-Absurd.Org.UK

Water

Books:
- *An Unreasonable Woman: A True Story of Shrimpers, Politicos, Polluters, and the Fight for Seadrift, Texas*, by Diane Wilson
- *Blue Gold: The Fight to Stop the Corporate Theft of the World's Water*, by Maude Barlow and Tony Clarke
- *Outgrowing the Earth: The Food Security Challenge in an Age of Falling Water Tables and Rising Temperatures*, by Lester R. Brown
- *Rainwater Harvesting for Drylands: Guiding Principles to Welcome Rainwater Into Your Life and Landscape*, by Brad Lancaster
- *Troubled Water: Saints, Sinners, Truth and Lies about the Global Water Crisis*, by Anita Roddick, Brooke Shelby Biggs, Robert F. Kennedy, Jr., and Vandana Shiva
- *Water Follies: Groundwater Pumping and the Fate of America's Fresh Waters*, by Robert Jerome Glennon
- *Water Wars: Privatization, Pollution, and Profit*, by Vandana Shiva

Documentary:
- *Thirst*, by Alan Snitow and Deborah Kaufman, ThirstTheMovie.Org

M any people have been under the illusion that water is an unlimited resource. But today we see rivers running dry, ice caps melting, underground aquifers depleted, and some of the most common sources of water poisoned. Now there are billions of dollars being spent to build reservoirs, to build dams, and to find safe sources of water, including by sending spaceships to investigate the possibility of sufficient amounts of water on other planets to support human colonies.

Who would ever have thought people would be paying money for drinking water, which is the common practice in many areas of the world today?

Millions of people around the world rely on snow and ice in the mountains to provide water. As the glaciers continue to melt without being replenished, the concern about access to water is becoming more urgent. At the same time water systems are being purchased by corporations, putting a price on and limiting access to water for hundreds of millions of people.

The water in many parts of the world has become so polluted that humans cannot drink it, animals get sick from it, and fish and other water life die from being in it. Every level of the food supply for wildlife and humans is threatened by water pollution. The water in the oceans is becoming so acidic from absorbing air pollution caused by the burning of fossil fuels that the coral reefs are dieing and shellfish may become extinct sometime in the next several decades. This would greatly accelerate the extinction of species.

According to a United Nations report in 2006, more young children die from consuming dirty water every year than die of HIV/AIDS, war, traffic accidents, and malaria combined. They estimated that 1.8 million children under the age of five die every year from contaminated water.

While Americans use an average of 40 gallons of water per day and spend about $10 billion per year on 7.5 billion gallons of bottled water, globally people spend about $100 billion on water and about 1.1 billion people don't have access to clean water on a daily basis.

In 1996 one of the hot new entrepreneurial products in Southern California was to open up a store to sell purified water to people who couldn't afford home delivery of drinking water. Customers bringing in their own bottles to these water stores paid for a gallon of tap water put through a reverse osmosis water filter. Other than the stores selling water there are vending machines where people can purchase filtered water, and delivery services that charge several dollars for a five-gallon container of water.

We now see water suppliers franchising the way fast-food restaurants did during the 1960s and 1970s. An International Bottled Water Association has been established for those in the business of selling bottled water, and a trade magazine called Beverage World features information on the bottled water business. Some say that wars will soon be fought over water.

The amount of money being spent on bottled water is considered to be a problem because it is the people who have money who are spending it on bottled water. Some say that money would have otherwise gone to the infrastructure to keep tap water safe. The water systems around the world are degrading, and the poor people are left without access to clean water.

Bottled water is also causing a problem in the way it is producing millions of tons of plastic trash every year. The drink companies that are producing much of the world's bottled water products are those that are involved in manufactured food that produces millions of tons of more trash. They included Coca Cola, Danone (Dannon Yogurt), Nestle, and PepsiCo.

Various communities around the world have been involved in protests and lawsuits against bottled water companies that are pumping from springs and wells that affect the water locals depend as their own water sources. Other bottling companies take the water directly from municipal water supplies, or from sources that are not of the best quality. Some bottled water has been found to contain industrial chemicals and bacterial contaminates.

The Food and Drug Administration created definitions for water products such as purified water, spring water, distilled water, and other varieties. The Environmental Protection Agency has set standards for allowable levels of contaminants in tap water. Whole city water systems have been shut down after unacceptable levels of contaminates have sickened people exposed to the water, such as what happened in Milwaukee, Wisconsin, in 1993 when thousands of people became sick from an outbreak of a protozoa called cryptosporidium.

Making fun of Beverly Hills people drinking bottled Perrier was a common subject of humor among comedians in the 1970s, but today it is common to be drinking purchased bottled water. Many studies have concluded that tap water has been contaminated with a variety of poisons in the form of industrial, pharmaceutical, and agricultural chemicals. The community where I live cannot use the wells beneath us for drinking water because aquifer has been contaminated with petroleum additives, which has resulted in a lawsuit involving hundreds of millions of dollars.

Some municipal water companies oxidize their water supply to disinfect it. Many cities and counties have been adding chemicals to their water systems to kill off microorganisms. Anyone would have to wonder what these chemicals that are designed to kill off living organisms will do to the humans who ingest the chemical-contaminated water.

It is a wonder why so many communities are adding chlorine and other chemicals to their water supply. Who is benefiting from the sale of these chemicals to the municipalities? What did the lawmakers get out of the decision to add the chemicals to the water supply? Did the company that sells the chemicals help to finance the campaigns of the politicians? How much money are the municipalities spending on the chemicals? How much money did the chemical companies spend to lobby the politicians of the municipalities to make the decision to add the chemicals to the water supplies? These questions should be on the minds of the people who live in these water districts where chemicals are being added to the water supplies.

The process of creating and using the chemicals to treat the water creates more water pollution. A byproduct of chlorination, trihalomethane, is regulated by the Environmental Protection Agency because it is considered to be a potential carcinogen. Another drawback of chlorine is that it reacts with naturally-occurring organic compounds and forms organochlorines, which cause a number of health problems, from asthma to genetic mutation, cholesterol oxidation, cancer, birth defects and fertility issues.

Fluoride is another chemical used in many municipal water systems. This neurotoxic chemical is a byproduct of aluminum, copper, and iron manufacturing and has been used as a rat poison and insecticide. It was first used in the water system of Grand Rapids, Michigan. The reason given for adding it to water supplies is that it has been found to prevent tooth decay. A study often cited in support of adding it to water supplies was one conducted by Alcoa, a manufacturer of aluminum. In 1947 an attorney working for Alcoa, Oscar Ewing, was appointed as head of the federal department of Public Health Services. Ewing worked with a public relations professional and Sigmund Freud's nephew Edward L. Bernays to promote water fluoridation throughout the country. Bernays considered his way of molding public opinion to be "the engineering of consent." What they did is get many municipalities to allow their water systems to be fluoridated by using unfounded studies. Fluoride has been linked to a variety of health issues, including skeletal fluorosis, cancer, damage to the pineal gland of the brain; thyroid disorder, and mental health problems. In addition to fluoride, Bernays was known to ignore scientific studies to promote the health benefits of cigarettes and bacon.

It is frightening that pollution has brought people to the point of putting so much effort and concern into simple drinking water, water that humans and all life forms on Earth depend on for survival. Without a constant supply of water, we would all die.

You should each take a look at how much water pollution you are responsible for and take action to reduce that impact on the water pollution in your community.

"Water belongs to the Earth and all species and is sacred to life, therefore, the world's water must be conserved, reclaimed, and protected for all future generations and its natural patterns respected.

Water is a fundamental human right and a public trust to be guarded by all levels of government, therefore, it should not be commodified, privatized, or traded for commercial purposes. These rights must be enshrined at all levels of government. In particular, an international treaty must ensure these principles are noncontrovertable.

Water is best protected by local communities and citizens who must be respected as equal partners with governments in the protection and regulation of water. Peoples of the Earth are the only vehicle to promote Earth democracy and save water."
— The Cochabamba Declaration, Cochabamba, Bolivia; December 8, 2000

Ways to reduce water pollution include:

- Using biodegradable soaps in all areas of the household and work area. Natural foods stores sell biodegradable soaps and cleaning detergents.
- Not dumping hazardous chemicals down the drain. Call your local city hall to find out where you can take hazardous chemicals for proper disposal.
- Getting your local government to ban the fluoridation of the water system.
- Becoming vegan.

It takes less water to produce a pound of vegetables, fruits, grains, or beans than it does to produce a pound of meat. As detailed in various areas of this book, the meat industry, and all the industries that support it, cause huge amounts of land, water, and air pollution.

The animal farming industry, and the farming needed to create the food to feed the farm animals is the leading cause of depletion of the Ogallala aquifer. The aquifer is America's largest source of underground water and rests under part of at least eight states, from Texas to South Dakota. Because the cattle and corn industries have used so much of the water, parts of the aquifer have been pumped dry. The use of synthetic farming chemicals (largely used to grow feed for farm animals) as well as nitrates from livestock feeding operations is also polluting the aquifer.

• Eating organic produce.

The chemicals used on most farms introduce billions of pounds of chemicals into the water, ground, and air. By buying organic produce you are reducing the use of these dangerous chemicals, and supporting businesses that work to do the same.

• Promoting organic agriculture in your region.

• Not using bottled water, unless absolutely necessary. Using a high-grade water filter, or other using ways of filtering your water.

• Using a stainless steel or other safe water container to carry your drinking water – rather than disposable containers.

• Where possible, creating an above-ground rainwater collection cistern system to use as your community water source.

• Washing full loads of laundry rather than small loads. Only use biodegradable, nonpetroleum laundry soaps.

• Riding a bike, walking, skating, or skate-boarding instead of driving a car or other motorized vehicle.

Not only do the oils and fuels used to run a motor contribute to water pollution, but the wear on the tires, brake pads, and belts spreads little bits of rubber and other material throughout the surrounding air and land. If you do drive a car, motorcycle, or other motorized vehicle, make sure the tires are inflated correctly to reduce tire wear and improve fuel use.

• Legalizing industrial hemp farming.

American Rivers, 1101 14th Street NW, Ste. 1400, Washington, DC 20005; 202-347-7550; AmericanRivers.Org

Corporate Accountability International, 46 Plympton St., Boston, MA 02118; StopCorporateAbuse.Org

Environmental Justice Coalition for Water, 645 13th St., Oakland, CA 94612; EJCW.Org

HarvestingRainwater.Com

H$_2$O for ME, Maine's Water Dividend Trust, Fryeburg, ME;

WaterDividendTrust.Com

International Rivers Network, Berkeley, CA; IRN.Org

Natural Resources Defense Council, NRDC.Org

RainwaterHarvesting.Org

Riverkeeper, 828 S. Broadway, Tarrytown, NY 10591; RiverKeeper.Org

Sierra Club Water Privatization Task Force, 85 Second St., 2nd Fl., San Francisco, CA 94105; SierraClub.Org/CAC/Water

Sweetwater Alliance, POB 44173, Detroit, MI, 48244; WaterIsSweet.Org

Tennessee Clean Water Network, Knoxville, TN; TCWN.Org

United Nations Educational, Scientific, and Cultural Organization, Water Portal, UNESCO.Org/Water

United States Environmental Protection Agency Local Drinking Water Information, EPA.Gov/SafeWater/DWInfo.htm

Urban Alliance for Sustainability, SFUAS.Org/Node/175 Information about the Greywater Guerillas.

WaterFilterComparisons.Net

Waterkeeper Alliance, 50 S. Buckhout, Ste. 302; Irvington, NY 10533; Waterkeeper.Org

World Health Organization Water, Sanitation, and Health, WHO.Int/Water_Sanitation_Health/Index.htm.

WorldWaterCouncil.Org

Waterlife Protection

Also see:
• Animal Protection
• Environmental Protection
• Trees

Book:
• *50 Ways to Save the Ocean*, by David Helvarg

Videos:

- *Lethal Sound*, narrated by Pierce Brosnan, about high intensity sonar sound blasting being used in the oceans by the military and by oil companies, killing sea mammals, and rupturing their ears.
NRDC.Org/Wildlife/Marine/SonarVideo/Video.asp

- *Oasis of the Pacific: Time is Running Out*, 58 minute documentary goes underwater to reveal humanities impact on Hawaii's waterlife. "Some of the world's most unique creatures are in danger of being lost forever."
ZeroImpactProductions.Com

Threatening the life of the World's seas, lakes, rivers, marshlands:

- Fishing of all sorts (all fish are overfished)
- Fish farms, the chemicals they use, and the sea life they kill to protect the farmed fish. Enormous amounts of shrimp-like water creatures called krill are harvested from ocean waters to fee farmed fish. This is one of the main reasons why some populations of penguins have been reduced by more than half; the krill they feed on is being taken to feed farmed fish.
- Recreational craft
- Military craft pollution
- Killing sea turtles for their meat and eggs. All sea turtles are endangered. Large numbers of them are killed every year by the fishing industry.
- Garbage dumped from cruise ships, military ships, fishing ships, yachts, and industrial shipping
- Pollution runoff from cities
- Dumping of industrial solvents, automobile oils, and other toxic chemicals
- Plastics that are mistaken for food by wildlife and kill off many thousands of sea turtles, millions of water birds, hundreds of thousands of sea mammals, and other waterlife every year.
- Jetliner pollution as jets fly over the world's oceans, lakes, and rivers hundreds of thousands of times every year the exhaust is often absorbed into the water, creating more problems for the oceans.
- Coral reef damage from poachers using bleach and cyanide to stun fish
- Poaching of ocean life for souvenirs: coral, starfish, and other solid forms of waterlife
- Burning of fossil fuels: coal and petroleum

ActForDolphins.Org

Algalita Marine Research Foundation, Algalita.Org

American Oceans Campaign, AmericanOceans.Org

American Rivers, 1101 14th Street NW, Ste. 1400, Washington, DC 20005; 202-347-7550; AmericanRivers.Org

America's Wetland, POB 44294; Baton Rouge, LA 708-4249; AmericasWetland.Com

Amigos para la Conservación de Cabo Pulmo (Friends for the Conservation of Cabo Pulmo), PulmoAmigos.Org

Aqua Geo Graphia, Journal of Ichthyology & Aquatic Biology, Aquageo.Com/AquaIssues/About.html

ARCHELON, the Sea Turtle Protection Society of Greece; Archelon. GR

The Association for the Protection of the Environment and the Marine Turtle in Southern Baja, MexOnline.Com/Tortuga.htm

Australian Institute of Marine Science, AIMS.Gov.AU

Australian Marine Conservation Society, AMCS.Org.Au

The Barbados Sea Turtle Project, DiveFree.Net/Species/Project.htm

BeachCombers.Org

BeautifulOceans.Com

BlueVentures.Org

Bristol Bay Alliance, POB 231985, Anchorage, AK 99523-1985 907-276-7605, BristolBayAlliance.Com
"The State of Alaska and the Canadian mining company, Teck Cominco, want to create North America's largest open pit gold mine and a 896-square-mile mining district in the headwaters of Bristol Bay. At the same time, the Bureau of Land Management is trying to open 3.6 million acres of vital fish and wildlife habitat in the Bristol Bay Watershed to hardrock mining.
    What most people don't know is that the hard-rock mining industry is the single largest source of toxic releases and one of the most destructive industries in America.
    The proposed Pebble Mine may pose the greatest single threat to this area's salmon-bearing rivers. Similar open pit mines have devastated entire watersheds and surrounding fisheries throughout the United States and around the world. The Pebble complex would sit just 15 miles north of Alaska's largest body of fresh water, Lake Iliamna. If the mine is allowed to

open, this lake could easily be contaminated with cyanide as well as with heavy metals, including mercury, arsenic, and selenium. Waters from this lake eventually drain into Bristol Bay. This whole region is considered to be more sensitive than the Alaska National Wildlife Refuge."

California Coast Keeper Alliance, CaCoastKeeper.Org

Canadian Ocean Habitat Protection Society, POB 13, Newellton, Nova Scotia, BOW 1PO Canada; AtlantisForce.Org/COHPS

Caribbean Conservation Corporation & Sea Turtle Survival League, CCCTurtle.Org

Cayman Turtle Farm, POB 645 GT, Grand Cayman, British West Indies; 345-949-3894; Turtle.KY

Center for Marine Conservation, CMC-Ocean.Org

Cetacea Defence, CetaceaDefenceUK@Yahoo.CO.UK

Chesapeake Bay Foundation, CBF.Org

Clean Water Network, CWN.Org

Coral Reef Alliance, CoralReef.Org

CoralReefWatch.NOAA.Gov

CousteauFoundation.Org

CryOfTheWater.Org

The Dolphin Society of Australia, DolphinSoc.Org

The Endangered Species Coalition, 1101 14th St., NW, Ste. 1400, Washington, DC 20005; 202-682-9400; StopExtinction.Org

Environmental Protection Agency, EPA.Gov/OWOW/Estuaries/Guidance/

EuroTurtle.Org

FishingHurts.Com

Friends of the Sea Otter, SeaOtters.Org

Goa Foundation, GoaCom.Com/GoaFoundation

Gray's Reef National Marine Sanctuary, GraysReef.NOS.NOAA.Gov

Greenpeace.Org

Gulf Restoration Network, HealthyGulf.Org

HarpSeals.Org

Hawaiian Islands Humpback Whale National Marine Sanctuary, HIHWN-MS.NOS.NOAA.Gov

Heal the Bay, 3220 Nebraska Ave., Santa Monica, CA 90404; 310-453-0395; 1-800 HEAL BAY (in California only); HealTheBay.Org

HealTheOcean.Org

HumboldtBayKeeper.Org

Indian Ocean – South-East Asian Marine Turtle Memorandum of Understanding, IOSeaTurtles.Org/ProjectDB.php

INitrogen.Org

Institute for Tropical Marine Ecology, ITME.Org

International Ocean Noise Coalition, AWIOnline.Org/Whales/Noise/IONC/Index.htm

International Rivers Network, 1847 Berkeley Wy., Berkeley, CA 94703; 510-848-1155; IRN.Org

The Leatherback Trust, Leatherback.Org

The Living Oceans Society, 207 W. Hastings St., Ste. 515, Vancouver, BC V6B 1H7; FarmedAndDangerous.Org

Lophelia.Org
    Focuses on deep cold water ocean reefs

Los Angeles Times "Altered Oceans" article, LATimes.Com/Oceans

MangroveRestoration.Com

Marine Conservation Biology Institute; MCBI.Org

MarineDebris.NOAA.Gov

Mauritius Marine Conservation Society, Pages.Intnet.Mu/MMCS

Mediterranean Association to Save the Sea Turtles, MedAsset.Org/Medas.htm

MillenniumAssessment.Org

National Marine Sanctuaries, Sanctuaries.NOS.NOAA.Gov

Natural Resources Defense Council, NRDC.Org

NorthCoastWaterNetwork.Org

NYNJBayKeeper.Org

Oceana.Org

OceanEnvironment.Com

The Oceanic Resource Foundation, ORF.Org

Ocean Portal, IOC.Unesco.Org/OceanPortal

TheOceanProject.Org

OceanSpirits.Org

Ocean Watch Foundation, OceanWatch.Org

Planetary Coral Reef Foundation, PCRF.Org

ProtectSeals.Org

> "Each year, fishermen club and shoot baby seals in the North Atlantic, just to earn a few extra bucks by selling seal skins. In 2005, it is estimated that 98.5 percent of the seals killed were two months of age or younger – and veterinary reports indicate that many seals have been skinned while still conscious and able to feel pain."

ReefCheck.Org
> "15 percent of the world's reefs have been lost over the past decade."

Reef Guardian International, ReefGuardian.Org

ReefRelief.Org

Reseau d'Information sur les Turtues Marines d'Outremer; Reseau-Tortues-Marines.Org

Responsible Cruising in Alaska, ResponsibleCruising.Org
   Deals with protecting Alaskan waters from cruise ships dumping trash, untreated sewage, oil, industrial solvents, and toxic waste.

RiverKeeper.Org

RiverNetwork.Org

Santa Monica Baykeeper; POB 10096, Marina del Rey, CA 90295; 310-305-9645; SMBayeeper.Org

Save Ningaloo Campaign, Save-Ningaloo.org

Save Our Sea Turtles in Tobago, Churchill.de/de/SeaTurtles.html

Save the Manetee Club, 500 N. Maitland Ave., Maitland, FL 32751; 800-432-join; SaveTheManatee.Org

SeaAroundUs.Org

SeaCology.Org

Sea Shepherd Conservation Society, POB 2616, Friday Harbor, WA 98250; 360-370-5650; SeaShepherd.Org
   Committed to the eradication of pirate whaling; poaching of sea life; the annual Canadian harp seal slaughter; shark finning; unlawful sea life habitat destruction; and violations of established laws in the world's oceans.

Sea Turtle Conservation Bonaire, BonaireNet.Com/Turtle/Turtle.htm

Sea Turtle Conservation Network of the Californias, Baja.SeaTurtle.Org

SeaTurtle.Org

Scripps.UCSD.Edu

The Starving Ocean, FisheryCrisis.Com

Surfrider Foundation USA, POB 6010, San Clemente, CA 92674-6010; Surfrider.Org

Surfrider Foundation of Australia, Surfrider.Org.AU

Swamp Watch Action Team, SwampWatch.Org

The Turtle Foundation, Turtle-Foundation.Org

Turtle Trax, Turtles.Org

Water Keeper Alliance, WaterKeeper.Org

TheWatershedProject.Org

Wider Caribbean Sea Turtle Conservation Network, WideCast.Org

WindowsOnOurWaters.Org

Weddings

BambuHome.Com
Biodegradable bamboo plates.

Conscious Clothing; 505-982-7506; GetConscious.Com
Creates hemp/tencel-blend wedding dresses.

Evite.Com
Invitations through the Net, instead of using paper.

MarcalPaper.Com
Recycled paper napkins

OrganicWeddings.Com

Rawganique.Com
Hemp tableclothes and napkins

Regards.Com
Invitations through the Net, instead of using paper

TwistedLimbPaper.Com
Recycled, hand-crafted invites

Vickerey.Com
Recycled and tree-free invites

Weight: Losing It and Gaining It

Most people eat not only unhealthful foods, they also eat way too many calories, don't get enough exercise, and lead a life that is far below their potential.

Today obesity is an increasing problem. There are more people on the planet who are suffering from being overweight than there are of people who are suffering from a lack of food. This is an indication of how many people are living unhealthful lives, not eating properly, not getting enough exercise, and not experiencing true health. It also reveals how people are using more than their share of Nature's gifts – which greatly damages their karma, and the planet.

People began to get fatter with the mass production of automobiles and refrigerators. They stopped walking and riding bikes and began driving everywhere. They stopped the physical labor that was involved in growing their food, and began instead to rely on stores to supply them with their food. Then the mass production of television sets, together with the introduction of processed foods and television commercials, caused people to become more stagnant. Then came mega-superstores where people can do all their shopping in one stop (buying more stuff they don't need, including more stuff to make their lives cozier, and lazier). This resulted in more dependency on international companies to create and sell everything a person needed and wanted to create their home. Even fewer calories were being used to finish chores. With the mass entertainment use of the Internet and computer games, people have become even heavier. Not only do they not grow their food, not build the things in their homes, and not go out to do the chores that required some physical activity, they are also increasingly dependent on the Internet to do their shopping. Instead of going to the store, they can now sit in a chair and do their shopping (purchasing more stuff that they don't need) with a few strokes of the computer keys. Children who used to be outside playing games and climbing trees now sit in chairs playing with their computer games and chatting with each other on the Internet – which doesn't even use the calories it takes to hold a phone to the ear. In offices people no longer walk to the next department to communicate, instead relying on email and remaining at their desk. So now the mass media is filled with stories of how fat everyone is getting, and the fad diet book authors and diet product manufacturers are stuffing loads of money into their bank accounts.

Recent studies have concluded that the obesity problem in America is going to cancel out all the advances in health and medicine experienced in the last few decades, and will cause more problems in society than the combined effects of cigarette smoking, alcoholism, and automobile accidents.

If you want to get healthy: Turn off your TV. Stop paying attention to TV characters that are simply a figment of the imaginations of scriptwriters, producers, and marketing wizards in Hollywood and Manhattan. Spend time talking with people rather than staring at a TV with them. Walk, jog, run, ride a bike, or rollerskate to get places. Unplug from your wires. Stop buying things that you don't need. Realize that health does not come in a bottle of diet drinks or diet pills. Stop eating candy, smoking cigarettes, and drinking soda pop and/or brewed alcohol. Don't eat processed foods, or foods that are cooked and/or contain animal products.

If you want to get healthy: Eat foods as they are presented to us from Nature – living raw fruits, vegetables, herbs, nuts, seeds, flowers, and water vegetables.

As you simplify, purify, and make your life healthier through Sunfood nutrition and the principles within this book, you will start to understand how much nonsense you put yourself through by living a toxic life in a society so driven by commercials and dependent on fossil fuels. You will have more energy, will feel better, and will experience clarity of thought.

Some people have told me that after they have switched their diet to a raw vegan diet they have experienced a radiance that they had never known and they feel as if their senses have been amplified. Hopefully this will be your situation, and you will feel alive and radiant.

When you compare human health to the health of wild animals, you can see the great difference between a being following an unhealthful diet and a being eating only what is natural. Animals in the wild are amazingly fit. In comparison, humans who eat processed foods and spend much of their time sitting down as they live in a commercial society are commonly overweight.

The Sunfood diet puts you in tune with the most healthful way of eating, pushes you to make physical activity part of your daily experience, and does not cause the obesity seen in those people who are eating the unhealthful commercial foods sold in stores and restaurants.

"To lose weight, specifically minimize – and preferably eliminate – cooked fats from your diet (these include heated oils in fried and sautéed food; pasteurized milk and cheese; cooked eggs; and meat [including fish and fowl]). Also eliminate cooked starches (these include bread, cakes, cereal, cookies, crackers, doughnuts, pasta, popcorn, potatoes, and pretzels, as well as rice and other cooked grains). And do not consume any processed sugars (these include what may be listed on ingredient labels as barley malt, beet sugar, brown sugar, cane sugar, corn syrup, corn sweetener, fructose, rice syrup, rice malt, and white sugar).

Cooked fats, starches, and sweeteners put extra pounds onto the body. Cooked starch is essentially sugar, and if this sugar is not used as fuel, or urinated away, it is converted to fat.

Cooked fats are devoid of lipase, the fat-splitting enzyme, and they accumulate in the body, as they are difficult to metabolize, which results in weight gain. Pizza, which contains high doses of both cooked starch and cooked fat, is particularly fattening.

Raw fats, such as that contained in avocados and olives, actually help a person to lose weight. This is because raw fats contain lipase, which the body can use to metabolize residues of cooked fats."
— **David Wolfe**

The raw vegan diet can also be used to gain weight. There are certainly enough fatty foods you can eat on a raw vegan diet to get some extra weight on your body. Nuts, seeds, olives, oils, and various foods, such as hummus, nut butters, pesto sauces, salad dressings, sauces, and raw vegan desserts can increase weight. To assist the weight gain, the fatty foods should be accompanied by greens. This is because the minerals and amino acids in the greens will be assimilated into the body with the fats to build mass.

Reasonable amounts of Sun exposure is also key for someone who wants to gain weight. This is because the vitamin D that is formed in the skin when it is exposed to Sun, and the release of hormones that is triggered by exposure to Sun help to build strong tissues.

Juicing vegetables, which is done to make the raw soups in many of the raw vegan recipe books, increases the caloric value of the meal because the system uses fewer calories to digest the juice. Juicing vegetables also extracts the contents of the cells into the system by directly infusing their nutrients, including enzymes and minerals needed for weight gain.

It is unlikely that obesity can be experienced on a Sunfood diet. When a body is being supported with the high-quality nutrients found in the raw vegan diet, and is exercised regularly, it will naturally be at a more healthful weight. Any additional weight and muscle mass desired can be had by combining the right foods, and doing the right assortment of exercises. When you eat a highly nutritious Sunfood diet you will naturally have more energy, and exercise will be a welcome adventure rather than something to be dreaded, as it is by people who are so laden with toxic substances in their bodies from eating junk that even walking becomes a burden.

> "The secret to gaining strength and weight by following a Sunfood diet is to eat green-leafed vegetables and plant fats together, while eating fewer sweet fruits. More nonsweet fruits may be included as well. "
> — David Wolfe

Muscle mass can be increased on a raw vegan diet. You only have to look at the gorilla or the race horse to see the capabilities of being muscular on a diet of raw plants.

The "body builders" who hang out lifting weights at their local gym could learn from the diet of gorillas. Gorillas are not sitting around in the jungle guzzling protein powder drinks and injecting themselves with the toxic weight-building drugs that are so commonly used by body builders. Pound per pound, gorillas are the strongest land mammals. And they subsist on vegetation – most of which is green leaves.

> "All the building blocks necessary to construct and energize your body are present in plants. Out of the 22 amino acids found in the body, 8 must be derived from food. The body is capable of recycling and manufacturing the other 14 amino acids. All 8 essential amino acids are packaged in abundance in raw plant foods, especially in green leaves and superfoods (spirulina, blue-green algae, bee pollen, maca, goji berries, wolfberries, and hempseeds)."
> — David Wolfe

Those having problems gaining weight on a raw vegan diet might not be eating enough fattening foods. Or they may not be eating the right combination of fats with greens. Or they have intestinal plaque left over from eating cooked foods; or they have parasites that are robbing them of nutrients and calories. They may also have the type of body that simply does not get above a certain weight.

Wheatgrass and Barleygrass Juice

Also see:
• Sprouting

Books:
• *Living Foods for Optimum Health: Staying Healthy in an Unhealthy World*, by Brian Clement and Theresa Foy Digeronimo

• *The Wheatgrass Book*, by Ann Wigmore

Wheatgrass, rye grass, kamut grass, and barleygrass juices are loaded with vitamins, minerals, enzymes, amino acids, chlorophyll, and other phytonutrients (plant nutrients). Along with water algae (wild blue-green, spirulina, and chlorella), these grasses are excellent sources of chlorophyll, the substance in plants where photosynthesis takes place.

Grass juices can be particularly helpful in reversing enzyme and mineral deficiencies and help a person transition into a more healthful diet. They assist the body in eliminating toxins, especially residues from exposure to drugs, pollution, and low-quality food.

Grass juices can be blended with green vegetable juices to infuse the system with alkalizing nutrients. One way to do this is to juice cucumber and celery, and then blend this with kale, collard greens, spinach, and green grass juice. This is an excellent drink prior to athletic or other physical activity because the alkaline minerals in greens will improve muscle and neural performance.

> "Chlorophyll is the blood of plants, just as hemoglobin is the blood of the body. The only difference between the two molecules is that chlorophyll is centered on magnesium, while hemoglobin is centered on iron. Eating green-leafed food is a transfusion of Sun energy to blood energy within the body."
> — David Wolfe

Obtain your seeds for grass juices from an organic source.

To start sprouting wheat berries (wheat seeds) and barley, simply soak them in a bowl for up to several hours. This breaks through and shuts off the enzyme inhibitors, and triggers cell growth. Or you can spread them across very moist soil at the end of the day, preventing Sun from drying them out. Then keep them moist by misting or sprinkling them with water about twice a day. In several days you will have grass ready to be trimmed and put through a juicer.

Many people will grow juicing grasses on trays with a thin layer of soil spread across them. Make sure the soil you use is organic and free of chemicals, and that it is in a tray that allows for excess water to drain out from the bottom.

You can often get free trays from natural foods stores that dispose of them after use. Or you can make a wood frame of four pieces of wood, and then staple or tack a natural cloth (such as hemp canvas) on the bottom. This creates what is essentially a very shallow box with a cloth bottom that is perfect for drainage. Spread about a quarter to a half inch of soil across this to use as the bed for the seeds to grow on.

After the seeds have begun to sprout, it is good to continue growing the grass in indirect Sun light. When the grass has reached its ideal height (about five inches), expose the grass to direct Sun light to ignite the chlorophyll and nutrient factory within the leaves, greatly increasing the nutrition of the grass. Trim with scissors and put through a juicer. Drink the fresh juice within a few minutes for ultimate nutritional infusion.

There are also green grass powders that you can purchase at natural foods stores. These can be helpful if you don't have a place to grow grasses, are traveling, or lead a lifestyle that doesn't allow access to fresh grass juice.

HippocratesInst.Org/html/Wheatgrass2.htm

InnerGardenWheatgrass.com

Mumm's Sprouting Seeds, Sprouting.Com

Sunfood Nutrition, Sunfood.Com
Sells green nutritional powder that contains low-heat dehydrated grasses.

WheatGrassDirect.Com

WheatGrassKits.Com

Wild Foods

Books:
- *Basic Essentials, Edible Wild Plants & Useful Herbs*, by Jim Meunick
- *Edible and Useful Wild Plants of the United States and Canada*, by Charles Francis Saunders
- *Edible Wild Plants: A North American Field Guide*, by Thomas Elias, Peter Dykeman
- *Edible Wild Plants and Herbs: A Pocket Guide*, by Alan M. Cvancara
- *Field Guide to Edible Wild Plants*, by Bradford Angier
- *A Field Guide to Edible Wild Plants: Eastern and Central North America*, by Lee Allen Peterson (photographer), Roger Tory Peterson (series editor)
- *Neighborhood Forager: A Guide for the Wild Food Gourmet*, by Robert K. Henderson

- *Stalking the Healthful Herbs*, by Euell Gibbons
- *Wild Edible Plants of Western North America,* by Donald R. Kirk

"What is a weed? A plant whose virtues have not yet been discovered."
— **Ralph Waldo Emerson**

"We would be better off nutritionally if we threw away the crops we so laboriously raise in our fields and gardens and ate the weeds that grow with no encouragement from us."
— **Euell Gibbons, *Stalking the Healthful Herbs***

One way to avoid eating unnatural foods, such as those that are chemically grown, or that have been genetically altered, is to eat wild foods. These are foods that grow in the wild, such as various herbs, greens, fruits, vegetables, berries, flowers, and other edible plant substances, such as sea vegetables (arame, dulse, kombu [kelp], hijiki, nori, and sea palm). Many of these are more nutritional than items you will find in your local market's produce section.

Eating the wild, natural plants from your region is good for the body because wild plants carry a strong electric charge and hold nutrients that are what you need for the environment where you live. In other words, eating wild foods from your region connects you to Nature as it adjusts your system and energy frequency to your environment. Eating the wild plants and honey from your region can also help alleviate seasonal allergies.

For most of the history of humanity, the plants people ate consisted of those growing in their region of the world, and much of that consisted of what they foraged on day hikes. Even when our ancestors began growing plants from other areas, they would eat them only after they were grown in their region. If they didn't have greenhouses, they could only grow and eat plant substances that survived in their region, and only in the season in which they would grow.

Everything changed with refrigeration; with the creation of large greenhouses heated by electricity or gas; and with the invention of the engines that allow for shipping food to distant lands.

Today not only do people not eat wild foods from their region, they often subsist on diets that mostly consist of foods grown in other regions of the world, and foods that are not grown in a healthful manner.

Except for a few years of unhealthful eating, one thing that I have enjoyed throughout my life is not only growing some of my own food and sharing it with others, but also discovering the edible plants that grow in the regions where I have lived. From my earliest childhood I was able to locate wild berry bushes, fruit trees, and vegetables. I have found food plants in the some of the most unlikely areas.

Where I grew up there were many apple, cherry, plum, pear, and peach trees growing in the woods and fields. These, along with wild tomatoes, grapes, and berries provided many meals for me as I spent time outside in the late spring, summer, and early fall. Climbing a tree to reach the fruit at the top is certainly one way to connect with Nature.

When I was a small boy I made friends with various hoboes and random travelers who would camp in the woods near the railroad tracks. Sometimes when I showed them where the wild fruits grew I had to remind myself that some adults don't know how some of the most common food plants look. I realized back then that some people go through their entire lives without harvesting their own food.

Wild fruits are generally lower in sugar than commercially and chemically grown fruit. Part of the reason for this is that only the more hardy seeds will survive to fruit in the wild where they are not treated with fertilizers, fungicides, herbicides, and pesticides. Because they are not treated with fertilizers, the roots of wild fruit and nut trees as well as wild fruit vines and berry bushes will often grow deeper into the ground to reach for nutrients. This results in fruits and berries that have a higher mineral content, are naturally better balanced, are more vibrant, and carry a stronger frequency than fruit and berries grown chemically.

If you see fruit or other wild food growing on private land, contact the owner and see if he or she will allow you to harvest some of it.

Wild Food Adventures, John Kallas, Ph.D., director, 5036 Southeast Mitchell St., Portland, OR 97206; WildFoodAdventures.Com

Wood

Have you ever thought about how much wood is being thrown away every day? People often throw away an entire piece of furniture because one part of it is broken. In addition, old houses, apartment buildings, and other structures are continuously being razed and bulldozed into heaps of broken wood that end up in trash dumps.

Now consider what can be done with that wood instead of trashing it.

A growing trend among artists and woodworkers is to recycle wood by gathering broken furniture, by "harvesting" wood from structures that are about to be demolished, and to create new furniture and new structures using this old wood. This prevents the wood from being wasted, and prevents the cutting down of trees.

There is a never-ending supply of free materials out there for the creative woodworker. And much of it is of the best types of wood that can be used to create amazing pieces.

Want to start a business? Begin to collect broken furniture, beams and wood from structures that are being remodeled or demolished. Also, go into Nature and look for fallen trees that can be used in woodworking. Gather nonelectric carpentry tools of old and teach yourself the old-fashioned art of carpentry. Then refashion this freely gathered wood into something useful, and finish it with a natural, nontoxic finish.

Take on an apprentice or two to teach them carpentry using reclaimed, reharvested, and fallen wood. If the pieces you create are of good quality, you will have developed yourself a business that helps prevent the cutting down of new trees.

Yoga

Also see:
• Thinking

Yoga is effective in improving health on all levels. It involves a combination of various movements to loosen the body; postures (asanas) to strengthen and focus the body; deep-breathing techniques (pranayamas); relaxation; and meditation to help clarify intention. Although yoga is considered to be an ancient Hindu practice, some form of yoga-like exercise has been practiced in a variety of cultures around the world for thousands of years.

You do not have to be any religion, or nonreligion, to practice yoga. It is a healthful activity that is open to all varieties of people.

From books to magazines to yoga teachers and music, there are many resources a person can utilize to learn about yoga; so many that they are beyond the scope of this book.

Yoga has become very popular around the world, and it seems as if there are yoga studios everywhere. But you don't have to go to a fancy studio or invest in expensive clothing or props to do yoga; all you need is your body and mind.

In yoga people learn that breathing helps to stabilize the functions of the body and mind.

A main part of practicing yoga is to control the breath, to breathe out frustration and other unwanted emotions and feelings, and to breathe in calm and control. Keeping control of the breathing pattern during yoga helps to eliminate the tension, unsteadiness, and other physical and mental feelings that may be experienced while holding certain yoga poses.

It is common to hear a yoga teacher say something similar to "breath into your pain." Those who regularly practice yoga understand this concept. Breathing can help to eliminate pain. Pain may be associated with a lack of oxygen (nutrient) in the area feeling the pain. Focused, intentional breathing can help the body and mind focus on particular issues being experienced, and help people guide themselves into a better state. Taken to heart, this yogic concept can be practiced in other areas of life that need attention (nourishment and/or nurturing in the form of words or actions). By being able to control the rhythm of the lungs a person can remain calm in stressful situations, and this will allow the person to think more clearly.

You can fool your body into experiencing different feelings simply by adopting the breathing pattern that typically appears during certain emotions. Actors are taught this to help them emote whatever feeling they are supposed to express in different scenes. By breathing as if they are going to cry helps the actor begin to cry. By breathing as if they are angry, the actor is more able to experience that feeling. The same concept helps singers express the feelings of their songs. Likewise, those who desire to be in the relaxed state that is conducive to being calm and steadfast should breathe slowly, which will help slow the heart rate and calm the mind and body.

Many animals have an understanding of breath and breathing. This includes the animals that dive under water, such as birds that hunt fish, as well as dolphin, elephants, hippos, seals, whales, turtles, and various other animals. Dogs who swim know when to hold their breath, and dogs that are taught to rescue people from burning buildings know to hold their breath in smoke. I have a friend whose dog has taught itself to jump and ring a bell. Before doing so the dog will stand for a moment and take some deep breaths before making the jump to ring the bell. Again, we can learn so much from animals if we would just start listening by observing.

Another form of exercise that is ideal for the body and mind is swimming. We spent the first months of our lives surrounded by liquid. Swimming is an excellent form of low-impact exercise that strengthens the muscles and bones, relaxes the mind, and relieves stress. Like yoga, swimming can be done into old age.

If stress is not released, the tension works against the body and illness is likely to settle in. Over a long term, stress may slow down the metabolism, resulting in weight gain and a body that is susceptible to toxic overload.

It is important to get exercise of some sort every day, especially in the morning. It not only relieves stress, but also helps prevent stress from gathering in the tissues, because exercise opens the tissues to the nutrients the cells in those tissues need to maintain health. Exercise also helps to move the fluids through the body that carry away toxic substances that clog the body and that contribute to stress.

Most of the retreats listed in the Healing Retreats section of this book include yoga classes as part of their program.

Look for yoga studios in or near your community. If there is not a yoga studio near you, start one! Make it affordable to all by establishing the classes as donation-only, with a suggested cost, but with only a box where people can donate after class. Yoga should not be about making money, it should be about enlightenment. Deny no one.

AdventuresOfYoga.Com
  Provides information on yoga for children.

Aquarian Times magazine, AquarianTimesMagazine.Com

ChildrensYoga.Com

International Kundalini Yoga Teachers Association, KundaliniYoga.Com

MatrikaYoga.Com
  A yoga magazine of art, poetry, fiction, truth, myth, and philosophy.

Natural High Lifestyle, NaturalHighLifestyle.Com
  Sells yoga supplies and clothes made from organic cotton, bamboo fiber, and hemp fabrics.

NeemKaroliBaba.Com

ProgressivePowerYoga.Com

MatthewSanford.Com

SoulYogaPractice.Com

Sunfood.Com
   Sells yoga videos and books attuned to the Sunfoodist lifestyle.

AshleyTurner.Org

WhiteTantricYoga.Com

YogaLifestyle.Com

YogaMovement.Com

Yoga.ResearchEasy.Com

YogaTimes.Com

Sunfood Living Index

F

M

Y

Z

About the Author

"Writing is a socially acceptable form of schizophrenia."
— E. L. Doctorow

John McCabe is the author of *Surgery Electives: What to Know Before the Doctor Operates*. First published in 1994, and now out of print, it was an exposé of the financial ties of the unethical and dangerous allopathic hospital, insurance, and pharmaceutical industries whose business practices and "health care" result in the deaths of thousands of people every year. The book received much media attention and was endorsed by all the patients' rights groups in North America as well as by members of the U.S. Congress.

McCabe has been a ghost co-writer on health-related books by other authors. He has also been a content and research editor on books written by David Wolfe, including the best selling raw vegan lifestyle book *The Sunfood Diet Success System*.

More recently McCabe is the author of *Hemp: What the World Needs Now*.

If there is information you think should be included in future editions of this book, send it to John c/o Caremania, POB 1272, Santa Monica, CA 90406-1272, or email Info@SunfoodLiving.Com.

See SunfoodLiving.Com

Also by John McCabe

Hemp: What the World Needs Now

"No time has passed when *Cannabis* has not been an integral part of the worldwide fabric of society. John McCabe has pointedly brought hemp's past into the eyes of the future. Understanding where the issues stem from that surround *Cannabis*, both industrial and medicinal, allows us to make the right decisions today for a better, more sustainable conscience tomorrow. It has been with much pride that I was able to share with John an American-Canadian hemp perceptive. Governmental recognition of this viable agricultural fiber and grain crop is plausible and necessary for the growth of the future fabric of today's worldwide society."
— Anndrea M. Hermann, Canadian Hemp Trade Alliance

"McCabe presents compelling evidence and then steps back – allowing the reader to personally consider the possible outcomes of re-introducing legal hemp agriculture in the United States as well as revising retributional drug policies worldwide."
— **Dave Thorvald Olson, Communications Director, HempLobby.Org; Author,** *Hemp Culture in Japan;* **Producer,** *HempenRoad*

"John McCabe has written a contemporary and politically relevant book that helps dispel and debunk many of the modern, government-created myths about the cannabis plant."
— **Allen St. Pierre, Executive Director, National Organization for the Reform of Marijuana Laws/NORML Foundation, Member, Board of Directors, Washington, DC**

"A very thorough and comprehensive overview of this amazing food, fuel, and fiber plant. I was left with the distinct opinion that our own American hemp history precludes the need for any further research... This book shines a bright light of truth, exposing the lie that is prohibition."
— **Cher Ford-McCullough, President, Women's Organization for National Prohibition Reform**

"I encourage the Tibetan people and all people to move toward a vegetarian diet that doesn't cause suffering."
— **Dalai Lama**

"Rest your head and keep your mind cheerful; shun wantonness, and pay attention to diet."
— **Leonardo da Vinci**

"The time has come when every individual must rise from the slumber of indifference, from the orthodox complacency of the standard rules and regulations of society, and break out, pioneering new fields of beautiful, ethical, and spiritual progress. It is now time to experience the incredible majesty of living."
— **David Wolfe**

To re-paraphrase Dorothy Parker... This book is not to be taken lightly; it is to be used as a tool to hurl your life forward with great force.

Plant mass quantities of native trees and wildflowers.
Grow organic food. Support organic farmers.
Outlaw genetic engineering of plants.
Legalize industrial hemp farming.
Enjoy peace on your path.
Share this book.
— **John, SunfoodLiving.Com**

About the Publisher

Davvid Wolfe, A Passionate Proponent of the Sunfood Lifestyle and publisher of *Sunfood Living*:
Born in 1970 to parents who are both medical doctors, David Wolfe grew up influenced by the world of Western medicine. This setting provided him with a unique perspective on health and healing.

Although he was a typical teenager playing sports and surfing, Wolfe's continual exposure to his parents' professions instilled in him a curiosity about why some people experience vibrant health while others seem to be stuck in cycles of perpetual illness.

At a young age, Wolfe began an intensive study of the medical and scientific books and trade journals in his parents' offices. His interests also spread into recognizing the dramatic health benefits of raw, plant-based nutrition as well as the area of philosophy focused on nurturing success through intentional thought, sharpening of the intellect, and use of natural talent.

Developing his own conclusions on what can lead a person toward experiencing vibrant health, success, and happiness, Wolfe began writing what became the best-selling book, *The Sunfood Diet Success System*. In the book, Wolfe shares his knowledge and discoveries about how a properly balanced raw plant-based diet infuses the body with life-force energy and vibrant health. He also describes his philosophy on what can bring about true happiness and success.

First published in 2000, *The Sunfood Diet Success System* continues to be a bestseller, inspiring people around the world to improve their lives on many levels. Wolfe is also the author of the insightful *Eating for Beauty*; and co-author of *Naked Chocolate*. The book by John McCabe, *Sunfood Living*, was specifically written to function as a companion book to Wolfe's *The Sunfood Diet Success System*. To satisfy demand from around the world, Wolfe's books are currently being translated into several languages.

In a quest to share his knowledge through seminars and literature, Wolfe founded the company, Sunfood Nutrition (www.sunfood.com). Through the company, Wolfe also develops and distributes raw superfood products grown under high ethical standards. Sunfood Nutrition was the first company to undertake the North American distribution of raw and organic: cacao beans (nibs), cacao butter, and cacao powder (raw chocolate), as well as goji berries, Incan berries, mangosteen, maca, and cold-pressed coconut oil.

In 2007 Wolfe's company relocated to a green environmentally-friendly building in Lakeside, California.

Wolfe has been a tireless international spokesperson for the natural, plant-based health and success lifestyle advocated in his books. He has conducted lectures and seminars in North, Central, and South America, as well as the South Pacific and throughout Europe. Because of his work, Wolfe is known as the world's leading authority on raw food nutrition and superfoods and one of America's leading herbalists and chocolatiers.

While continuing to host at least six health, fitness, and adventure retreats per year, Wolfe is taking time to write more books dealing with health, nutrition, and his success philosophy for helping not only individuals, but the planet as well.

Wolfe has degrees in mechanical and environmental engineering and political science. He has studied at many institutions, including Oxford University and the University of California at Santa Barbara. He concluded his formal education by receiving a Juris Doctor in Law from the University of San Diego. He now participates in higher education in the position of professor of nutrition for Dr. Gabriel Cousens' masters degree program on live-food nutrition at the Tree of Life Rejuvenation Center in Patagonia, Arizona.

As a defender of wildlife, the environment, food security, and human rights, Wolfe founded the nonprofit Fruit Tree Planting Foundation (www.ftpf.org). The Foundation is raising funds to plant billions of fruit trees around the planet in locations that benefit human nutrition, the environment, and wildlife.

As a man with many diverse interests, Wolfe practices yoga and is also the drummer in the rock group, The Healing Waters Band. The group's sound has been described as "carrying a classic surfer music sincerity of a bygone era mixed with an edgy, poetically mod lyrical tone, and a cleverly entertaining and enlightening in-your-face independent rock attitude."

For more information:

www.davidwolfe.com

www.ftpf.org (The Fruit Tree Planting Foundation)

www.thebestdayever.com (David Wolfe's online magazine).

www.sunfood.com

David Wolfe's Headquarters:

Sunfood Nutrition™ or www.sunfood.com (formerly Nature's First Law or www.rawfood.com)

11653 Riverside Drive, Lakeside, CA 92040, USA; 800-205-2350; 001-619-596-7979